ANGIOGRAPHY OF THE UPPER EXTREMITY

SERIES IN RADIOLOGY

VOLUME 7

ANGIOGRAPHY OF THE UPPER EXTREMITY

BLAGOJA K. JANEVSKI, M.D.

Department of Diagnostic Radiology,
Sint Annadal Hospital, University of Limburg,
Maastricht, The Netherlands

1982
MARTINUS NIJHOFF PUBLISHERS
THE HAGUE/BOSTON/LONDON

Distributors:
for the United States and Canada
Kluwer Boston, Inc.
190 Old Derby Street
Hingham, MA 02043
USA

for all other countries
Kluwer Academic Publishers Group
Distribution Center
P.O.Box 322
3300 AH Dordrecht
The Netherlands

Library of Congress Cataloging in Publication Data

Janevski, Blagoja K.
Angiography of the upper extremity.

(Series in radiology; v. 7)
Includes index.
1. Extremities, Upper–Blood-vessels–Diseases–Diagnosis.
2. Angiography. 3. Extremities, Upper–Blood-vessels–Radiography. 4. Hand–Blood-vessels–Radiography.
I. Title II. Series: Series in radiology; 7. [DNLM:
1. Arm–Radiography. 2. Angiography. 3. Hand–Radiography
4. Arm–Blood supply. 5. Hand–Blood supply. WG 500 J33a]
RC951.J36 616.1'3 82–6375
AACR2

ISBN 978-94-009-7596-5 ISBN 978-94-009-7594-1 (eBook)

DOI 10.1007/978-94-009-7594-1

Softcover reprint of the hardcover 1st edition 1982

FOREWORD

Over the last few decades, angiography has developed enormously and an extensive literature has been published on the subject. In the last few years, the number of publications has decreased because the applications of this diagnostic method seem to have been almost fully explored.

One of the applications for which this statement might not be true is angiography of the upper extremity. The clinical interest for this field has never been as great as for other parts of the body.

In Maastricht, Janevski was able to accumulate an unusually large amount of experience in the field of angiography of the upper extremities, and this book is the result of his experience. It contains a careful analysis of his angiographic findings and a very thorough description of vascular anatomy and its many variants. The extensive clinical material also enables him to indicate those circumstances in which angiography can make an important contribution to diagnosis.

This monograph deserves the attention of all who are interested in the anatomy and pathology of the arm and the hand, and is particularly intended for radiodiagnosticians and surgeons.

A. E. van Voorthuisen, M.D.

March, 1982
Leiden

DEDICATION

This book is dedicated to my children Lucienne, Lidia and Déjan
and to my wife Charlotte, whose love, patience and support
were my constant inspiration.

PREFACE

The purpose of this book is to acquaint medical specialists with the possibilities offered by angiography for diagnosis of disturbed circulation of the arm and hand. Three general areas are covered: radiological methods of examination, vascular anatomy and clinical and angiographic aspects of the most common pathological processes involving the upper extremity.

The arteriograms, all obtained by the subtraction method, are of patients investigated between 1970 and 1980 exclusively at the Department of Diagnostic Radiology of Sint Annadal Hospital in Maastricht. The case material described and illustrated stems mainly from the Department of Surgery and to a lesser extent from the other departments. It was my good fortune to work in this hospital where the surgical team had acquired considerable experience and intense interest in the ischaemic syndromes of the hand. As a vascular radiologist I soon became involved in the radiological investigation of the arteries of the arm and hand. During all of these years of research I have received total support from my radiological associates and the members of the surgical vascular team, to whom I am tremendously thankful. I wish to acknowledge with deep gratitude the aid provided by the surgeon Prof. H. A. J. Lemmens.

The job undoubtedly could not have been accomplished without the patience, support and suggestions of all of my fellow-workers.

I would like to acknowledge the help of the nurses, Miss Jeanne Crijns and Mrs. Anita Panis-Rousie, as well as all of the roentgen technicians who worked in the angiographic room. I particularly wish to express my greatful appreciation to our head radiographers, Miss Anny Mordant and Miss Hetty Nelissen, for their invaluable assistance during the examinations and especially to the latter for her help in recording and classifying the roentgenological and clinical data essential for the realization of this book.

The photographs which form such an important part of this book are entirely the work of Mr. C. Evers and his staff of the photographic department of Sint Annadal Hospital. The graphical illustrations were made by C. Voskamp and the subtraction films, which improve the quality of many of the radiographs, are the work of Mr. Th. Bieler and Mr. A. J. L. van der Groen. To all of them I am very greatful. I wish to thank also Mrs. Marie-Thérèse Finders-Velraad for typing and retyping the manuscript and Miss Yvonne Bessems for other secretarial work.

In acknowledging the various people who have helped in the realization of this study I would like to take this opportunity to express my appreciation to my colleagues Henk Sanches and Jan Zonjée for their encouragement and advice throughout the production of this book.

Finally I am particularly thankful to the professors of the University of Leiden, A. E. van Voorthuisen, radiologist; J. M. F. Landsmeer, anatomist and J. L. Terpstra, vascular surgeon, for their willingness to read the manuscript and especially for their critical judgement and constructive remarks.

Blagoja K. Janevski, M.D.

CONTENTS

Chapter 1

INTRODUCTION

The surgical team of St. Annadal Hospital has a tradition of great interest in the treatment of vascular disease. The radiological team shared this interest and has developed methods for optimal radiological investigations. This co-operation resulted in a considerable concentration of patients with vascular diseases in the hospital.

Vascular problems of the upper extremities became one of the subjects of common research and a great number of patients with these kind of problems were referred to us. The radiological examination techniques were standardized and the arteriographic examination of the hand was improved by the use of pharmacological vasodilators and the routine application of photographic subtraction.

Altogether in ten years 750 selective studies of the upper extremity were performed in more than 500 patients. This material is the subject of this book, which has the following objectives:

1. To present the optimal technical specifications for upper extremity angiography.
2. To present a thorough analysis of the arteriographic anatomy of the upper extremity.
3. To describe the angiographic symptoms of upper extremity pathology and to establish the value of angiography for diagnosis and treatment.

1.1 Outline of the Book

The book is divided into ten chapters. After a general introduction in chapter one, the subsequent chapters treat the following subjects.

Chapter 2 provides a short historical review of angiography as a whole and of arteriography of the hand in particular.

Chapter 3 deals with the method of percutaneous transfemoral catheterization of the arteries of the upper extremity and particularly the arteries of the hand, discussing the problems the angiographer encounters frequently, describing the angiographic complications which may occur and emphasizing the measures to keep them to a minimum.

The transfemoral approach for catheterization of the arteries of the upper extremity is considered to be a safe and easy method and has become the routine technique for investigation of these vessels. In cases where stenotic or occluded arteries are present and the introduction of a catheter is not possible another method for the visualization of the arteries of the forearm and hand is used. This method, the so-called direct brachial cut-down technique is described in detail. The advantages and disadvantages of the procedure are included.

Chapter 4 concerns vasospasm and pharmacoangiography, i.e. the use of vasodilators in hand angiography.

Confronted with the problem of vasospasm which prevented the proper filling of the small peripheral arteries with contrast material in the beginning of the study (1970) it was necessary to test several pharmacological agents for their potential value in brachial angiography. Tolazoline hydrochloride proved to have a strong vasodilatory effect, but the recommended dose was high and side-effects of the drug were frequently encountered.

For this reason we performed a second study

with the purpose of finding the optimal dose and timing for visualization of the arteries and veins on hand angiograms.

The results of this study are given at the end of the chapter.

Chapter 5 includes a short description of the embryological patterns persisting in the arteries of the arm in order to understand the congenital variations of the arteries of the upper extremity.

Chapter 6 is devoted entirely to the normal angiographic anatomy and its variations of the main arteries of the arm and hand. The study is based on an analysis of 323 aortic arch aortograms, 250 selective subclavian arteriograms and 500 hand arteriograms. It was found that the arteries of the hand show considerable variations in their distribution; therefore a new classification of different patterns of both palmar arches is made, accompanied by photographs and sketches. At the end of the chapter our results are compared with those of other authors.

The chapters seven, eight, nine and ten are devoted to the angiographic patterns and clinical aspects of the most common pathological processes involving the arteries of the upper extremity. A review of the literature is given and the results of our angiographic investigations of different arterial diseases are discussed. The chapters include illustrations that are considered to be representative of the kind of pathological changes seen in different morbid conditions. Special attention is paid to the correlation between angiography and pathology and to the indications for angiography of the upper extremity.

Chapter 7 comprises the acute and chronic traumatic lesions of the arteries of the upper extremity. A review of the literature is given. The role of angiography is described and the angiographic signs of different arterial injuries are emphasized.

Chapter 8 deals with congenital vascular lesions and vascular tumours. A short description of congenital stenosis, atresia, hypoplasia and aplasia of the arteries of the upper extremity is given. Arteriovenous malformation and arteriovenous fistulae are described more extensively. Our case material, illustrated with typical examples, is analysed.

Chapter 9 contains a detailed description of the thoracic outlet compression syndrome, including historical review, aetiology, clinical and physical signs and an analysis of a large number of cases. The optimal angiographic approach for this syndrome is discussed in detail.

Chapter 10 covers the pathology of arterial occlusive disease of the upper extremity beginning with arteriosclerosis and its many manifestations as well as the steal phenomena, such as the steal syndromes of the subclavian and innominate arteries and the thyrocervical trunk. A special type of vasospastic disorder, i.e. Raynaud's disease, is briefly discussed.

Other arterial occlusive diseases such as embolism and thrombosis, fibromuscular hyperplasia, thromboangiitis obliterans and collagen diseases are also considered.

At the end of the chapter a general conclusion on acquired vascular diseases is given.

The abnormalities of the venous system of the upper extremity and the treatment of the arterial diseases are not discussed.

Chapter 2

THE HISTORY OF ANGIOGRAPHY OF THE UPPER EXTREMITIES

The history of upper extremity arteriography and angiography, as a whole, starts with the history of roentgenology. Wilhelm Konrad Röntgen discovered X-rays on November 8th, 1895; four weeks later, two Austrians, E. von Haschek and O. T. Lindenthal, residents under Prof. Franz Exner of the Second Institute of Physics and Chemistry in Vienna, demonstrated upper extremity arteriography before a small audience, including W. K. Röntgen. Their vascular contrast study was obtained by injection of a chalk-containing solution into the arterial system of an amputated arm. The specimen was obtained from Prof. Julius Tandler, head of the Institute of Anatomy at the same university. The report on this first arteriogram of the upper extremity was published in an article entitled 'Ein Beitrag zur praktischen Verwertung der Photographie nach Röntgen' (Haschek *et al.*, 1896).

The available X-ray apparatus was primitive and it was necessary to use an exposure time of nearly thirty minutes. Because of these technical limitations this first vascular study did not show many details. In the same year, similar experiments were carried out by McIntyre in England and by Destat and Berard in France, who confirmed the observations of their Austrian colleagues.

Since that time research has constantly been directed towards improvement of the diagnostic instruments and development of the least toxic contrast medium.

Early in the second decade of this century, after the discovery of the contrast medium *Lipiodol* (iodized poppyseed oil), phlebography became practicable on a clinical basis. This contrast substance was injected into the antecubital vein of a living human subject in France by Sicard and Forestier (1923), who fluoroscopically followed the flow of the contrast fluid through the right cardiac chambers into the pulmonary arteries.

In the same year, Berberich and Hirsch obtained the first peripheral angiogram of a living patient, by injecting *strontium bromide* into the arteries and veins of the arm and hand.

The first successful arteriogram of a lower extremity was carried out by Brooks (1924), in a patient under general anaesthesia, by means of surgical exposure of the femoral artery near the groin. He injected *sodium iodide* as a contrast medium. His procedure remained for many years the standard method for examination of the arteries of the leg.

Then, since visualization of the superficial and peripheral arteries and veins was possible with success and relative safety, the deeply situated vessels of the body and the cranium became a challenge to the diagnostician.

One year later the first successful aortogram was performed by Dos Santos, Lamas and Pereira-Caldas in Portugal. They began their work in 1925 and reported their results in 1929. These authors used the translumbar needle puncture technique and demonstrated the abdominal aorta with all its branches by means of an injection of opaque medium. Ten years later, Robb and Steinberg showed that the thoracic aorta could be demonstrated satisfactorily by the introduction of a contrast medium into peripheral veins. That same year (1939), Castellanos and Pereiras of Cuba described the retrograde brachial injection of contrast media for opacification of the thoracic aorta.

The injection of a contrast medium into the lumbar aorta through a catheter was described for the first time by Farinas in 1941. He used the method of surgical exposure of the femoral artery which was then punctured with a trochar; the catheter was subsequently passed through the opening and threaded into the abdominal aorta. Radner in 1948 obtained opacification of the thoracic aorta following open retrograde catheterization of the radial artery.

Ten years after Farinas, in 1951, Peirce introduced a catheter into the femoral artery through a needle. The modification of this technique by Seldinger (1953) permitted the development of percutaneous transfemoral angiography, widely used at the present time.

REFERENCES

BERBERICH, J. und S. HIRSCH: Die Röntgenographische Darstellung der Arterien und Venen im lebenden Menschen. *Klin. Wchnschr. 49: 2226, 1923.*

BROOKS, B.: Intra-arterial Injection of Sodium Iodide. *JAMA 82: 1016, 1924.*

CASTELLANOS, A. and R. PEREIRAS: Counter-current Aortography. *Rev. Cubana cardiol. 2: 187, 1939.*

DOS SANTOS, R.: Phlebographie d'une veine cave inférieure suturée. *Jour. urol. Paris, 39: 586, 1935.*

FARINAS, P. L.: A New Technique for the Arteriographic Examination of the Abdominal Aorta and Its Branches. *A., J. Roentgenology., 46: 641, 1941.*

HASCHEK, E. und O. T. LINDENTHAL: Ein Beitrag zur praktischen Verwertung der Photographie nach Röntgen. *Wien. klin. Wchnschr., 9: 63, 1896.*

LAMAS, A. C. et R. DOS SANTOS, P. CALDAS: L'arteriographie des membres de l'aorte et de ses branches abdominales. *Bull. Soc. Chir., Paris, 55: 587, 1929.*

PEIRCE, E. C.: Percutaneous Femoral Artery Catheterization in Man With Special Reference to Aortography. *Surg. Gynec. & Obst., 93: 56, 1951.*

RADNER, S: Thoracal Aortography by Catheterization From the Radial Artery. *Acta radiol. 29: 178, 1948.*

ROBB, G. P. and I. STEINBERG: A Practical Method of Visualization of the Chambers of the Heart, the Pulmonary Circulation and Great Vessels in Man. *Jour. Clin. Investigation, 17: 507, 1938.*

RÖNTGEN, W. C.: Über eine neue Art von Strahlen. *Erste Mitt. Sitzber. Phys.-Med. Ges. (Würzburg), 137, 1895.*

SELDINGER, S. I.: Catheter Replacement of Needle in Percutaneous Arteriography; a New Technique. *Acta Radiol., 39: 368, 1953.*

SICARD J. et G. FORESTIER: Injections intravasculaires d'huile iodée sous controle radiologique. *Compt. rend. Soc. Biol., 88: 1200, 1923.*

Chapter 3

EXAMINATION TECHNIQUE

There are different techniques used for subclavian and brachial angiography at the present time:

- transfemoral catheterization technique (Seldinger)
- brachial cut-down technique
- percutaneous brachial artery puncture
- retrograde axillary puncture with antegrade positioning of the catheter (Hawkins and Hudson).

It is up to the radiologist to decide what kind of technique to use in each individual case.

Percutaneous transfemoral catheterization by the Seldinger technique is the preferred method for upper extremity angiography. When severe peripheral atherosclerotic changes are present and the femoral artery pulses are diminished on both sides, then surgical exposure and retrograde needle puncture of the brachial artery is the method of choice.

The so-called retrograde axillary puncture with antegrade positioning of the catheter in the ipsilateral brachial artery, as described by Hawkins and Hudson (1974), is only possible when the distal axillary artery is easily palpated. Relatively short and small polyethylene catheters (French 4 and 5) are used for this technique. The advantages of this method, according to the authors, include not only the reduced risk of arterial injury, because small catheters are easily advanced, but also the possibility of good brachial plexus anaesthesia and local vasodilatation via an additional injection of local anaesthetic slightly proximal to the arterial puncture site. This procedure has never been used in our department.

In the majority of cases subclavian and hand angiography are performed by passing the catheter percutaneously via the right, or the left, femoral artery. In a very small number of cases (in our experience less than 2%), usually involving older patients with tortuous atherosclerotic arteries or stenosis and occlusion of the femoral and iliac vessels or even the subclavian and axillary arteries, surgical exposure of the brachial artery is required.

3.1 Preparation of the Patient for Upper Extremity Angiography

The preparation of the patient for subclavian and hand angiography does not differ from the preparation for any other catheterization by the Seldinger technique. The patients should not be dehydrated, but food should be withheld for the preceding six to ten hours. In most instances, angiography can be carried out under local anaesthesia with adequate pre-operative analgesia and sedation.

Arterial injections of contrast media cause transitory pain and a sensation of heat in the area of distribution of the artery. These symptoms are particularly severe following injections into the peripheral circulation of the arms. In such cases, involuntary movement on the part of the patient may blur the films and spoil the examination. As a result, catheterization may become prolonged and cause discomfort and increasing anxiety to the patient. These factors together with the mental stability of the patient and his physical condition must all be taken into account when deciding whether to use general or local anaesthesia.

Subclavian and hand arteriographic examinations of very young or mentally disturbed persons are usually best performed under general anaesthesia. For these individuals the pre-anaesthetic medication should be left to the anaesthetist.

3.2 Premedication for Angiography Under Local Anaesthesia

The following list is not complete but includes many of the drugs used for the preparation of patients for angiography under local anaesthesia. For effective action sufficient time must be allowed between administration of the drug and the actual examination. Any interaction with drugs prescribed for medical treatment of the patient should be avoided.

Unless otherwise stated the dose recommended is that for the average adolescent and average adult.

An intramuscular injection of *pethidine* and *atropine* is the pre-medication of choice for subclavian and hand angiography.

For all adults over 16 years of age, the usual dosage is 75 mg pethidine and ½ mg atropine sulfate. Adolescents between 10 and 16 years old receive 50 mg pethidine and ¼ mg atropine. Both drugs have to be administered together intramuscularly 30 to 60 minutes before the examination.

If the examination is prolonged and the patient becomes distressed, analgesia may be enhanced by the slow intravenous injection of an additional 25 to 50 mg pethidine. The patient may become pale and perspire but hypotension is not usually a complication.

Pethidine is used because of its analgesic properties. It has considerably less potency as an analgesic than morphine, but is usually adequate to control the degree of pain caused by angiographic examination and it has few side-effects.

Atropine sulfate has a strong vagolytic action and is generally used in a similar dose when there is a potential hazard of vasovagal attack. It is an anti-sialagogue and has uncomfortable side-effects such as dryness of the mouth.

There are numerous other drugs used for premedication in angiography because of their sedative and analgesic effects. The most common are: diazepam (Valium); promethazine hydrochloride (Phenergan); trimeprazine tartrate (Vallergan); morphine and barbiturates.

3.3 Instruments, Equipment and Contrast Media

3.3.1 Catheters

The choice of the catheter is based on softness, lack of recoil during injection, and flow capacity. We use a single end-hole Cook (French 7) radiopaque polyethylene catheter with torque control, specially shaped for selective catheterization of the subclavian arteries and the cerebral vessels: the so-called Headhunter (nrs. 1 and 4).

These catheters are designed mainly for selective and superselective angiographic procedures. The trademark *Torcon* (torque control) expresses the ability to control precisely rotation of the catheter tip. The major advantage of these catheters, namely superior torque control and manoeuvrability, has been achieved by encapsulating a stainless steel wire braid between the smooth external and internal catheter walls. The braiding also enables the catheters to withstand high injection pressures (up to 1000 PSI). The other advantages of these catheters are that the curves remain constant and are not affected by the introduction procedure or body temperature.

3.3.2 Needles and Guide Wires

Needles for percutaneous catheterization were originally developed by Seldinger. They are a complex triple puncture set, consisting of an outer blunt-ended cannula and an inner fitted needle and/or fitted stylet with bevelled point. The cannula is tapered 3 mm from the tip. The needle and the stylet are 3 mm longer than the cannula. The outer diameter of the cannula is 2 mm; it is available in different lengths (70 mm; 90 mm; 100 mm).

The guide wires are made of stainless steel and the core, which passes through the entire spiral, is soldered at both ends with nontoxic silver solder to avoid electrolytic action and destructive chemical effects.

The guide wires should have a smooth outer

surface and an inner safety core to facilitate manipulation and easier sliding of the catheter. They are also available in different lengths. For selective catheterization of the subclavian and brachial arteries, a guide wire 120 to 150 cm long should be used. Every single guide wire is sterile when packed and should be used only once, in order to avoid pyrogenic or toxic reactions to organic clotting due to inadequate cleaning.

3.3.3 Equipment

In our department equipment produced by Philips Medical Systems is used. An angio-diagnost catheterization table is supplied by a double-focus Super *Rotalix* X-ray tube (0.6/1.5 mm and 100 kw) and a high output 12-valve X-ray generator, the *Maximus* M 150.

The films are exposed by serial film changer (Elema-Schönander = AOT).

3.3.4 Local Anaesthesia

At the site of the puncture of the femoral artery a local anaesthetic (10 ml 1% lidocaine) is injected.

3.3.5 Contrast Media

There are different water-soluble contrast agents available for angiography at the present time. Since the methylglucamine salts of the contrast media have been shown to be less toxic to the central nervous system than sodium salts they are usually used for subclavian and brachial angiography.

It is also known that the pain and heat sensation occurring in peripheral arteriography are essentially attributable to the high osmotic pressure of the contrast medium. Therefore the use of contrast agents with low osmolarity is advisable.

Up to now we have carried out all investigations with conventional ionic methylglucamine salts such as:

1. Methylglucamine metrizoate (Isopaque Cerebral) with an iodine concentration of 280 mg/ml and an osmolarity of 1,460 milliosmoles/kg.
2. Methylglucamine ioxitalamate (Telebrix 30) with an iodine concentration of 300 mg/ml and an osmolarity of 1,490 milliosmoles/kg.
3. Recently methylglucamine sodium ioxaglic acid, in the proportions 2:1 (Hexabrix), with an iodine content of 320 mg/ml and an osmolarity of 580 milliosmoles/kg became available; it was used for several of the angiographic examinations presented in this thesis.

The important properties of Hexabrix, as far as our investigations are concerned, are its high iodine concentration and its relatively low osmotic pressure, which considerably reduce the pain occurring during angiography.

The only available non-ionic contrast medium metrizamide (Amipaque) has an osmolarity of 470 milliosmoles/kg at a concentration of 280 mg/ml. Because of its price it was not used in our department for upper extremity angiography.

In subclavian arteriography special attention must be paid to the neurotoxic effect of the contrast medium. Because of the proximity of the vertebral artery and thyrocervical trunk to the catheter tip during contrast injection the danger exists that a large volume of contrast material will reach the central nervous system. In order to prevent this a total volume of 16-18 ml contrast medium is injected at a rate of 8 ml per second for subclavian arteriography and 4-5 ml per second for brachial arteriography. In our experience these injection rates permit complete filling of the arteries and rarely cause reflux of the contrast medium into the proximal branches of the subclavian artery.

3.4 Technique of Catheterization

After transfemoral introduction of the catheter into the abdominal aorta under fluoroscopic control, heparin (Thromboliquine) is administered to prevent fibrin embolus formation along the surface of the catheter (Wallace *et al.*, 1972). For the same reason frequent and forceful flushing of the catheter with physiological saline is necessary. The heparin is diluted with 10 ml normal saline and injected intra-arterially through the catheter itself. For patients over 50 kg bodyweight, 75 mg (1500 I.U.) heparin are administered. Infants and adults between 20 and 50 kg bodyweight generally receive 50 mg heparin. For children under 20 kg an average of 20-30 mg heparin is usually sufficient.

From the lumbar aorta, the catheter usually advances easily in the ascending aorta without a guide wire. In patients suspected of having a dissecting aneurysm or a large thoracic aneurysm, a 'J' guide wire has to be advanced beyond the catheter to lead the catheter through the deformed lumen around the aortic arch into the ascending aorta (White Jr., 1976) After removal of the guide wire, a forceful flushing of the catheter with physiological saline is necessary.

Selective catheterization of the subclavian arteries begins actually when the catheter reaches the aortic arch. The method of catheterization is slightly different for the right and left subclavian artery.

Usually the left subclavian artery can be catheterized by simply turning the tip of the catheter to the left, craniolateralwards with respect to the aortic arch. The entrance of the catheter into the left subclavian artery can easily be observed under fluoroscopy. In younger individuals the catheter usually enters the subclavian artery directly from the descending aorta.

For catheterization of the right subclavian artery, the catheter has to be advanced into the ascending aorta. Than it is repeatedly withdrawn while the tip is rotated until the origin of the innominate artery has been reached. Once the innominate artery is entered, the tip of the catheter has to be rotated in the direction of the subclavian artery (Fig. 1). Very often a 'J' guide wire is needed to avoid selective catheterization of the right common carotid artery or the right vertebral artery. The guide wire usually provides enough stability to permit easy advance of the catheter into the right subclavian artery. The catheter and the guide wire have to be advanced as one unit. The final position of the catheter is confirmed by a test injection of a small amount of contrast medium.

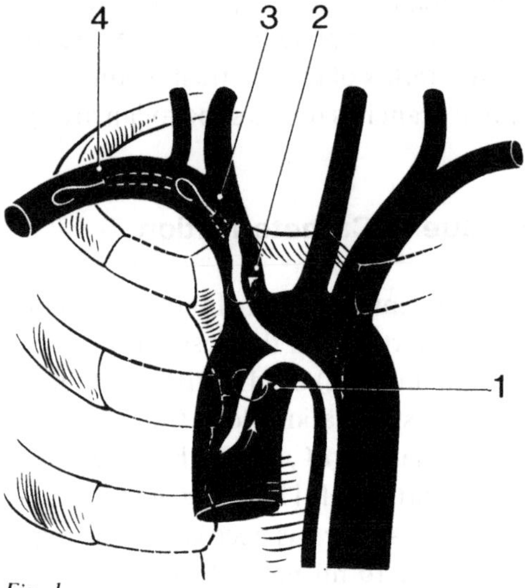

Fig. 1
Sequential steps for selective catheterization of the right subclavian artery.
1. Headhunter catheter in ascending aorta;
2. After withdrawal and rotation, catheter positioned in innominate artery;
3. Rotation of the catheter tip in the direction of the subclavian artery;
4. With or without a 'J' guide wire, advancing of the catheter in the right subclavian artery.

In elderly patients with dilatation and elongation of the aortic arch and a sharply angled brachiocephalic vessel, selective catheterization of the right subclavian artery can be a serious problem (Fig. 2).

In such cases the catheter technique described by Simmons, Tsao and Thompson (1973) who use a sidewinder Ducor catheter is helpful. This catheter was specifically designed for this type of aortic arch.

Since most subclavian artery stenoses occur at, or distal to, the first rib and subclavian compression develops at the same site, the catheter has to be left just proximal to the first rib. Immediately prior to angiography the position of the catheter has to be checked again.

Radiographs are first taken of the upper chest and shoulder in a neutral position with the upper arm parallel to the thoracic wall. Sixteen cubic centimeters of contrast medium are injected at a rate of 8 ml per second over a period of 4 seconds. In our department a *Medrad-IV* pressure injector is used; the roentgenograms for this examination, six in total, are made with a serial film changer (Elema-Schönander = AOT) at a frequency of two exposures per second for the first two seconds and one exposure per second for the following two seconds. If proximal subclavian artery stenosis is present and the collaterals are not clearly visualized, the serial study has to be repeated; the exposures are then taken over a longer period of time.

In patients with thoracic outlet compression syndrome, a second series of radiographs has to be taken with the upper arm in a provocative position. Sixteen to eighteen ml of contrast medium are injected at a rate of 8 ml per second. Two radiographs per second are obtained for three seconds, and one per second for the next two seconds. Eight films are generally sufficient for this study.

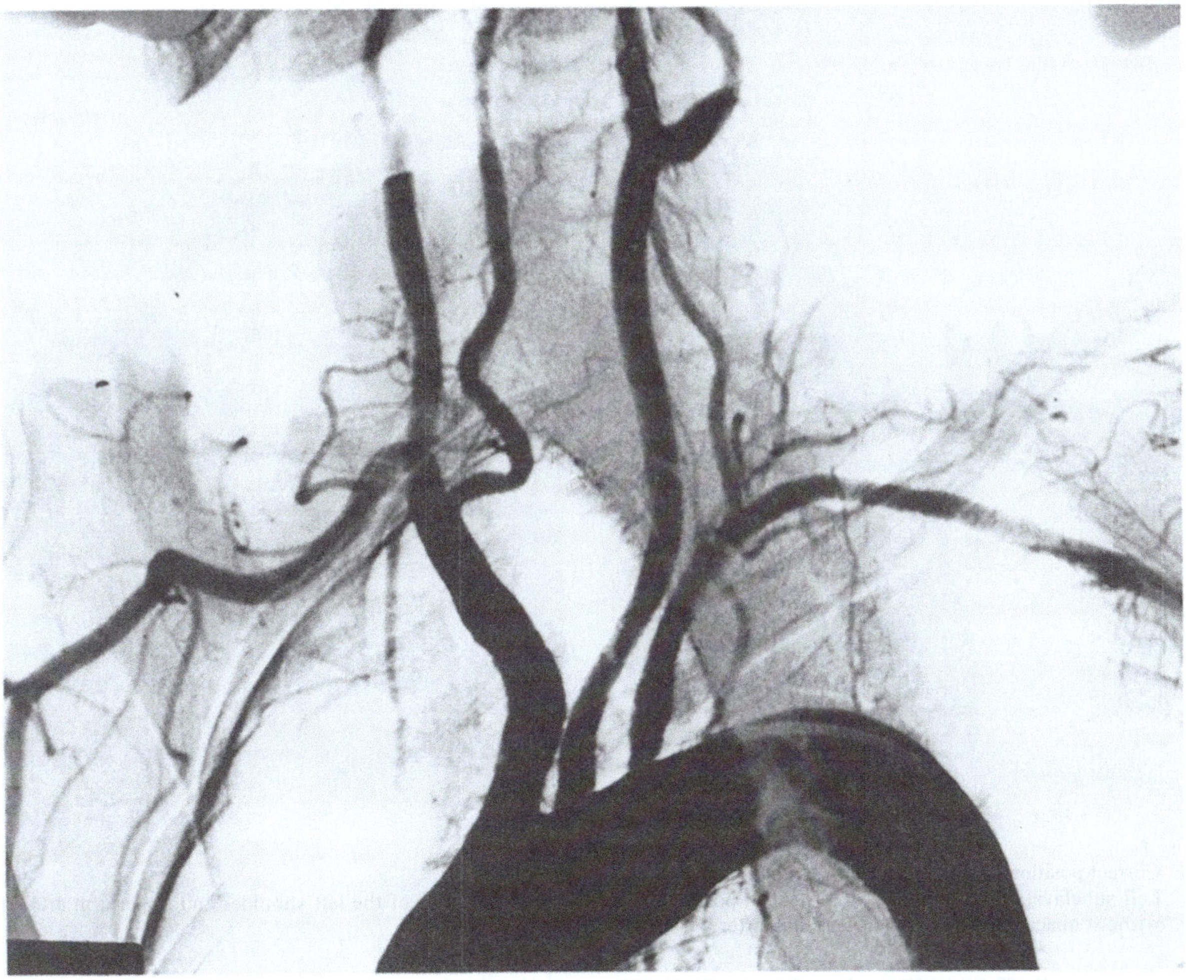

Fig. 2
Elongation and moderate dilatation of the aortic arch. The brachiocephalic vessels arise at a sharp angle from the anterior and superior portion of the ascending part of the arch. Pattern commonly seen in elderly individuals.

In view of the marked neurotoxicity of roentgen contrast media, all precautionary measures have to be taken before the pressure injection into the subclavian artery. A test injection of contrast material has to be administered to determine the final position of the catheter tip, which must lie distal to the origins of the vertebral artery and thyrocervical trunk (Figs. 3A and B). The stability of the catheter is controlled under fluoroscopy by forceful manual injection of physiological saline. With good stability, the catheter tip remains in the same place in the lumen of the subclavian artery during this injection.

If a severe compression or complete obstruction of the subclavian artery exists, as will be observed on the fluoroscope during the test injection, the total volume of contrast medium should be diminished. Otherwise, because of the obstruction, a large volume of contrast medium will go to the cerebral vessels (Figs. 4A and B). In such instances a volume of 10-12 ml contrast medium is sufficient to demonstrate the location and extent of the compression (Figs. 5A and B). After the exposures are made, the patient is asked to slowly put his arm back in the previous position. The catheter is flushed with physiological saline and remains in the subclavian artery until the X-ray films have been developed and inspected.

3.4.1 Catheter Flushing

Most complications related to catheter angiography are caused by emboli. Systemic heparinization by intra-arterial injection of heparin (Thromboliquine 1500 I.U.) and frequent vigorous flushing of the catheter with heparinized physiological saline

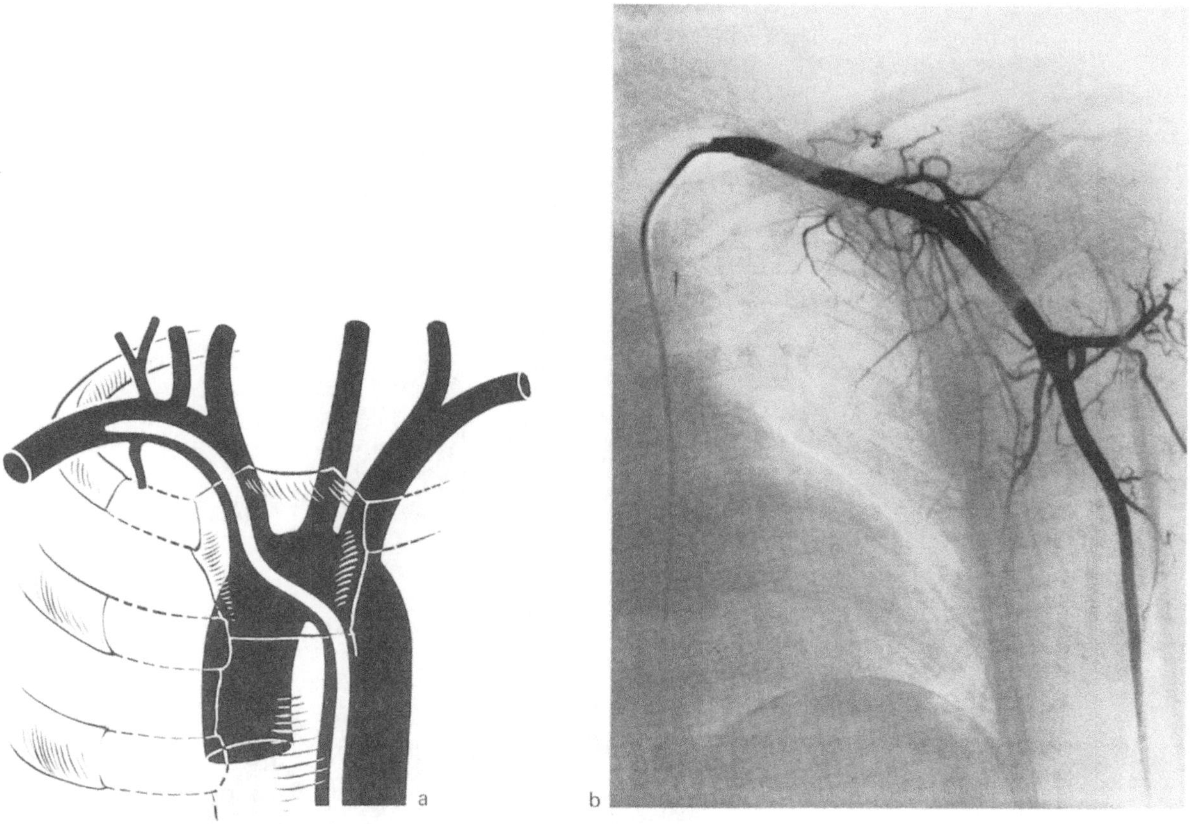

Fig. 3
A. Correct position of the catheter in right subclavian arteriography.
B. Left subclavian arteriogram; arm in neutral position. Note the optimal filling of the left shoulder and upper arm arteries without opacification of the left vertebral artery.

during the entire examination can prevent these complications. The catheter has to be flushed every 2-3 minutes, particularly after the test injections, and after aspiration of blood from the catheter.

Before any injection into the catheter, slight aspiration is necessary to clear air bubbles that are frequently present at the connection between the syringe and the catheter stopcock. At the end of every injection, the stopcock is immediately closed to prevent reflux of blood into the catheter tip.

3.5 Catheter Technique for Hand Angiography

3.5.1 Introduction of the Catheter

As in subclavian arteriography a single end-hole catheter (French 7; Cook Headhunter 1) is used for this study.

Introduction of the catheter into the brachial artery is possible only after angiographic or fluoroscopic examination by means of test injections of the subclavian and axillary arteries. If local occlusive diseases are excluded the catheter has to be advanced as far as possible, usually to the distal part of the brachial artery: the catheter tip is positioned just beyond the origin of the deep brachial artery, 10-12 cm above the antecubital fossa (Fig. 6). In this position the catheter is distal to all large arteries of the shoulder and upper arm. Occasionally the catheter cannot be advanced into the brachial artery because it has entered a side branch. In such cases the catheter should be repositioned in the main artery under fluoroscopic control, and a J-tipped guide wire should be used to facilitate easy catheter passage through the subclavian and axillary arteries. The flexible tip of the J-guide wire must be free in the arterial lumen and the stiff portion of the wire has to protrude 0.5 to 1 cm beyond the catheter tip. This usually provides enough stability of the catheter to permit

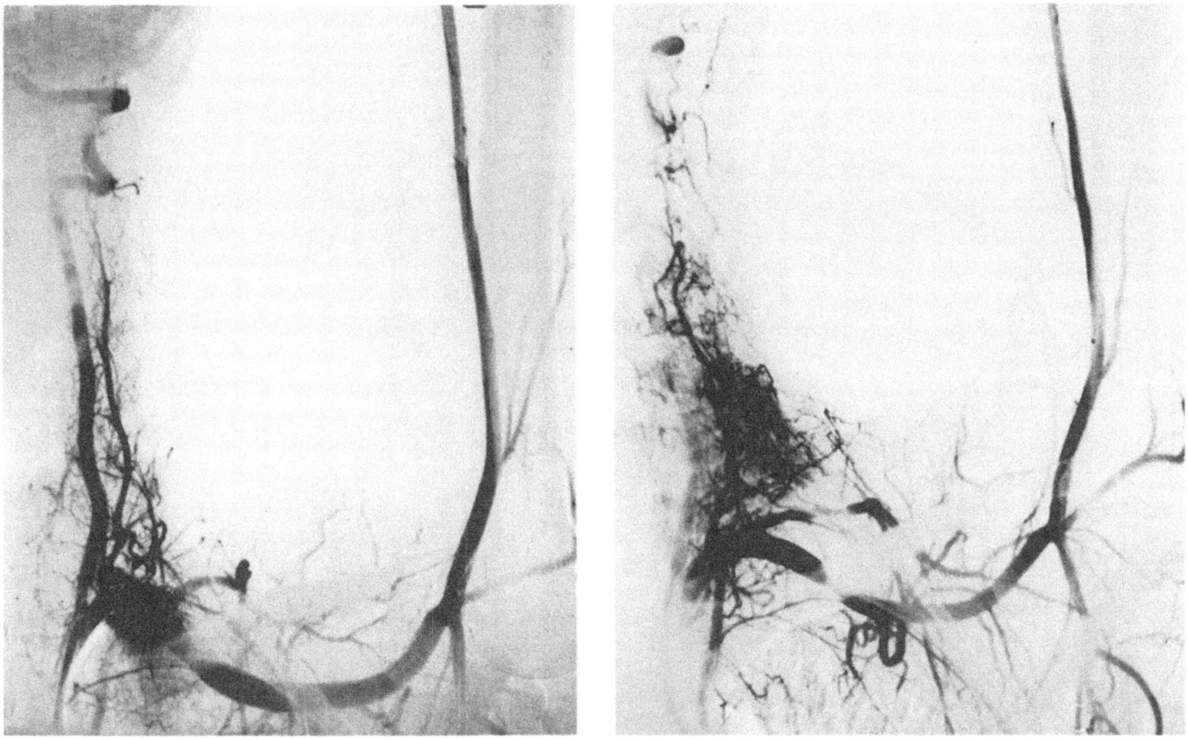

a b

Fig. 4

Left subclavian arteriograms of two patients with moderate (A) and severe (B) costoclavicular compression of the subclavian arteries; a large amount of contrast medium goes to the vertebral artery and the thyrocervical trunk due to the compression (4B reproduced from J. M. Greep *et al.*, Pain in Shoulder and Arm, chapter 3. Martinus Nijhoff, The Hague, Boston, London 1979).

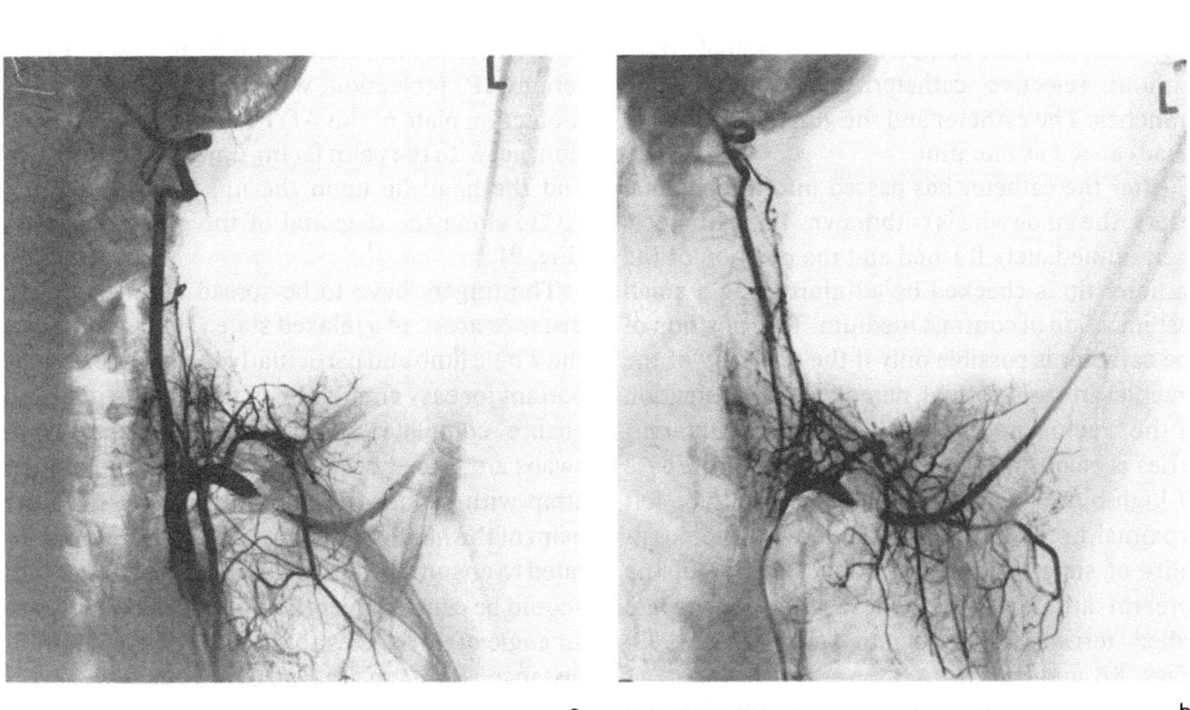

a b

Fig. 5

Selective subclavian arteriograms, taken with small amounts of contrast medium, of two patients with severe costoclavicular compression. In case A, 12 ml and in case B 10 ml of methylglucamine ioxitalamate were used.

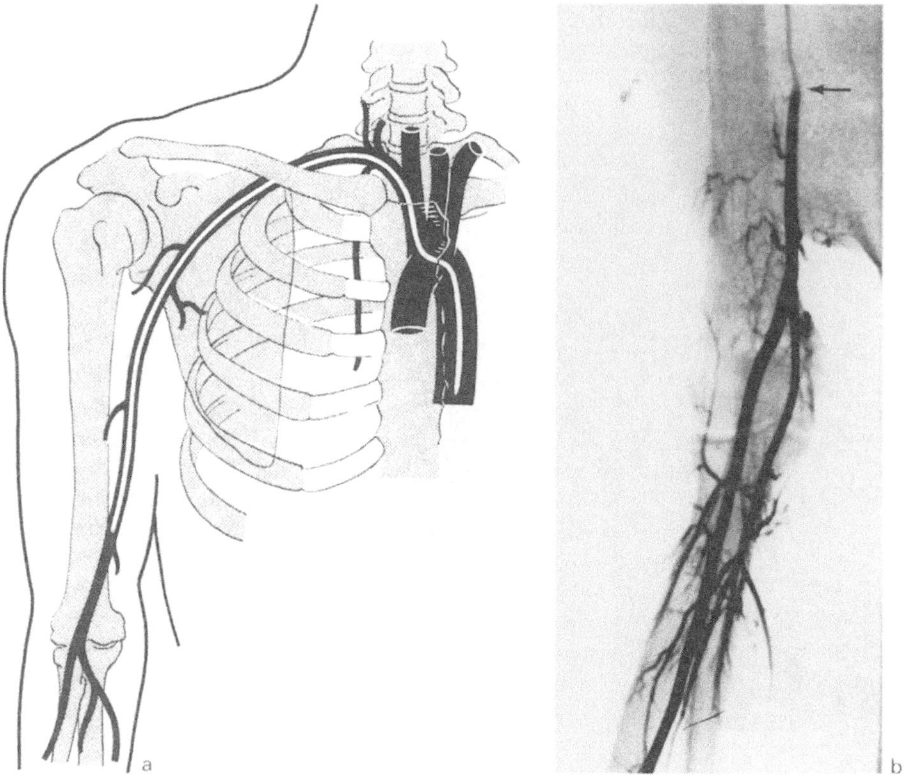

Fig. 6
A. Final position of the catheter in right brachial angiography.
B. Catheter tip (arrow) positioned 10-12 cm above antecubital fossa.

easy passage of the catheter in the brachial artery without selective catheterization of the side branches. The catheter and the guide wire have to be advanced as one unit.

After the catheter has passed into the brachial artery, the guide wire is withdrawn. The catheter is then immediately flushed and the position of the catheter tip is checked by administering a small test injection of contrast medium. This position of the catheter is possible only if the anatomy of the brachial artery is normal, namely if the bifurcation of the brachial artery into the radial and ulnar arteries is below the elbow joint (Fig. 7). In the case of high bifurcation the catheter tip has to be left proximal to the bifurcation; otherwise the possibility of superselective injection into one of the forearm arteries exists. These arteriograms are called territorial arteriograms (Janevski, 1979) (Figs. 8A and B).

For angiographic examination of the forearm and hand the AOT serial changer is placed beside the catheterization table, to the right or the left of the patient in accordance with the catheterization site. The X-ray films are taken in the anterior-posterior (AP) projection, with the arm lying on the protection plate of the AOT in the supinated position, i.e. with the palm facing upward. The forearm and the hand lie upon the upper surface of the AOT, along the diagonal of the protection plate (Fig. 9).

The fingers have to be spread out a moderate distance apart, in a relaxed state. The relaxation of the whole limb and particularly of the fingers is important for easy circulation of the blood. Finally, to ensure complete immobilisation of the hand, swabs are placed between the fingers and a linen strap with sandbags at the ends is put over the palm of the hand. The X-ray tube is shifted and rotated to ensure correct focussing. The X-ray beam should be centred over the midline of the wrist, at an angle of 90 degrees to the film. The focus-film distance is 100 cm (Fig. 10).

Prior to angiography a vasodilator has to be injected intra-arterially. For this purpose we use 20 mg tolazoline hydrochloride (Priscol; Priscoline) di-

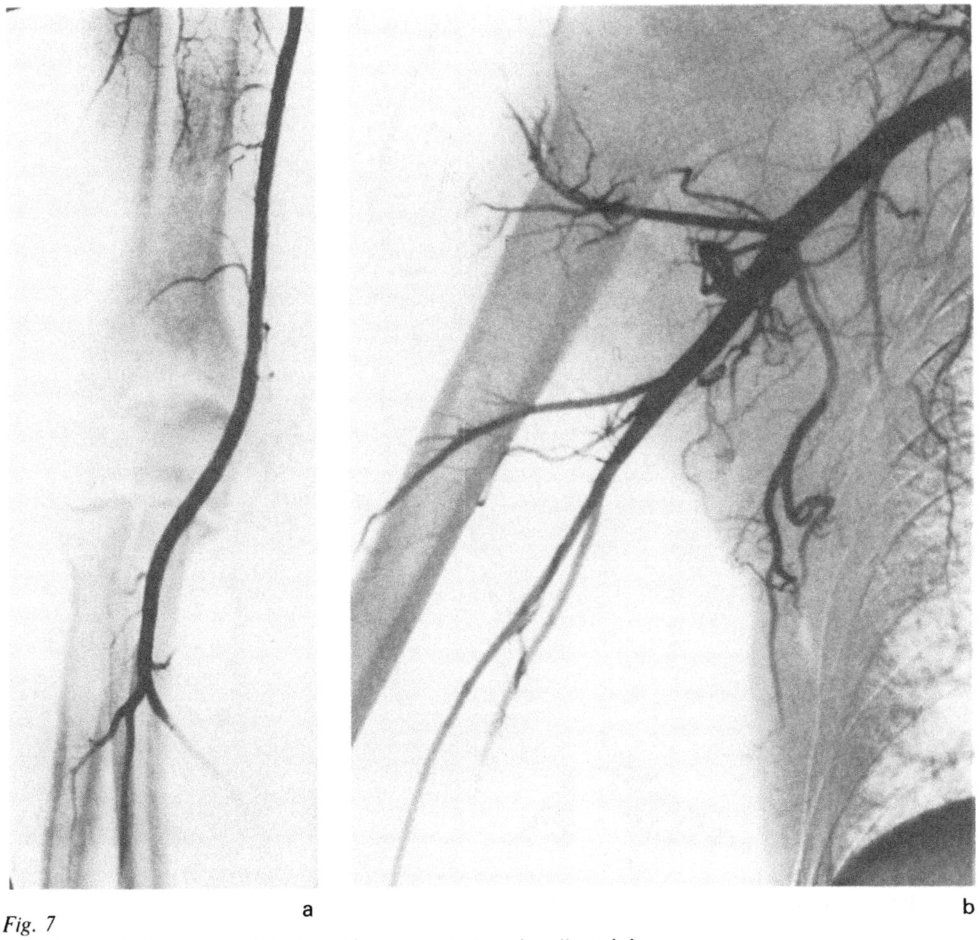

Fig. 7
A. 'Normal' bifurcation of the brachial artery, below the elbow joint.
B. High bifurcation of the right brachial artery.

luted with physiological saline to 20 ml per injection. A maximum dosage of 75 mg per patient should not be exceeded. The vasodilator has to be injected very slowly through the catheter, usually over a period of 100-120 seconds. Following the intra-arterial injection of the Priscoline a characteristic local reddening of the skin is observed. The patient feels a slight warmth over the forearm, the palm and the fingers. The injection of contrast medium has to be given when the warm feeling reaches the fingertips; this occurs about 10-15 seconds after the end of the tolazoline injection.

Usually a total volume of 18 ml of contrast medium is injected at a rate of 5 ml per second and the films are exposed over a period of 8 seconds.

3.5.2 Roentgenography

The arteriograms are routinely studied by the subtraction technique. Normally the roentgenograms are taken in the frontal (AP) projection, as described above; occasionally other projections are needed (right and left oblique or, very rarely, lateral). The roentgenograms are taken in rapid succession at a rate of three films per second for the first 3 seconds, and one film per second for the next 8 seconds.

With this series of films optimal angiography of the hand is usually obtained, with good filling of the arteries, capillaries and veins.

3.5.3 Postangiographic Care

After the angiograms are found to be satisfactory, both technically and for diagnostic purposes, the catheter is pulled back to the aortic bifurcation and 5 ml (50 mg) protamine sulfate are injected through it to insure complete neutralization of the

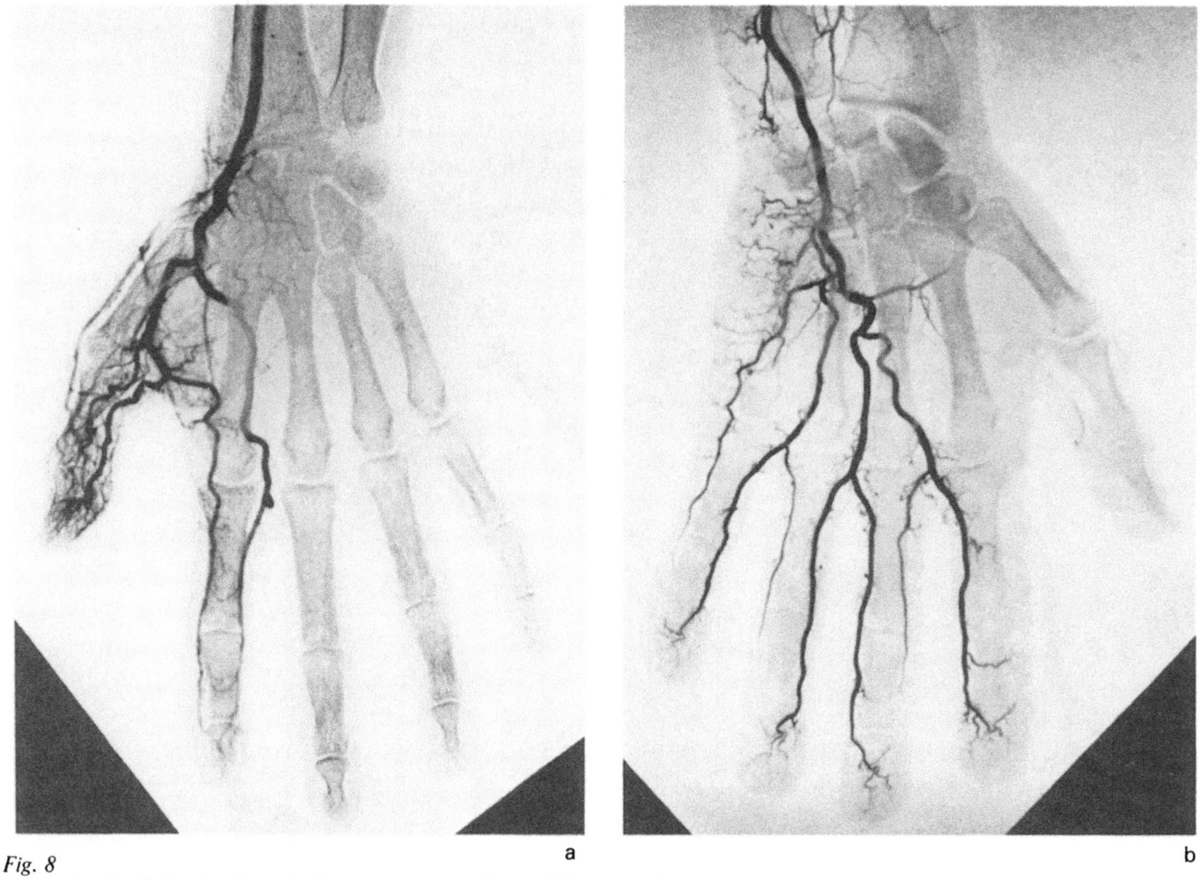

Fig. 8
Superselective injection into the forearm arteries of two different patients (territorial arteriography).
A. radial territory.
B. ulnar territory.

heparin. The catheter is then removed and manual pressure is applied to the femoral artery at the puncture site for approximately 5 to 10 minutes. More time may be required for hypertensive patients. The pressure should be adequate to stop bleeding, but not so forceful that the vessel is completely occluded. This latter point is particularly important in children and thin patients. During manual compression the posterior tibial artery and the dorsal pedal artery pulses should be checked regularly.

When complete haemostasis is achieved a firm dressing is applied to the puncture site, and the patient is transported in bed back to his ward.

In all instances the patient must remain at least 24 hours in hospital and, particularly for the first two hours, is watched closely for any evidence of bleeding or other complications.

Almost all of the postangiographic complications appear within the first few hours after the examination.

3.6 Another Method for Hand Angiography
(Direct Brachial Angiography)

As mentioned before, our preferance for hand angiography is the catheterization technique via the femoral artery with selective injection into the distal part of the brachial artery. When introduction of the catheter into the brachial artery is not possible because of severe aortofemoral or subclavian arteriosclerosis, cut-down brachial angiography can be a useful alternative. In our department, this technique, originally introduced and developed by Lemmens (1971), is always carried out under general anaesthesia. It consists of surgical exposure of the brachial artery in the antecubital fossa or in the lower part of the upper arm and insertion of a blunt-ended cannula into the vessel.

The method allows direct injection of the contrast material into the brachial artery at the in-

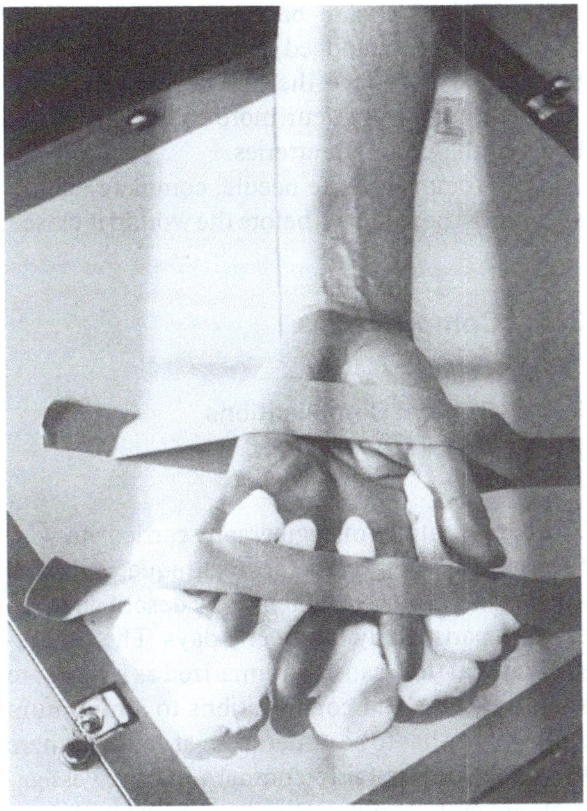

Fig. 9
Correct positioning of the hand prior to angiography.

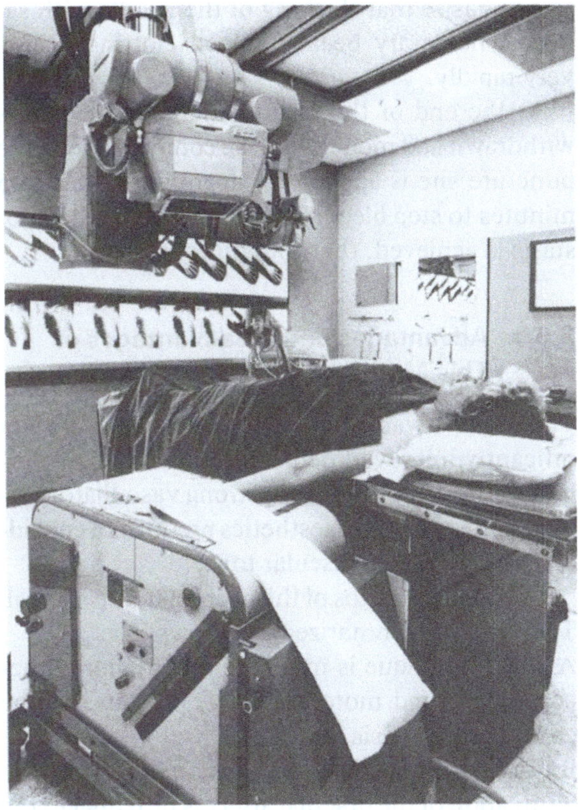

Fig. 10
Positioning of the patient for left hand angiography.

volved site, and generally provides excellent opacification of the hand arteries.

A special small puncture needle set, consisting of a blunt cannula (1.40 × 70 mm) and a pointed stylet, is used for this technique. In addition transparent polythene tubing 30 cm long is needed for connection of the needle to the syringe. Two syringes are also required, one filled with contrast material and the other filled with physiological saline.

After a small transverse incision is made in the antecubital fossa and the distal part of the brachial artery is carefully exposed, retrograde puncturing of the vessel is carried out. The needle is introduced through the skin distal to the incision, advanced towards the anterior wall of the artery, and slowly introduced into the arterial lumen.

The angle between needle and skin should be as small as possible to enable the needle to pass through a large area of soft tissue and thereby ensure adequate fixation.

A free backflow of blood indicates proper positioning of the needle tip within the lumen of the vessel. The blunt-ended cannula is then carefully advanced farther proximalwards in the arterial lumen. In this position the needle has good stability and the contrast injection can take place immediately after the administration of a vasodilator (usually a solution of 20 mg tolazoline in 20 ml physiological saline).

The retrograde manual injection of the contrast medium is performed 10-15 seconds after the intra-arterial injection of the vasodilator. A single dose of 16 ml contrast medium will usually be sufficient to produce a satisfactory examination with optimum filling of the forearm and hand arteries.

The positioning of the hand and the frequency of the exposures are exactly the same as in catheter angiography.

Immediately after administration of the contrast material, the second syringe filled with physiological saline is attached to the Teflon connecting tube, and the needle is flushed until the X-ray films are developed and inspected. It is important to emphasize that flushing of the needle with saline is necessary because blood clotting occurs very rapidly.

At the end of the examination, the needle is withdrawn and moderate swab compression of the puncture site is applied for approximately 3 to 5 minutes to stop bleeding. After complete haemostasis is achieved, the wound is sutured.

3.6.1 Advantages and Disadvantages of This Method

The major advantage of this technique is the significantly improved demonstration of small peripheral arteries, because the strong vasodilatory effect of the general anaesthetics produces a considerable decrease in vascular tone.

The disadvantages of this technique are several. They can be summarized as follows.

A. The technique is more traumatic, more time-consuming and more expensive, because of the general anaesthesia.

B. In cases of anatomical variation, e.g. when the bifurcation of the brachial artery is proximal to the antecubital fossa, complete opacification of the hand arteries is not possible. In such cases a second higher incision in the upper arm is necessary or separate injections into the radial and the ulnar arteries have to be made. These angiograms, as we said before, are called *territorial arteriograms* (Figs. 8A and B).

C. In the event that repositioning becomes mandatory, the patient's arm cannot be moved without the risk of damaging the arterial wall with the puncture needle. The needle tip may strip the intima from the media, particularly if saline or contrast medium is injected into the arterial wall, resulting in actual occlusion and thrombosis of the brachial artery. The use of a small-sized puncture needle set with a blunt cannula and the experience of the examiner are the major means of preventing these accidents. There is little doubt in the literature that general anaesthesia adds to this risk, since extravasation or subintimal injection may not be suspected until the X-ray films are developed and inspected. If the patient is examined under local anaesthesia his reactions and subjective symptoms may provide immediate warning of such mishaps and prevent further injections.

To avoid serious complications, no more than two injections should be administered into the brachial artery. Prolonged cannulation should also be avoided to reduce the risk of arterial spasm. This is thought to occur more frequently in the brachial than in other arteries.

After removal of the needle, complete haemostasis must be achieved before the wound is closed.

3.7 Complications

3.7.1 General Complications

Literature

The complications of angiography carried out with the transfemoral catheter technique are well known and have been extensively described in literature, particularly in its early days. The conclusions at that time can be summarized as follows: to keep accidents and complications to a minimum angiography has to be undertaken at centres where this procedure is fairly common. The investigations are best conducted by a radiologist with considerable training and experience in this field (Sutton, 1969).

General complications such as acute anaphylaxis or minor allergic reactions (urticaria, coughing, sneezing) after administration of contrast medium are still a potential risk and may occur during any angiographic examination. Local complications of the transfemoral catheter technique, such as injury of the intima, a pseudo-aneurysm or A-V fistula at the puncture site, thrombosis, local infection, plaque occlusion, impaired circulation and gangrene, are at the present time rare. Minor complications, e.g. haemorrhage at the puncture site or postangiographic perivascular haematomas, oedema and arterial spasm, are still often seen.

The complications and disadvantages of the direct brachial cut-down technique were discussed in the section on this method.

The complications of the transaxillary and transbrachial catheter techniques will be discussed very briefly, because these techniques were seldom used in our department.

Peripheral nerve injury as a complication of percutaneous axillary catheterization is well known in the literature. The high rate of neurological complications in transaxillary arteriography is caused by the anatomical relationship of the axillary artery to the brachial plexus at the puncture site. Neurological complications include: pain, transitory or permanent paraesthesia, and, in the event of severe injury of the brachial plexus or one of its branches, complete or partial paralysis of the arm (Staal *et al.*, 1966; Dudrick *et al.*, 1967; van Voorthuisen, 1967; Lyon *et al.*, 1975).

Complications originating at the site of catheterization are most frequent and severe with the transaxillary approach. These include axillary artery thrombosis with ischaemic symptoms in the hand, false aneurysm and uncontrollable bleeding from the puncture site. This is related to the small size and location of the axillary artery, which make haemostasis difficult. Pseudoaneurysms occur with the greatest frequency in the axillary artery (Hessel *et al.*, 1981).

In brachial percutaneous arteriography the main complications are thrombosis and the formation of aneurysms at the puncture site (Eriksson *et al.*, 1970). Postangiographic pseudo-aneurysms are more rare than thrombosis. The problem of postangiographic arterial complications in brachial arteriography has been described by several authors (Lang, 1963; Bergentz *et al.*, 1966; Chiavacci *et al.*, 1976). After performing 4,000 brachial arteriograms McBurney *et al.* (1973) reported complications, either thrombosis or a false aneurysm in the brachial artery, in 22 patients.

Other complications, such as bleeding, expanding haematoma, dissection, dislodging of arteriosclerotic plaques and spasm, are well-recognized risks of percutaneous brachial puncture. Formation of an arteriovenous fistula after retrograde brachial catheterization is also described in the literature. This complication was reported by Shine *et al.* in 1967 and by Kanshepolsky *et al.* in 1971.

Recently a report was published by Hessel *et al.* (1981) about the complications of angiography, including the transfemoral, transaxillary and translumbar approaches. The complications were analysed that occurred in the period from July 1974 through June 1975 in 514 U.S. hospitals, where a total number of 118,591 angiographic examinations were performed by more than one thousand radiologists.

The analysis revealed an inverse relationship between complication rate and annual number of arteriograms obtained. The transfemoral route carried a significantly lower risk of complications than the transaxillary approach. The overall arteriographic complication rates were: transfemoral 1.73%, translumbar 2.89% and transaxillary 3.29%. Thirty deaths were reported, 27% of which were caused by aortic dissection or rupture of an aneurysm. Five patients died of unspecified cardiac causes, and only two of the 30 deaths (7%) were attributed to drug reactions (Hessel *et al.*, 1981).

For further understanding of the problem of angiographic complications, this recent publication is highly recommended.

3.7.2 Angiographic Complications Our Experience

Over the past ten years, in which we have performed 592 aortic arch aortograms, 750 selective subclavian and brachial arteriograms and over 2000 angiograms of all other types, excluding cerebral angiograms, there were no deaths or any other serious complication in our department. One case of brachial artery thromboembolism developed in a young female two hours after selective angiography of the left brachial artery.

Thrombosis at the puncture site did not occur in any patient. Bleeding at the puncture site was seen in 21 patients (0.5%). In two patients bleeding was sufficiently severe to necessitate transfusion. All complications are summarized in Table I. Minor complications such as spasm and postangiographic haematomas at the puncture site are not included.

3.7.3 Neurological Complications Related to Catheter Angiography of the Brachiocephalic Vessels

Literature

The value of the catheter technique for selective opacification of the brachiocephalic vessels and its branches by introduction of the catheter from either the brachial, axillary or femoral artery is now well established. Transfemoral catheterization is favoured, because it causes only minor discomfort to the patient. Furthermore, it permits selective catheterization of the external and internal carotid arteries after demonstration of the common carotid artery and permits the examination of more than one vessel in the same sitting (Cronqvist *et al.*, 1970).

Neurological complications related to catheter angiography of the brachiocephalic vessels may occur regardless of the way in which the catheter is introduced into one of these arteries. About 80-90% of the neurological complications that develop after angiography are transient. Fatalities occurred in 0.7 percent of the cases in the series of Taveras (1976). Arteriosclerosis is a predisposing factor to these complications. The incidence of cerebral complications is four times higher for patients with cerebrovascular disease than for those having nonischaemic lesions (Taveras, 1976).

3.7.4 Neurological Complications Our Experience

Complications caused by the neurotoxic effect of contrast media may also occur in subclavian arteriography, particularly if excessive amounts of contrast fluid are used or the circulation of the subclavian artery is impaired. To avoid the administration of large amounts of contrast medium into spinal or cerebral arteries, attention should be directed to the relation between the injected dose and the capacity of the peripheral vascular system. Care is also required for patients with the thoracic outlet compression syndrome, when the injection is given with the arm in the hyperabduction position and severe compression of the subclavian artery exists, as discussed and illustrated in 3.4.

Other neurological complications associated with spasm of a cerebral artery, obstruction of the vessel lumen by the catheter, a clot embolism or an air embolus may also occur during the selective catheterization of the upper arm arteries.

In order to achieve a realistic representation of the incidence of neurological and other complications, the following analysis includes the complications of our subclavian, brachial and cerebral angiographies and all other types of angiographic procedure carried out in our department during the last ten years (see Table I).

In our series consisting of 549 vertebral and 664 carotid angiographies carried out with the catheter technique, severe complications related to the angiography occurred in only six cases (0.5%). One patient developed neurological symptoms of embolization of the right carotid artery directly after the injection of the contrast medium; in five other cases cortical blindness developed after vertebral angiography (Table I). In all of these cases the blindness was transient with a duration of six hours to three days. In the series of 750 subclavian and brachial angiographies, only one complication of short duration was observed. This complication occurred in a 50-year-old female patient with a renal transplant and septicaemia at the time of the examination. The patient history and physical examination revealed multiple surgically created arteriovenous fistulae in both forearms to permit chronic intermittent haemodialysis. An infected aneurysm in the involved arteries was suspected to be the underlying cause of the septicaemia. Selective brachial angiography was performed and revealed no evidence of such an aneurysm. Fourteen hours after angiography the patient became blind; loss of vision was transient with complete recovery within three days. It is uncertain whether

TABLE I

Angiographic Complications 1970-1980.

Type of angiography	*Number*	*Thrombo-embolism*	*Thrombosis at the puncture site*	*Bleeding at the puncture site*	*Cortical blindness*	*Percent*
Thoracic aorta	592			2		0.33
Carotid R + L	664	1		1		0.30
Vertebral	549				5	0.91
Subclavian-Brachial	750	1		2	1	0.53
All other types	2116			16		0.75
Total	4671	2		21	6	0.68
Percent		0.09%		0.45%		

this accident can be attributed to the angiographic procedure, but if this complication is added to the other five which occurred after vertebral angiography, the incidence of cortical blindness in our series of 1,213 cerebral and 750 subclavian and brachial angiographies carried out with the catheter technique is 0.3%. In vertebral angiography the incidence of this complication is almost one percent (see Table I).

REFERENCES

AMPLATZ, K.: Percutaneous arterial catheterization and its application. *Amer. J. Roentgenology, 87: 265, 1962.*

BERGENTZ, S. E., L. D. HANSSON and B. NORBACK: Surgical management of complications to arterial puncture. *Ann. Surg., 164: 1021-1023, 1966.*

CRONQVIST, S. and H. O. EFSING, E. PALACIOS: Embolic complications in cerebral angiography with the catheter technique. *Acta Radiol., 10: 97-107, 1970.*

CHIAVACCI, W. E., R. L. BUCCIARELLI and B. E. VICTORIA: Aneurysm of the Subclavian Artery: A Complications of Retrograde Brachial Artery Catheterization. *Cath. and Cardiovascular Diagnosis, 2: 93-106, 1976.*

DUDRICK, S., W. MASLAND and M. MISHKIN: Brachial plexus injury following axillary artery puncture. *Radiology, 88: 271, 1967.*

ERIKSSON, I. and H. JORULF: Surgical complications associated with arterial catheterization. *Scand. J. Thor. Cardiovascul. Surg., 4: 69-75, 1970.*

HAWKINS, I. F. and T. HUDSON: Priscoline in Bone and Soft-tissue Angiography. *Radiology, 110: 541-546, 1974.*

HESSEL, S. J., D. F. ADAMS and H. L. ABRAMS: Complications of Angiography. *Radiology, 138: 273-281, 1981.*

JANEVSKI, B.: Angiography of the Upper Extremity in 'Pain in shoulder and Arm', edited by Greep *et al. Martinus Nijhoff, The Hague, Boston, London, 3: 24-48, 1979.*

KANSHEPOLSKY, J., H. DANIELSON and R. E. FLYNN: Iatrogenic Arteriovenous Fistula After Retrograde Brachial Arteriogram. *Bull. Los Angeles Neurolog. Soc., 36: 126-130, 1971.*

LANG, E. K.: A survey of complications of percutaneous retrograde arteriography. *Radiology, 81: 257-000, 1963.*

LYON, B. B., B. A. HANSEN and T. MYGIND: Peripheral Nerve Injury as a Complication of Axillary Arteriography. *Acta Neurol. Scandinavica, 51: 29-36, 1975.*

MCBURNEY, R. P., L. LEE and J. R. FEILD: Thrombosis and Aneurysm of the Brachial Artery Secondary to Brachial Arteriography. *The Amer. Surgeon, 115-117, 1973.*

SIMMONS, C. R., E. C. TSAO and J. R. THOMPSON: Angiographic approach to the difficult aortic arch: A new technique for transfemoral cerebral angiography in the aged. *Am. J. Roentgenol. Radium Ther. Nucl. Med., 119: 605-612, 1973.*

SHINE, K. I., D. O'KEEFE and J. W. HARTHORNE: Arteriovenous fistula after retrograde brachial catheterization. *New England Journal of Medicine, 276: 1431-1436, 1967.*

STAAL, A., A. E. van VOORTHUISEN and L. M. van DIJK: Neurological complications following arterial catheterization by the axillary approach. *Br. J. Radiol., 39: 115-116, 1966.*

SUTTON, D.: Textbook of Radiology. *The Williams and Wilkins Co., Baltimore, 60: 1065-1118, 1969.*

SUTTON, D.: 'Arteriography of the Upper Extremities' in Abrams, H. L.: *Angiography vol. II, Second Edition, Little Brown and Co. Boston, 1971.*

TAVERAS, J. M.; E. W. WOOD: Complication of Angiography in Diagnostic Neuroradiology. *The Williams & Wilkins Co., 1: 486-490, 1976.*

VOORTHUISEN van, A. E.: Selectieve arteriografie van de arteria coeliaca en de arteria mesenterica superior. 1-6, 1967.

WALLACE, S., H. MEDELLIN, D. de JONGH and C. GIANTURCO: Systemic Heparinization for Angiography. *Amer. J. Roentgenol., 116: 204-209, 1972.*

WHITE, R. I. Jr: Fundamentals of Vascular Radiology. *Lea & Febiger, Philadelphia, 86-90, 1976.*

Chapter 4

VASCULAR TONUS AND PHARMACOANGIOGRAPHY

One of the most frequently occurring phenomena in peripheral angiography is vasospasm. Severe vasospasm does not permit optimal filling of the arterial lumen with contrast material and it makes a reliable diagnosis impossible.

To understand the mechanism of spasm a detailed knowledge of the anatomy, histology and physiology of the peripheral vessels is required.

Literature

4.1 General Anatomic and Histologic Considerations

The structure of arterial walls varies according to vessel function and size. Central large arteries are rich in collagen and elastin, which give tensile strength, pliability and elastic tension. As the vessel extends peripherally to terminate in the vascular beds of the extremities, there is a progressive reduction of collagen and elastin so that the smooth musculature provides most of the vascular tone of the arteries supplying the skin of the digits (Metzler and Silver, 1979).

All arteries are composed of three coats: 1. Internal or endothelial coat (tunica intima); 2. Middle or muscular coat (tunica media); and 3. External or connective tissue coat (tunica adventitia).

The tunica intima consists of a) an endothelial layer, with differently shaped cells (polygonal, oval and fusiform) all with round or oval nuclei; b) a subendothelial layer, consisting of connective tissue which is well-developed only in fairly large vessels; in arteries less than 2 mm across this layer consists only of a single stratum of stellate cells; and c) an elastic membrane or fenestrated layer, containing a network of elastic fibres extending mainly in the longitudinal direction.

Between the fibres are small elongated apertures, giving it a fenestrated appearance. This membrane or internal elastic layer provides the thickness of the inner coat. In minute arteries the elastic membrane is a very thin layer but in the larger arteries and in the aorta, it can be quite thick.

The tunica media consists generally of muscle fibres arranged in a transverse pattern. In the smaller arteries it contains mainly plain muscle fibres in fine bundles arranged in lamellae and distributed in circles around the vessel. The lamellae vary in number according to the size of the vessel; the small arteries have only a single layer, and the larger three or four layers. The thickness of the wall of the arteries is mainly determined by this muscular coat.

The tunica adventitia consists predominantly of connective tissue but, in all arteries – large and small, it also contains elastic fibres. The elastic tissue is much more abundant next to the tunica media, and it is sometimes described as a special layer between the adventitia and media, called the tunica elastica externa. This layer is most marked in medium-sized arteries. In the smaller arteries it consists of a single layer of connective tissue and elastic fibres, while in the smallest arteries, just before capillaries, the elastic fibres are absent. The connective tissue becomes more homogeneous as it approaches the capillaries and is gradually reduced to a thin membranous envelope, that finally disappears.

All arteries are supplied by nutrient vessels, called *vasa vasorum*. These blood vessels arise from a branch of the artery, or from a neighbouring vessel, close to the point where they are distributed. They ramify in the periadventitial tissue and are distributed to the external coat (adventitia). In man they do not penetrate into the tunica media.

The arteries are also supplied with nerves, which are derived from the sympathetic nervous system. They form a plexus upon the surfaces of the larger trunks, and run along the smaller arteries as single filaments or bundles of filaments which twist around the vessel and unite with one another in the form of a plexus. The branches derived from these plexuses (nervi vasorum) penetrate the adventitia and are distributed principally to the smooth muscle fibres of the tunica media, where the receptor is situated. There are two types of receptors, alfa and beta-adrenergic. In the muscular tissue of the arterial wall both types of receptor are present.

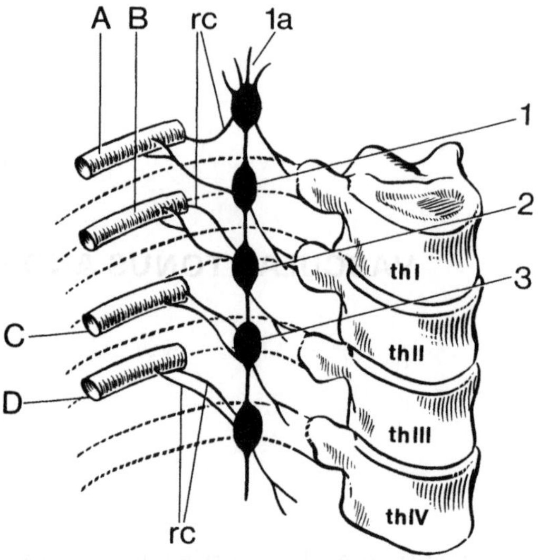

Fig. 11
Upper thoracic sympathetic trunk.
1a Stellate ganglion (Ganglion cervicothoracicum; – stellatum)
1, 2, 3 Upper thoracic paravertebral sympathetic ganglia (Ganglia thoracica superior)
rc Communicating rami (Rami communicantes)
A B C D Peripheral nerves.

4.1.1 Innervation of the Vascular System of the Upper Extremities

The vascular system of the upper extremity is innervated by the autonomic nervous system which includes all nerve cells (neurons) located outside the spinal cord and in the spinal cord as well as the nuclei of the brain stem. The nerve cells in the spinal cord and the brain stem are known as preganglionic neurons. The outlying nerve cells are arranged in aggregates and form the so-called autonomic ganglia. Some of these ganglia are incorporated in a pair of longitudinal cords, known as sympathetic chains or trunks (truncus sympaticus). The trunks with the ganglia extend from the base of the cranium to the coccyx on both sides of the spine. The thoracic portion of the left and the right sympathetic trunk lies ventral to the necks of the ribs and is covered by the pleura. It includes ten or eleven thoracic ganglia (Fig. 11).

In many instances the first thoracic ganglion is fused with the inferior cervical ganglion to form the cervicothoracic, or stellate, ganglion. In man, such a fusion may be found in fifty percent or more of the cases.

The autonomic innervation of the peripheral blood vessels is solely sympathetic. The sympathetic nerves which supply the arteries of the upper extremity originate in preganglionic nerve cells whose bodies lie in the corresponding lateral horns of the grey matter of the spinal cord (Fig. 12). The axons of these cells extend with the anterior nerve roots and the white communicating rami into the paravertebral sympathetic ganglia and form a synapse there with postganglionic neurons. Axons from the sympathetic postganglionic nerve cells

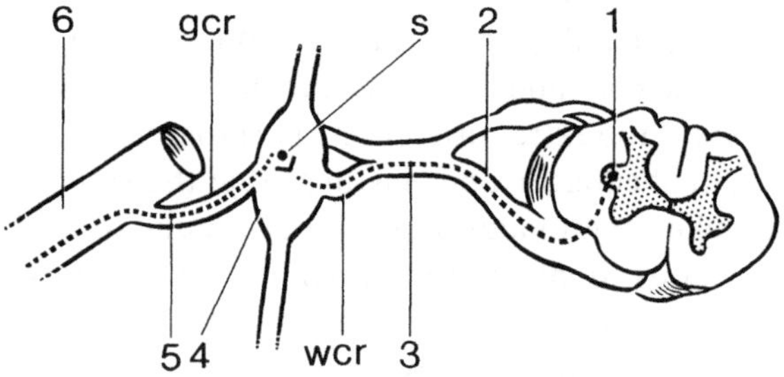

Fig. 12
Sympathetic pathways.
1. Preganglionic nerve cell
2. Anterior nerve root
3. Preganglionic axon
s Synapse
4. Paravertebral sympathetic ganglion
wcr White communicating ramus
gcr Gray communicating ramus
5. Postganglionic axon
6. Peripheral nerve.

pass through the gray communicating rami into the peripheral nerves of the brachial plexus and then down the arm to supply the skin and vessels of the upper extremity. In general each sympathetic trunk ganglion is connected with every spinal nerve on the same side through communicating rami; therefore a typical spinal nerve contains not only the somatic (motoric) efferent fibres and afferent (sensory) fibres, but also the autonomic efferent fibres.

The blood vessels of the upper extremity are innervated through nerve fibres (axons) arising from the sympathetic ganglion cells localized in the lower cervical and upper thoracic regions. For the innervation of the hand, the second and third thoracic segments are very important (Kuntz *et al.*, 1931). These sympathetic fibres join the brachial plexus and the second and third intercostal nerves. There are also sympathetic branches of variable dimensions, which derive from the second paraspinal ganglion and connect with the first and the second intercostal nerves. Other anatomical variations also exist.

The nerve fibres of the sympathetic system, which go together with the spinal nerves, reach the blood vessels through branches which join the vessels at intervals along their course. These nerve branches form plexuses upon the surfaces of the larger vascular trunks and run along the smaller arteries as single filaments, or bundles of filaments, which twist around the vessel and unite with one another in the form of a plexus in the superficial adventitial layers of the artery or vein. The branches derived from the plexus (nervi vasorum) penetrate the adventitia and are distributed principally to the smooth muscle fibres of the tunica media of the arteries.

The terms sympathetic or parasympathetic are important because they define the anatomical relations in the visceral nervous system. However, stimulation of the autonomic ganglion cells or their axons results in the liberation of chemical substances which play essential roles in the transmission of the nerve impulses from the nerve fibres to the effector tissues (Kuntz, 1953). The substance liberated due to stimulation of sympathetic ganglion cells, or sympathetic postganglionic fibres, has the properties of adrenalin. This substance has been called sympathin.

The substance liberated upon stimulation of parasympathetic ganglion cells, or postganglionic fibres, possesses the properties of acetylcholine. It has been called parasympathin. These two substances are released at the neuro-effector junctions. However, during stimulation some sympathetic ganglion cells do not release sympathin but an acetylcholine-like substance, which is probably identical to parasympathin; likewise stimulation of some parasympathetic ganglion cells results in the liberation of an adrenalin-like substance which probably is identical to adrenalin. These facts show clearly that sympathetic and parasympathetic ganglion cells cannot be separated by their function into two single categories. Those autonomic ganglion cells which liberate an adrenalin-like substance when stimulated have been classified as adrenergic, and those which liberate an acetylcholine-like substance as cholinergic.

The sympathetic efferent nerves of the blood vessels from the thoracic region include adrenergic (vasoconstrictor fibres) and cholinergic (vasodilator fibres) cells. In principle they cause the contraction and relaxation of the arterial wall, regulating the amount of blood sent to the distribution area of the artery.

4.2 Physiology of Vascular Tonus General Discussion

The smooth muscles of vessels undergo continuously asynchronic contractions through the activity of the sympathetic vasoconstrictive nerves. The summation of these contractions produces vessel wall tone. At the present time it is thought that the peripheral vessels of the extremity do not have vasodilatory innervation (Hertzmann, 1959). The muscular tone is also influenced by physical and chemical agents.

Cold stimulation produces digital vasoconstriction and heat stimulation produces vasodilatation. Response to cold is both a central, sympathetically mediated phenomenon and a local vascular phenomenon. For example, cold stimulus applied to one extremity produces digital vasoconstriction in both extremities, which is abolished by sympathectomy. However, the vasculature of a digit whose sympathetic innervation has been interrupted also responds with vasoconstriction to direct application of cold (Metzler and Silver, 1979).

Humoral agents present in the blood also affect the vascular smooth muscles. Circulating cathecholamines have only a vasoconstrictive effect on digital arteries (Conrad, 1972). Polypeptides such as bradykinin, kallidin and histamine have a vasodilatory effect on the smooth muscle fibres in the small vessels. The nicotine absorbed from smoking cigarettes has a peripheral vasoconstrictive effect by decreasing blood flow to the skin and increasing vascular resistance.

It has been shown in patients with vasospastic disorders that after smoking only two cigarettes blood flow to the skin of the feet is decreased by 40% and the vascular resistance is increased by 100% (Coffman, 1967). When the oxygen tension of the blood is decreased the ability of the smooth muscles of the vascular wall to contract is reduced. Elevation of carbon dioxide tension causes vasoconstriction of the arteries and simultaneous capillary dilatation. Finally, vasospasm may be induced by mechanical irritation of the muscle fibres of the arterial wall. For example, the puncture of an artery for catheterization may produce a vasospastic reaction of variable duration.

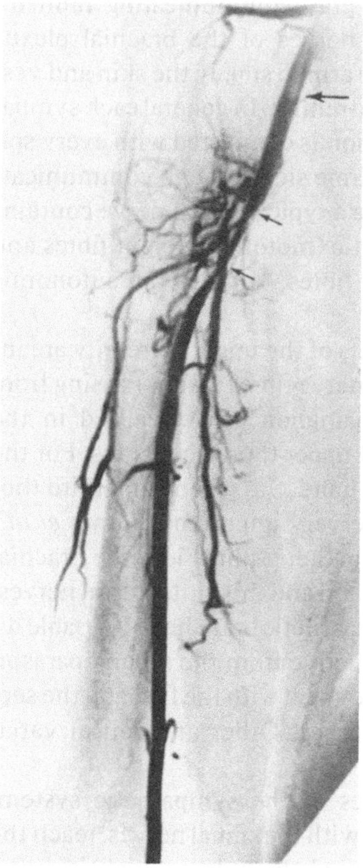

Fig. 13
Right brachial arteriogram of young female.
Iatrogenic spasm of the proximal portion of the brachial artery (small arrows) caused by catheter manipulation. Injection was administered after withdrawal of the catheter tip proximalwards to the nonspastic segment of the artery (large arrow).

Occasionally during catheterization an iatrogenic arterial spasm may be observed when the guidewire or the catheter is advanced too far distalwards in an artery of small calibre.

In such instances, an immediate withdrawal of the catheter is necessary. Iatrogenic vasospasm is particularly common in children and female adolescents. It tends to occur when the size of the catheter approaches the size of the vessel lumen.

In principle, every catheterization of a peripheral limb artery may lead to arteriospasm and impaired circulation in the extremity.

The contrast medium should never be injected into a spastic artery by means of a pressure injector. According to the author's own experience, withdrawal of the catheter tip into the nonspastic segment of the artery allows safe injection of the contrast medium (Fig. 13). If the spasm is severe, the filling of the peripheral vessels may be slow, and visualization of these vessels requires a prolonged series of roentgenograms. The volume of contrast medium injected should be as small as possible and additional projections should not be obtained unless they are absolutely necessary.

In conclusion it can be said that the peripheral vessels are subjected to a high degree of neurogenic (sympathetic) regulation but are also capable of local regulation, and that they react to cold and warmth, mechanical stimuli – either internal or external and to hormonal, chemical and metabolic vasoactive substances which may be present in the blood circulation.

4.3 Disturbed Vascular Tonus of the Extremities

There are different conditions which cause vasospasm of the arteries of the extremities. Arterial spasm after use of ergotamine has been described in the literature by many authors. Toxic reactions to ergotamine are usually caused by overdosage, but hypersensitivity to therapeutic doses is now also known.

Most cases of sensitivity or overdosage have occurred when ergotamine is given as an intramuscular injection or a suppository. However, there are several reports in the literature of arteriospasm following oral administration of ergotamine (Fuchs and Blumenthal, 1950; Glazer *et al.*, 1966; Imrie, 1973; Zicot *et al.*, 1978). In these cases the lower limbs have been affected predominantly. The spasm associated with ergotamine can occur at any stage of therapy. It may have an acute course or cause chronic haemodynamic disturbances in the extremities. It is generally admitted that recovery is rapid after withdrawal of the drug, but if an ischaemic neuropathy has developed it may be the source of chronic problems (Zicot *et al.*, 1978).

The effect of ergot alkaloids on the peripheral circulation is twofold. There is a direct stimulation of the vascular smooth muscles causing vasoconstriction and at the same time there is a contrary alpha-adrenergic blocking effect which tends to cause vasodilatation. When ergotamine is prescribed in therapeutic dosages, the vasoconstrictor effect predominates (Imre, 1973).

Methysergide is an ergot derivative, but has only a slight vasoconstrictor and oxytoxic effect. It is a most effective agent for the prophylaxis of migraine and other vascular headaches, but is not effective when given during acute attacks.

It is not certain whether the prophylactic benefit of methysergide is the result of central or peripheral activity.

Acute arterial spasm of the lower extremities after methysergide therapy was described by Raw and Gaylis in 1976. In 1977 Ameli *et al.* published an unusual case of a woman who suffered transient brachial artery occlusion after receiving methysergide for the treatment of headaches. It has been demonstrated that small or large doses of this drug may cause severe vasoconstriction of the middle-sized and small arteries in any part of the body. Fortunately, in all observed cases, the vasoconstriction disappeared after cessation of therapy with this drug. There are many other conditions associated with vascular spasm which have been described in the literature. An unusual case of nontraumatic toxin-induced peripheral arterial spasm which occurred after a bee sting was described by Karmody and Tsapogas in 1972. Five cases of transient vascular spasticity of the lower extremities following abdominal aortography were described by Cornell (1969). According to the author this spasm which is of unknown aetiology appeared approximately five minutes after the injection of contrast fluid by pressure injector. All of the patients noted numbness and stiffness of the legs, which they were unable to move. Immediate fluoroscopy after injection revealed no evidence of intramural or extravascular contrast medium accumulation. The authors stated that these aortograms did not differ, as far as any of the technical factors or the type and amount of contrast medium were concerned, from those of patients who did not experience vascular spasms in the lower extremity. Di Chiro and his associates described in 1967 transient lower extremity spasticity after abdominal aortography in patients with an arteriovenous aneurysm of the spinal cord, with the suggestion that the vascular anomaly may lower the threshold of the spinal cord to the neurotoxic effects of the contrast medium.

The patients described by Cornell were hypertensive and arteriosclerotic, but their records revealed no history of allergy or previous disturbances of the nervous system and there was no arteriovenous malformation in the lower spinal cord.

Five cases of unilateral painful vasospasm in the lower limbs of young women were described by Huygens in 1975. In all of these patients the symptoms were limited to one lower limb. The foot was affected with severe pain of spontaneous onset, described as burning or aching and lasting for periods varying from minutes to days. The pain was constant and could not be relieved with analgesics such as aspirin. In four patients the severity of the pain was such that they could walk only with discomfort. In all patients the pain disappeared when lumbar sympathectomy was carried out on the affected side. The aetiology of this unilateral arterial spasm, according to the author, was unknown. The absence of previous nerve injury excludes causalgia as the diagnosis.

Other primary vasospastic disorders, generally associated with Raynaud's disease, and secondary vasospastic disorders or Raynaud's syndrome associated with systemic, regional or traumatic diseases such as connective tissue disease, nerve in-

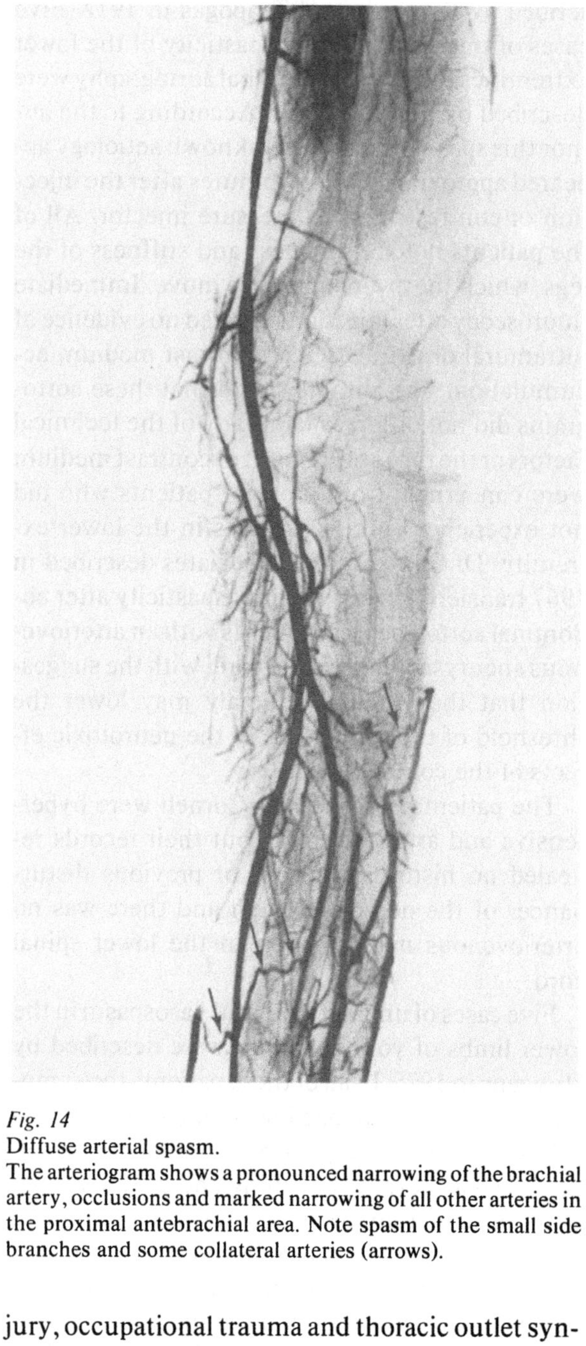

Fig. 14
Diffuse arterial spasm.
The arteriogram shows a pronounced narrowing of the brachial artery, occlusions and marked narrowing of all other arteries in the proximal antebrachial area. Note spasm of the small side branches and some collateral arteries (arrows).

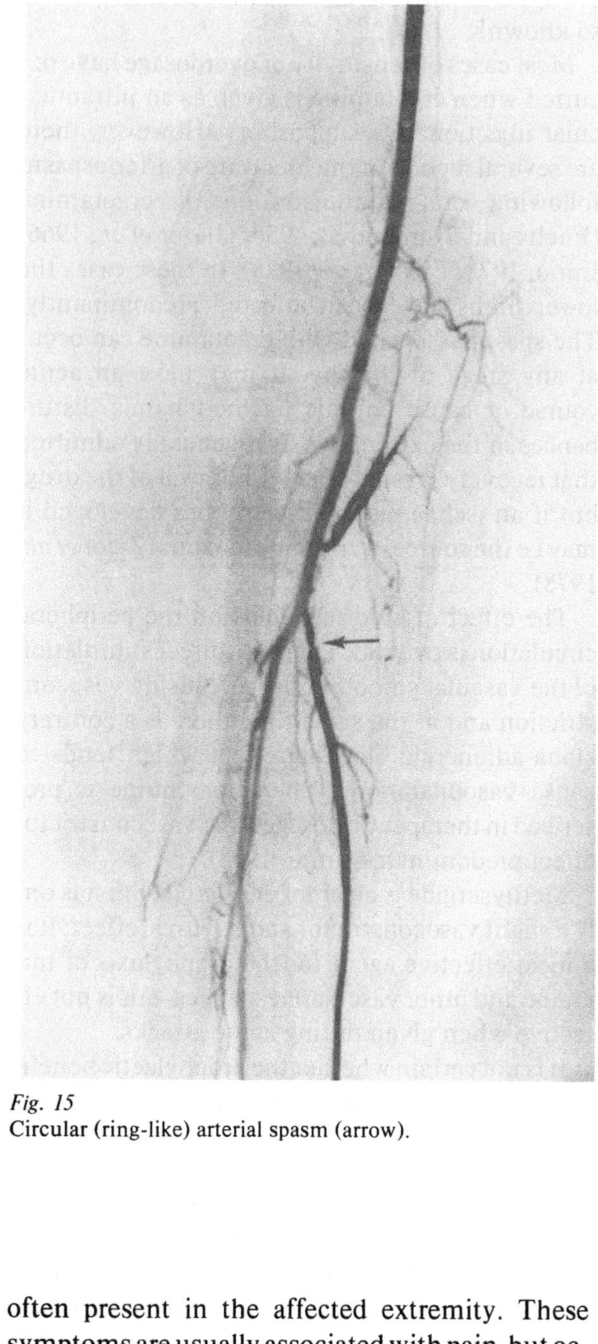

Fig. 15
Circular (ring-like) arterial spasm (arrow).

jury, occupational trauma and thoracic outlet syndrome will be discussed in the following chapters.

4.3.1 Clinical Manifestations of Vasospasm of the Extremities

Pain is a very constant symptom of lasting vasospasm and usually cannot be relieved with analgesics. Associated symptoms of cold and hot sensations, swelling of the extremity, numbness, tingling and colour changes (redness, blueness, or a mottled appearance involving both colours) are often present in the affected extremity. These symptoms are usually associated with pain, but occasionally they can occur independently.

Physical examination during an attack reveals decreased arterial pulses in the affected limb in comparison with those in the opposite limb.

4.4 Roentgenographic Manifestations of Arterial Spasm, Our Experience

On the basis of the angiographic pattern arterial

spasm can be divided into two groups: diffuse and local arterial spasm.

Diffuse arterial spasm refers to contraction of an arterial wall throughout the entire length of the artery and its branches. In such cases the lumen of the artery remains patent but is greatly diminished. The calibre of the affected arteries is determined by the degree of the spasm; this type of vasospasm is very often associated with arterial disease (Fig. 14).

Local arterial spasm means a segmental contraction of an arterial wall, which may be circular (ring-like) (Fig. 15) or longitudinal over a short segment of the artery. It is usually caused by a local mechanical irritation of the arterial wall. This type of arterial spasm tends to occur very often during catheterization of the brachial artery in young patients, when the catheter is advanced too far into the artery (Fig. 16).

Circular spasm is a local phenomenon, which

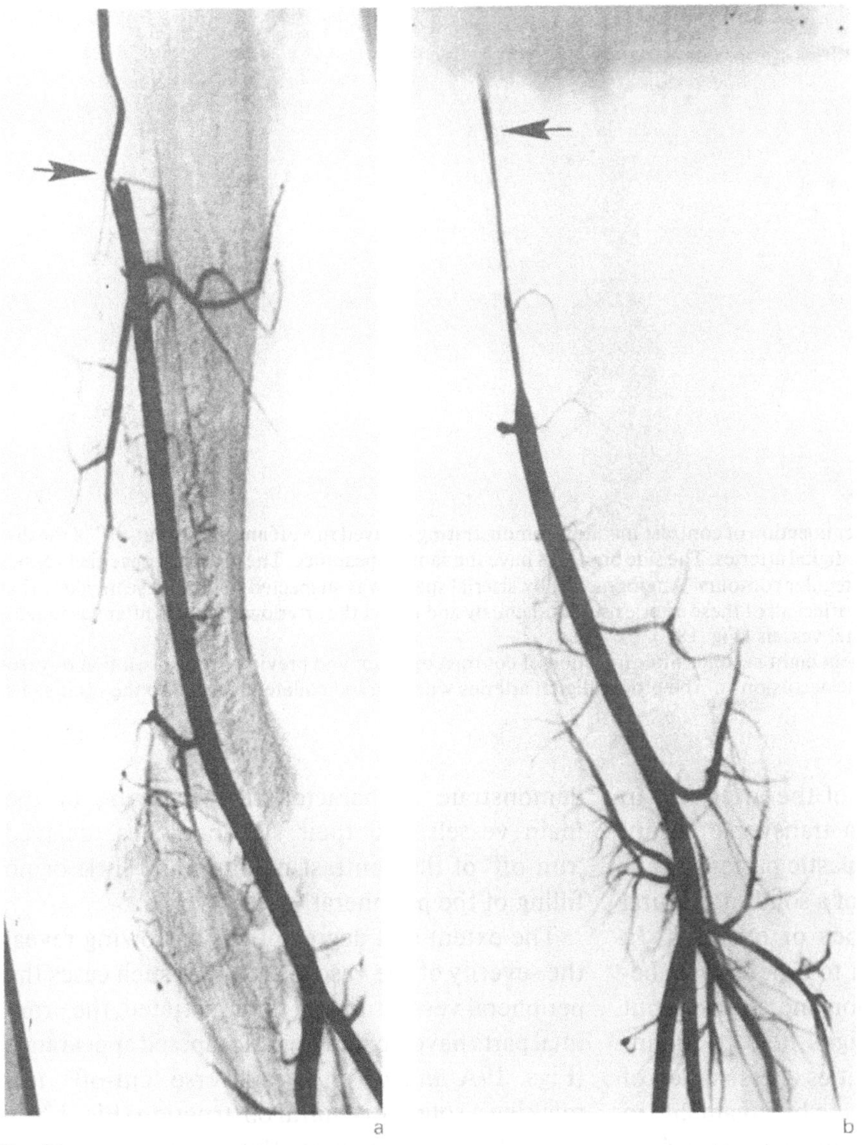

Fig. 16

A. The arteriogram demonstrates a normal brachial artery with the catheter in the proximal part (arrow), no evidence of spasm.

B. Brachial arteriogram of another patient shows a smooth extensive narrowing of the proximal segment of the brachial artery distal to the catheter tip (arrow). This is the typical angiographic appearance of a local longitudinal arterial spasm.

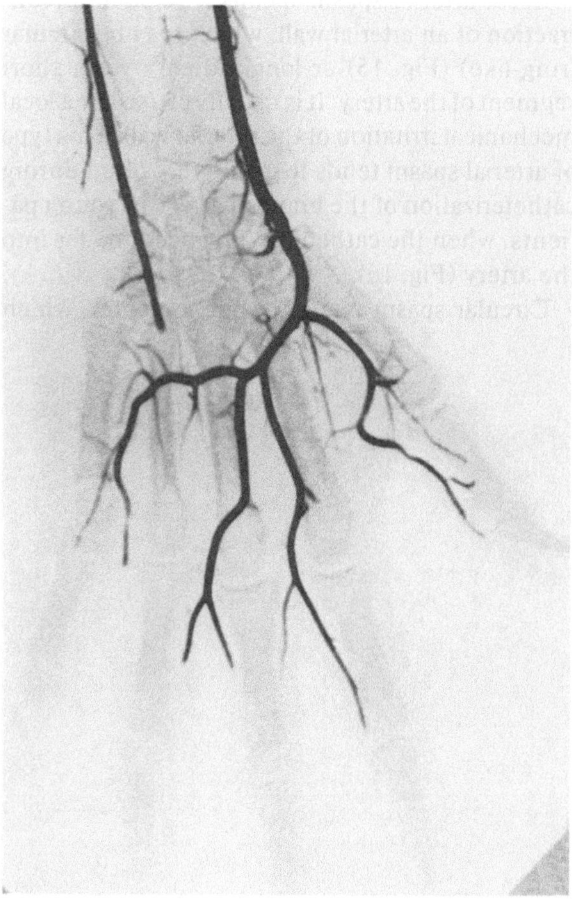

a

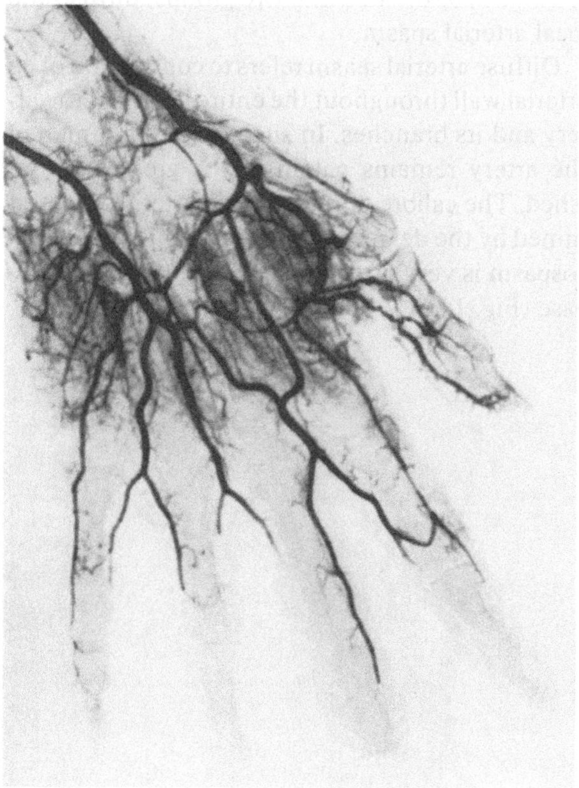

b

Fig. 17A and B

A. Hand arteriogram ten seconds after injection of contrast medium demonstrating delayed run off and sharp 'cut-off' of the distal ulnar artery as well as all proper digital arteries. The side branches have the same appearance. The proximal opacified vessels appear to be normal with smooth regular contours. Angiographically arterial spasm was suspected. It did not seem likely that thrombosis or an embolism could affect all of these arteries simultaneously and in fact the arteriogram taken after vasodilator was injected showed normal digital vessels (Fig. 18C).

B. Hand arteriogram of another patient eight seconds after injection of contrast medium and previous administration of vasodilator. There are multiple organic occlusions of the proper digital arteries with marked collaterals distal to the occlusions.

causes a ring-like narrowing of the artery or, in cases of severe vasospasm, a transverse abrupt 'cut-off' (Fig. 17). This vasospastic pattern is angiographically similar to that of a solid intramural obstruction due to a thrombus or embolus. In some cases it may be difficult to differentiate between organic arterial occlusion and a spasm, but usually other angiographic signs help to distinguish between these two entities. Persistance of collaterals, for example, seems to be invaluable in the diagnosis of organic occlusion of a vessel. Collaterals are never present in occluded spastic arteries (Figs. 17A and B).

In the majority of cases arterial spasm is easily recognisable on the angiogram. The arteriograms demonstrate a characteristic narrowing of the main vessels and their side branches, delayed 'run-off' of the contrast medium and little or no filling of the peripheral vessels.

The extent and degree of the narrowing reveal the severity of the vasospasm. If in such cases the peripheral vessels are not demonstrated, the proximal parts have a characteristic tapered appearance (Figs. 19A and B) or a transverse 'cut-off', mimicking a solid intramural obstruction (Fig. 17A).

Another diagnostic method used to recognize this spastic condition is to administer a strong vasodilator intra-arterially. Usually the vasospasm disappears or decreases within two to three minutes after the injection (Fig. 18C).

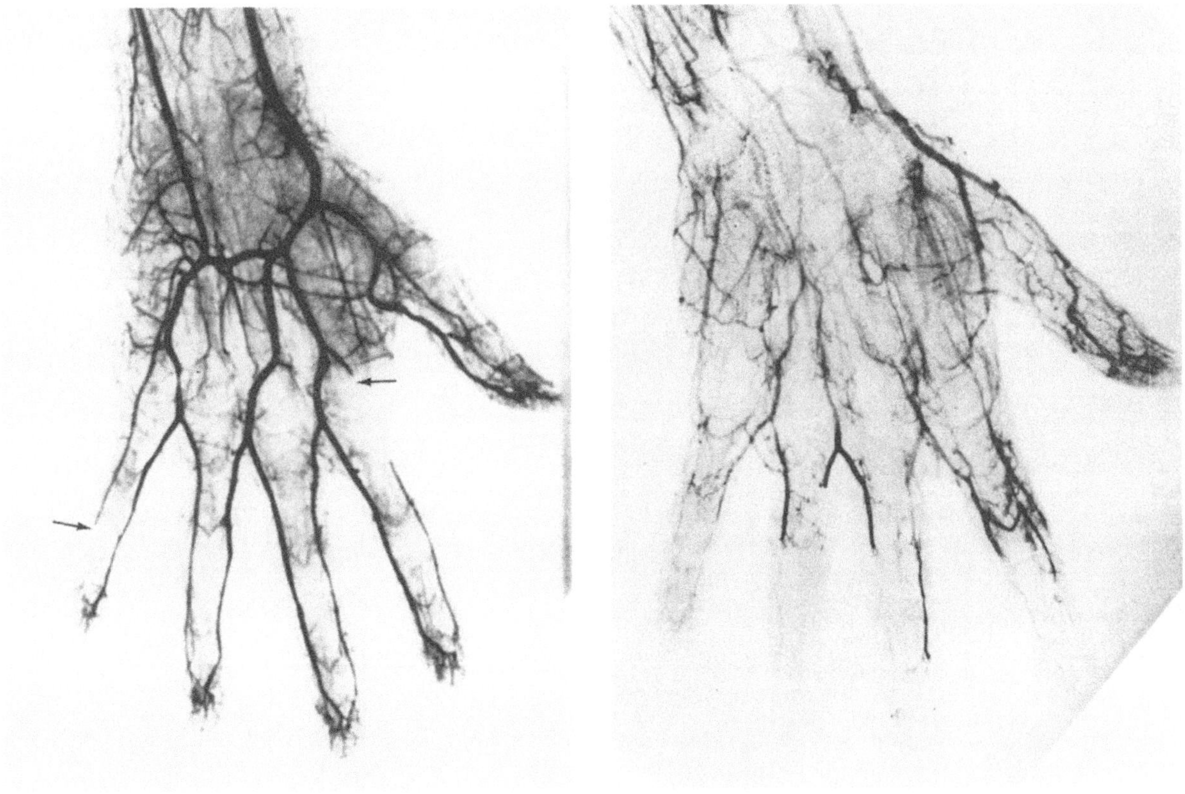

c d

Fig. 18C and D
Repeat arteriograms after intra-arterial administration of vasodilator; same cases as in Figs. 17A and B.

C. The same patient as in Fig. 17A. The film obtained ten seconds after injection of contrast medium demonstrates normal filling of the hand's arteries and side branches. The proper digital arteries are opacified up to the fingertips. Note a small spastic contraction of the proximal part of the arteria radialis indicis and the distal part of the proper digital artery of the fifth finger (arrows).

D. The same patient as in Fig. 17B. Latest film (11 seconds after injection of contrast medium) shows no progression of the contrast distal to the occlusions of the proper digital arteries. The proximal part of the hand arteriogram already shows the early venous phase.

4.5 Pharmacoangiography

Pharmacological agents, both vasodilators and vasoconstrictors, have long been used to enhance angiography. The intra-arterial injections of vasodilators have been used to enhance visualization of the portal and superior mesenteric veins, some hepatic metastases and the arterial, capillary and venous manifestations of bone and soft tissue lesions. In acute angiography vasodilators have been used to reveal the sites of bleeding or to demonstrate oesophageal varices. Moreover with the aid of vasodilators bronchial arteriography has recently become feasible; the dilatation of these vessels during angiography may afford the opportunity to demonstrate peripheral lesions.

Vasoconstrictor drugs have been used in angiography to demonstrate pathological neoplastic vessels in small carcinomas of the kidney and are often given via superselective intra-arterial injection for therapeutic purposes, e.g. to control some types of gastrointestinal haemorrhage.

4.5.1 Vasodilators Used in Peripheral Angiography: Review of Literature

The use of intra-arterial vasodilators for peripheral arteriography was first reported in 1937 by Sgalitzer who used papaverine, apparently without much success. In the same year Ratschow found that the reactive hyperaemia following arterial compression is useful for opacification of the peripheral vessels. The latter author also used diathermy and a sympathetic blockade by application of a local anaesthetic. He achieved some improvement in his angiographic studies, but frequently the va-

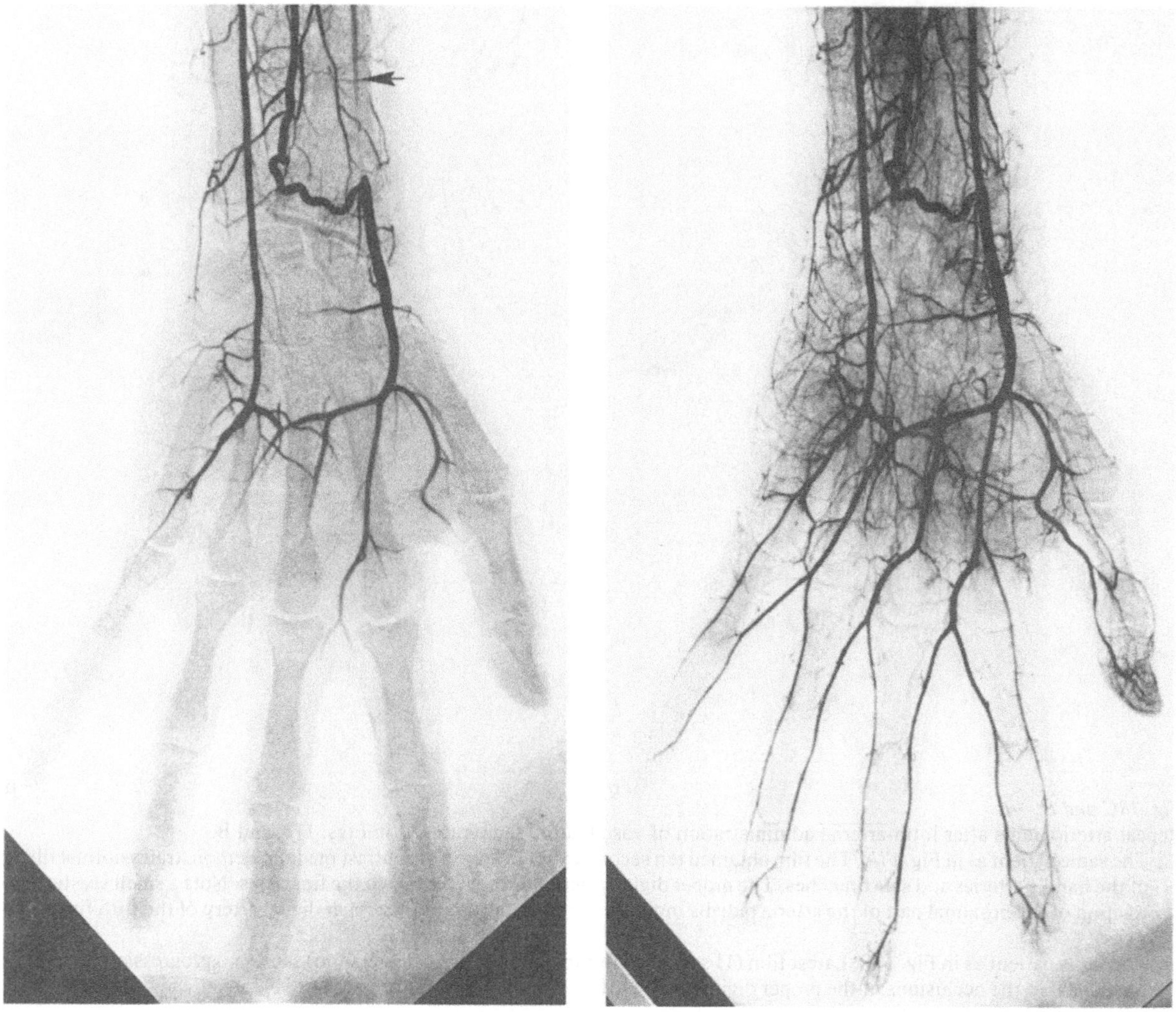

Fig. 19 a b

A. Hand arteriogram of a sixteen year old female; 10 mg tolazoline were injected intra-arterially prior to contrast injection. Eight seconds after contrast injection, the arteriogram shows severe spasm of the radial artery proximal to the large collateral (arrow). Note typical spastic tapering of the third and fourth metacarpal and proper digital arteries of the thumb and index finger. Tapering also of all side branches.

B. Repeat arteriogram after intra-arterial administration of additional 20 mg tolazoline. Six seconds after contrast injection the arteries appear to be normal, except for a small spastic narrowing of the distal digital arteries. The radial artery has completely regained its normal calibre.

sodilatory effect was not sufficient to visualize the small peripheral arteries.

In recent years Kahn and Callow (1965), in their study of 35 lower and 7 upper extremity arteriograms, showed that tolazoline hydrochloride (Priscol) and reactive hyperaemia are most successful in improving visualization of peripheral vessels, while papaverine and lidocaine are not effective.

Hishida (1963), in an extensive series, found tolazoline hydrochloride much less effective than his method of reactive hyperaemia; however, there is some doubt whether he injected the drug sufficiently slowly to produce maximum local action. Jacobs and Hanafee published their experience with tolazoline in peripheral arteriography of the lower extremities in 1967. Bron, Stilly and Shapiro (1971) used tolazoline to enhance renal arteriography. Sherry, Crummy and Ahlstrand (1973) published their successful results with tolazoline in 250 peripheral arteriograms of the lower and upper extremities. Hawkins and Hudson (1974) found tolazoline hydrochloride to be a most effective vasodilator for visualization of tumour vascularity on 64 bone and soft tissue arteriograms. Goldstein, Thaggard, Wallace and Neiman (1976) used tolazoline hydrochloride as an important adjunct to hepatic angiography for evaluation of space-occupying lesions in the liver. It's vasodilatory effect on the small blood vessels of the liver enhanced visualization of neoplastic vessels on previously negative hepatic angiograms.

4.5.2 The Use of Tolazoline Hydrochloride in Peripheral Brachial Angiography

At the present time surgical correction of diseased arteries is carried out in many cases farther distalwards; therefore preoperative evaluation of patients with peripheral vascular diseases necessitates visualization of the arteries distal to the site of obstruction.

The reason for insufficient opacification of the small arteries is certainly the slow blood flow through many of these vessels due to a certain degree of vasospasm.

To produce vasodilatation and increased blood flow and to obtain maximal visualization of the small arteries vasodilator drugs can be given before the injection of contrast medium.

A strong vasodilator often used in peripheral angiography is tolazoline hydrochloride.

4.5.3 Tolazoline Hydrochloride

(Syn: Benzazoline hydrochloride; Tolazoline chloride; Priscol; Priscoline; 2-Benzyl-2-imidazoline hydrochloride.)

It is a white, or almost white, odourless crystalline powder with a bitter taste. A 1% solution in water has a pH of 5 to 7.

Tolazoline hydrochloride is a strong adrenolytic and sympatholytic agent acting upon the alpha receptors of the postganglionic fibres. Apart from its adrenergic blocking action, it has a direct dilator effect on the peripheral blood vessels, especially the arterioles and capillaries, and increases the peripheral blood flow. It has little effect on the blood pressure and is of no value for the treatment of hypertension. Local intra-arterial administration causes a sensation of warmth, which is greater and more prolonged than that experienced after such vasodilators as histamine, nicotinic acid or carbachol.

Tolazoline is mainly used in the treatment of peripheral vascular disorders due to arterial spasm, such as acrocyanosis and Raynaud's disease.

Diagnostically, it has been used to assess the potential value of sympathectomy and to enhance angiography.

The usual dose is 25 to 75 mg.

4.5.4 Toxic Effects

Minor side-effects of tolazoline hydrochloride include gooseflesh and flushing; more serious side-effects are tingling, cold, shivering, nausea, vomiting and epigastric pain. In peripheral arteriography Sherry *et al.* (1973) have described side-effects such as tachycardia and headache of short duration. One of their patients developed haemoglobinuria for 24 hours following the administration of 100 mg tolazoline and a large volume of contrast medium, but the aetiology of this complication remained uncertain.

4.5.5 Contra-Indications

Collapse and shock are absolute contra-indications for the use of tolazoline. Care should also be taken when it is given to patients with coronary insufficiency, cardiac arrhythmia and severe diabetes.

4.6 Our Investigations

4.6.1 Selection of Proper Drug

The purpose of this part of Chapter IV is to describe our experience with the vasodilator tolazoline which was used in 730 selective studies of the arteries of the hands of more than 500 patients. Confronted with the problem of vasospasm which prevented the proper filling of the small peripheral arteries we tested several pharmacological agents to determine their potential value in routine brachial arteriography.

In 1970 a preliminary study was performed in 25 patients of different ages, using one or more of the followings drugs and doses: tolazoline (50-60 mg); histamine (0.1-0.2 mg); papaverine hydrochloride (30 mg) and lidocaine hydrochloride (60 to 100 mg). Each of the medications was diluted to 20 cc with physiological saline. In all cases brachial angiography was performed under local anaesthesia using the transfemoral catheterization technique. Before the injection of contrast material one of the drugs was administered slowly through the catheter.

The analysis of these twenty-five angiographic comparative studies indicated that the best vasodilatation was achieved with tolazoline.

The arteriograms obtained after a slow injection of tolazoline were superior to those made after a rapid injection. The major advantages were a significantly improved visualization of the small peripheral vessels, a considerable increase in the size of the small arteries of the hand and a slight vasodilatory effect on the large arteries of the forearm.

4.6.2 Time-Dose Relation in the Use of Tolazoline

To establish a standard technique for brachial angiography a second study was performed.

The purposes of this study were:

a. To detect the time of maximum dilatation of the peripheral vessels in order to determine the moment when the contrast should be injected.
b. To find the minimal dose of tolazoline necessary for optimal visualization of the arteries and veins on the hand angiograms while avoiding the side-effects of the drug, and
c. To demonstrate the relation between size of the small arteries and the dose of tolazoline.

Twenty-nine patients were studied (50 extremities). In eight patients one extremity and in the remaining 21 patients both extremities were investigated. There were 17 females and 12 males; their ages ranged from sixteen to sixty-eight years. Eight patients had symptoms on only one side. Five of the 29 had minor symptoms, and only two of the 29 patients were asymptomatic.

4.6.3 Technique

In all cases the transfemoral catheterization technique was employed. Under local anaesthesia a 100 cm Headhunter, French 7 polyethylene catheter was introduced through the femoral artery and the catheter tip was positioned selectively under fluoroscopic control in the brachial artery, just distal to the origin of the deep brachial artery, at a point 10 to 12 cm above the antecubital fossa. The forearm, the palm and fingers were placed in the supine position over the Schönander film changer. An intra-arterial injection of 20 mg tolazoline diluted to 20 ml with physiological saline was given over a period of two minutes. Eighteen ml contrast medium were injected at a rate of 5 ml per second. The serial films were made over a period of 11 seconds (Table II).

TABLE II

Technical Data for Tolazoline Injection

Tolazoline	*Injection Time*	*Contrast total volume*	*Contrast inj. rate*
20 mg (in 20 cc physiological saline)	120 sec.	18 ml	5 ml/sec.

Before starting the intra-arterial injection of vasodilator the whole procedure was explained to the patients, emphasizing that during the administration of the drug a transitory hyperaemia of the skin and a sensation of warmth distal to the site of injection would be experienced. Each patient was requested to indicate when this sensation was no-

TABLE III

Warm Sensation and Reddening of The Skin in 50 Extremities.

	Elbow				*Wrist*				*Fingers*			
Time in seconds	*W*	*%*	*R*	*%*	*W*	*%*	*R*	*%*	*W*	*%*	*R*	*%*
0- 30	25	50	19	38	4	8	2	4	–	–	–	–
30- 60	10	20	9	18	20	40	12	24	–	–	–	–
60- 90	15	30	12	24	21	42	18	36	–	–	–	–
90-120	–	–	10	20	5	10	10	20	8	16	3	6
120-150	–	–	–	–	–	–	8	16	37	74	42	84
> 150	–	–	–	–	–	–	–	–	5	10	5	10

ticed at the level of the elbow, the wrist and the tips of the fingers.

The time of the warm sensation and reddening of the skin at the level of the elbow, wrist and fingers were noted. The results of this study are given in Table III.

With this combination of subjective and objective criteria it was possible to follow the effect of the vasodilator in successive steps from the elbow to the tips of the fingers. The optimal moment for contrast injection was determined by the sensation of diffuse warmth throughout the whole forearm and the appearance of intense reddening of the skin from the elbow to the fingertips, indicating maximum vasodilatation of the small arteries and capillaries.

As is shown in Table III, in 90% of the cases this moment appears to be 20 to 30 seconds after the end of the intra-arterial injection of the drug, or 140-150 seconds after the start of intra-arterial administration of tolazoline.

This was confirmed by intra-arterial monitoring of the pressure in the distal part of the brachial artery before and after administration of the vasodilator (Fig. 20).

The intra-arterial catheter was connected to a Gould Statham Model P 23 ID pressure transducer and the signal displayed on an electronic oscilloscope (Hewlett Packard, Model 7803-B) which indicated the blood pressure before injection of 20 mg tolazoline and immediately afterwards. The systolic pressure fell for 20-30 seconds to its lowest level which was maintained for 2.5 minutes; it then gradually increased again, reaching the pre-injection level after 5 minutes. This corresponds to the time period within which most of the skin discolouration disappears. The diastolic pressure remained unchanged. The skin colour and the blood pressure of the contralateral arm were unchanged indicating a local action of the drug.

This was confirmed by measuring the blood pressure in the opposite arm of ten patients before the administration of the drug, immediately afterwards and ten minutes later. In all instances the blood pressure remained unchanged.

The drop in the systolic pressure of the injected arm, however, indicates the phase of maximum vasodilatation in the extremity. It is obvious that for optimal visualization of the small peripheral vessels of the hand the contrast medium should be injected between 0.5 and 2.5 minutes after the end of the administration of tolazoline.

To find the minimal dose of tolazoline necessary for optimal visualization of the small digital vessels and for demonstration of the dilatation of the small arteries with different doses of tolazoline, an additional study of 40 extremities was carried out using intra-arterial injections of 10, 30, 40 and 50 mg tolazoline. The technique for these arteriograms was the same as that described for the previous study. The results of these examinations can be summarized as follows:

a. Arteriograms made after injection of 10 mg of tolazoline did not visualize the peripheral vessels sufficiently in all cases. In patients without spastic complaints visualization of the peripheral arteries was possible, but opacification was delayed and the arteries were small in calibre. In these cases, an injection of an additional 20 mg tolazoline in the same extremity produced a

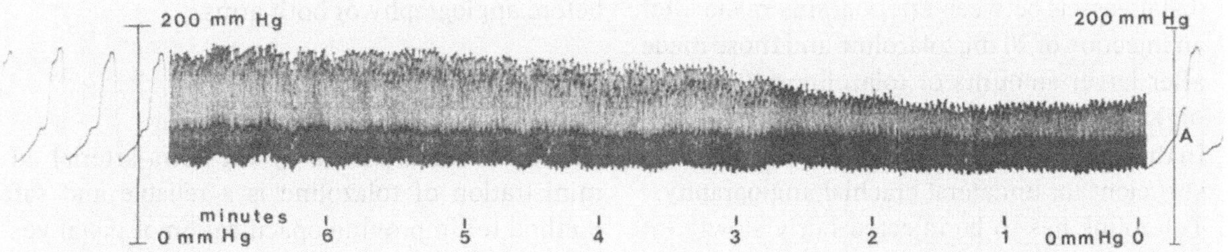

Fig. 20
Point A indicates the end of the intra-arterial injection of 20 mg of tolazoline and reconnection of the catheter to the pressure transducer and oscilloscope.
The intra-arterial pressure in the distal brachial artery was recorded continuously for several minutes (from right to left). Lowest systolic pressure occurs between 0 and 2.5 minutes indicating the phase of maximal vasodilatation. Between 2.5 and 5 minutes systolic pressure gradually increases to pre-injection level.

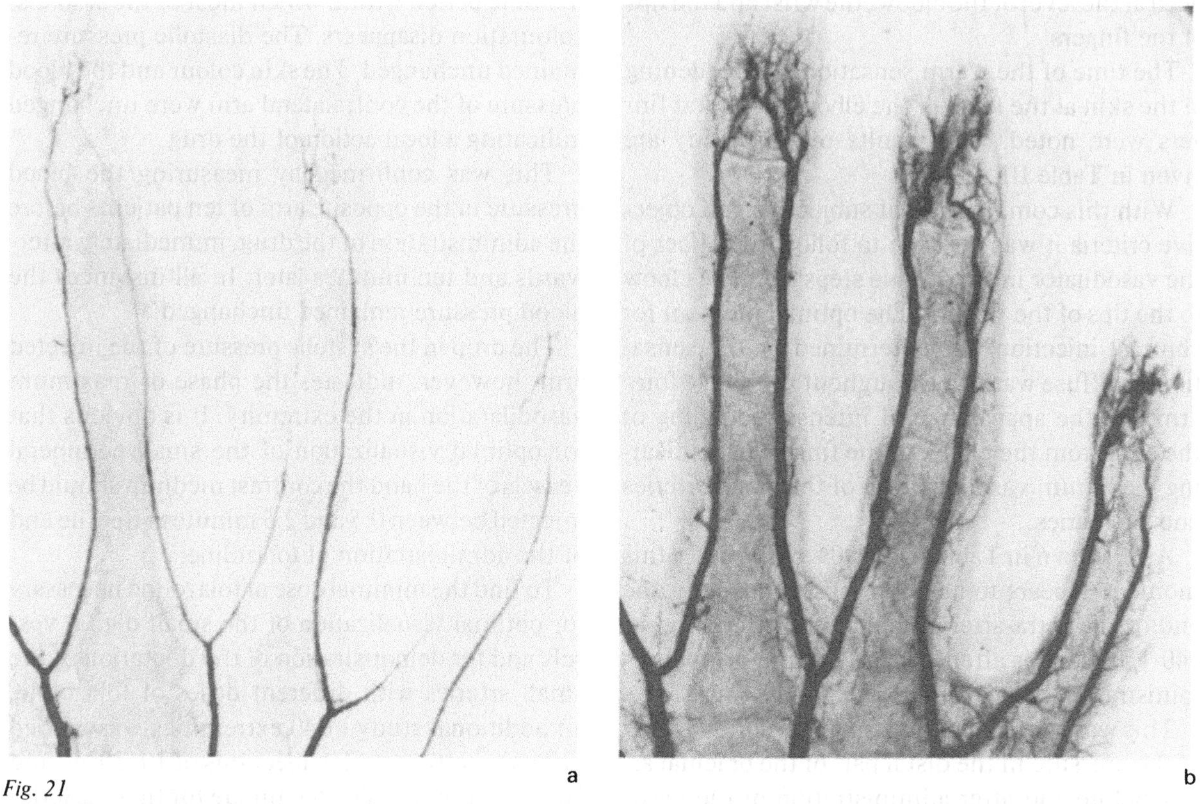

Fig. 21

A. Maximal visualization of the digital arteries after injection of 10 mg tolazoline intra-arterially; roentgenogram taken 10 seconds after injection of 18 ml methylglucamine ioxitalamate at a rate of 5 ml per second.

B. Similar contrast injection after administration of additional 20 mg tolazoline in the same brachial artery 15 minutes later. Serial film taken 8 seconds after injection of contrast medium shows an obvious dilatation and remarkable increase in the size of the arteries.

remarkable increase in the size of the digital arteries (Fig. 21).

b. The roentgenograms obtained after 30, 40 and 50 mg of tolazoline, however, did not differ considerably from the first series of roentgenograms produced after a 20 mg tolazoline injection.
c. No consistent difference was demonstrable in the time when the contrast fluid appeared in the distal vessels between arteriograms made after an injection of 20 mg tolazoline and those made after larger amounts of tolazoline (40 and 50 mg) are given.
d. In the majority of cases 20 mg tolazoline is quite sufficient for unilateral brachial angiography.
e. Tolazoline has to be injected fairly slowly (at least 120 seconds) to produce maximum local action.

The technique of injecting the tolazoline seems to be more important than the dose itself.

A fast bolus injection of tolazoline intra-arterially reaches the systemic circulation rapidly and generally gives rise to systemic reactions such as tachycardia, hypotension and headache. These reactions are seen more often when a large amount of the drug is used. More serious complications such as collapse may be seen when the permissible dose (75 mg) is exceeded. We have seen this complication only once: in a hypotensive young female patient 100 mg tolazoline was administered before angiography of both arms.

4.6.4 Conclusions

Vasodilatation induced by the intra-arterial administration of tolazoline is a reliable and safe method for improving opacification of distal vessels in peripheral brachial angiography. In the last ten years more than 500 patients underwent arteriographic examination of the upper extremities in our department; tolazoline was used for 730 selective arteriograms of the hand.

Tolazoline decreases the circulation time and

permits visualization of small vessels and collaterals. The opacification of small digital arteries is improved in the vast majority of patients regardless of the state of run-off.

The ease and simplicity of intra-arterial administration of the drug are definite advantages.

A dose of 20-30 mg tolazoline diluted to 20 cc with physiological saline is sufficient for unilateral angiography.

Slow injection is necessary for optimal local effect.

REFERENCES

AMELI, F. M., M. NATHANSON and I. ELKAN: Methysergide Therapy causing Vascular Insufficiency of the Upper Limb. *The Canadian Jour. of Surgery, 20: 159-161, 1977.*

BRON, K. M., J. W. STILLY and A. P. SHAPIRO: Renal Arteriography Enhanced by Tolazoline. *Radiology, 99: 295-297, 1971.*

COFFMAN, J. D.: The Attenuation by Reserpine or Guanethidine of the Cutaneous Vasoconstriction caused by Tobacco Smoking. *Am. Heart J., 74: 229-234, 1967.*

CONRAD, M. C.: Circulation of the Skin, in Functional Anatomy of the Circulation to the Lower Extremities. *Chicago, Year Book Medical Publishers Inc., p. 90, 1972.*

CORNELL, S.H.: Spasticity of the Lower Extremities Following Abdominal Aortography. *Radiology, 93: 377-379, 1969.*

DI CHIRO, G., J. DOPPMAN and A. K. OMMAYA: Selective Arteriography of Arteriovenous Aneurysm of Spinal Cord. *Radiology, 88: 1065-1077, 1967.*

FUCHS, M. and L. S. BLUMENTHAL: Use of Ergot preparations in migraine *JAMA, 143: 1462-1464., 1950.*

ERIKSON, U., G. HELMIUS, A. HEMMINGSSON: On the Use of Bradykinin in Arteriography of the Arm. *Australasian Radiology, 18: 345-349, 1974.*

GOLDSTEIN, H. M., A. THAGGARD, S. WALLACE and H. L. NEIMAN: Priscoline-Augmented Hepatic Angiography. *Radiology, 119: 275-279, 1976.*

GLAZER, G., K. A. MEYERS and E. R. DAVIES: Ergot Poisening. *Postgrad. Med. J., 42: 562-568, 1966.*

GRAY, H.: Anatomy of the Human Body. *Philadelphia, Lea & Febiger, 24th ed. 545-642, 1944.*

HAWKINS, I. F. jr. and T. HUDSON: Priscoline in Bone and Soft-tissue Angiography. *Radiology, 110: 541-546, 1974.*

HISHIDA, Y.: Peripheral Arteriography Using Reactive Hyperemia. *Jap. Circ. J., 27: 349-358, 1963.*

HUYGENS, H.: Unilateral Painful Vasospasm in the Lower Limbs of Young Women. *Austr. N.Z. Jour. Surgery, 45: 147-151, 1975.*

IMRIE, C. W.: Arterial Spasm Associated with Oral Ergotamine Therapy. *Brit. J. Clinical Practice, 27: 457-460, 1973.*

JAKOBS, J. B. and W. N. HANAFEE: The Use of Priscoline in Peripheral Arteriography. *Radiology, 88: 957-960, 1967.*

KAHN, P. C. and A. D. CALLOW: Selective Vasodilatation as an Aid to Angiography. *Am. J. Roentgenology, 94: 213-220, 1965.*

KARMODY, A. M. and M. J. TSAPOGAS: Arterial Spasm of Rare Etiology. *Angiology, 23: 464-473, 1972.*

KUNTZ, A. and D. I. FARNSWORTH: Distribution of Afferent Fibers Via the Sympathetic Trunks and Gray Communicating Rami to the Brachial and Lumbosacral Plexuses. *J. Comp. Neur., 53: 389-, 1931.*

KUNTZ, A.: The Autonomic Nervous System, in *Ciba Collection, vol. I, sec. 4: 80-99, 1953.*

KUNTZ, A: Afferent Innervation of Peripheral Blood Vessels through Sympathetic Trunks: Its Clinical Implications. *South. Med. J., 44: 673-679, 1951.*

LANG, E. K.: A Survey of the Complications of Percutaneous Retrograde Arteriography (Seldinger Technique). *Radiology, 81: 257-263, 1963.*

METZLER, M. and D. SILVER: Vasospastic Disorders. *Postgrad. Med., 65: 79-84, 1979.*

RATSCHOW, M.: Leistung und Bedeutung der Vasographie als Funktionsprüfung der peripheren Blutgefässe. *Fortschr. a. a. Geb. d. Röntgenstrahlen, 55: 253-266, 1937.*

RAW, K. and H. GAYLIS: Acute Arterial Spasm of the Lower Extremities after Methysergide Therapy. *S. Afr. Journal, 50: 1999-2001, 1976.*

SGALITZER, M.: Unterscheiding funktioneller und organischer Erkrankungen der Extremitätenarterien durch die Röntgenuntersuchung. *Fortschr. a.d. Geb. d. Röntgenstrahlen, 56: 387-404, 1937.*

SHERRY, J. J., A. B. CRUMMY and R. A. AHLSTRAND: A Technique of Peripheral Arteriography using Tolazoline. *Australasian Radiology, 17: 308-312, 1973.*

SUTTON, D. and B. J. PRESTON: Angiography in Peripheral Ischemia due to Ergotism. *Brit. J. Radiol., 43: 776-777, 1970.*

SUTTON, D.: Textbook of Radiology. *Baltimore, The Williams and Wilkins Co., 60-1065-1118, 1969.*

WILNER, H. I., R. KAY and B. A. EISENBREY: Pharmacologic Aids in Angiography of the Upper Extremity. *Radiology, 121: 150-154, 1974.*

ZEITLER, E.: Zur sicheren Darstellung von Digitalarterien an Händen und Füssen in Lokalanästhesie nach oraler Alkoholgabe. *Fortschr. Geb. Röntgenstr. Nuklearmed., 123: 67-68, 1975.*

ZICOT, M., F. GRANDFILS and D. HONORE: Prolonged Arterial Hemodynamic Disturbances in the Lower Limbs After Oral Use of Ergotamine. *Angiology, 29: 495-496, 1978.*

Chapter 5

EMBRYOLOGY OF THE ARTERIES OF THE UPPER LIMB

The congenital anomalies of the arteries of the upper extremity seem to be caused by an inhibited development of the vessels in different stages of the embryonic growth (Singer, 1933). To understand the primitive conditions persisting in the arteries of the upper extremity a complete knowledge of the embryological development of the entire vascular system is required. As the scope of this subject is very large and many factors in the different stages of its embryological development are not yet completely understood, this chapter is restricted only to a short description of the embryology of the arteries of the arm.

The arteries of the arm can be recognized for the first time in an embryo of 4-7 mm. The innominate artery or brachiocephalic trunk is derived from the fourth primitive aortic arch. It represents a common trunk from which the right common carotid and right subclavian arteries originate. According to Congdon (1922), the stem of the right subclavian artery is formed by a portion of the right fourth aortic arch, the dorsal aorta caudal to it and the right sixth (sometimes called the seventh) intersegmental artery.

The left subclavian artery represents the most proximal part of the hypertrophic sixth (seventh) intersegmental branch of the left primitive dorsal aorta, near the point where the latter is joined by the left fourth arch artery.

According to Senior (1926), in the embryonic development of the arteries of the upper limb, five stages can be recognized. In Figure 22 the charac-

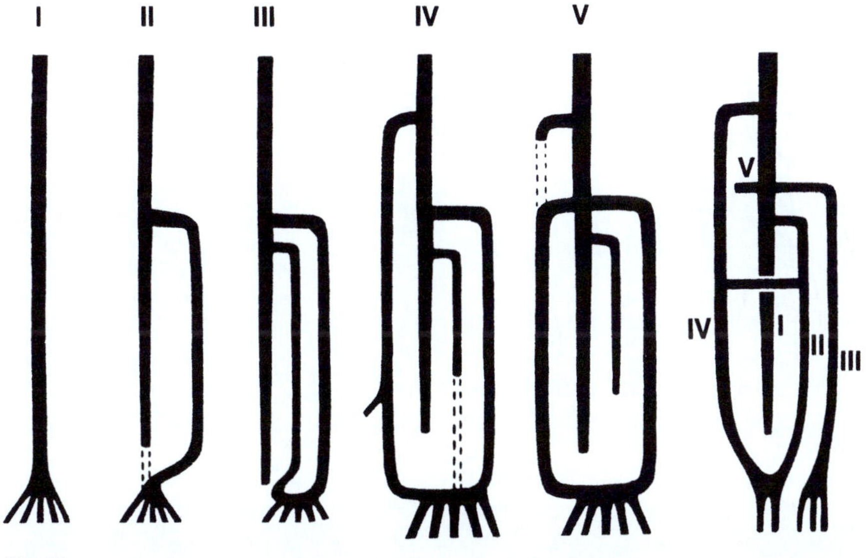

Fig. 22
Diagrams illustrating the five stages of development of the arteries of the arm (after Piersol), and a similar diagram to explain the anomaly illustrated in Fig. 23.

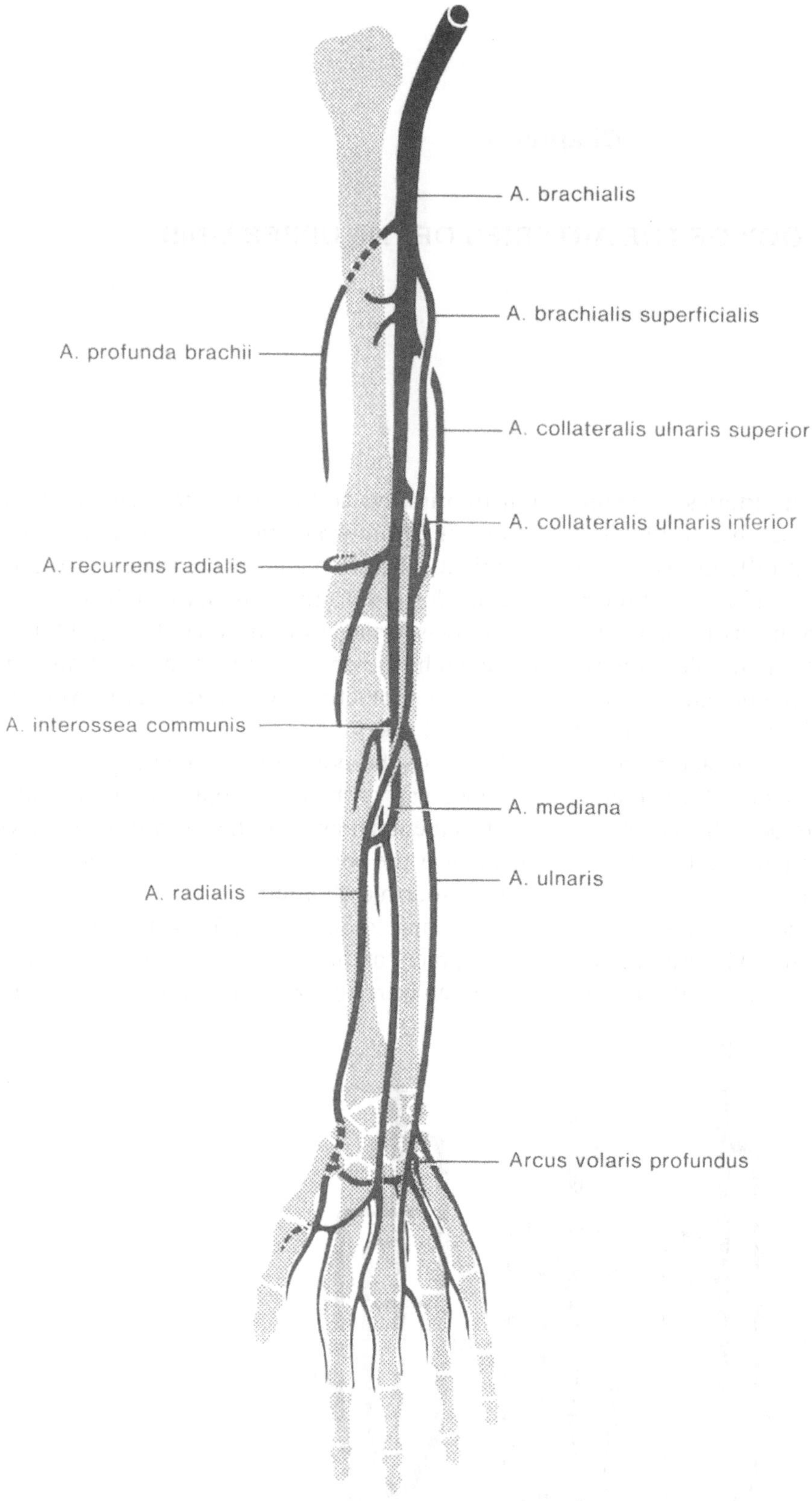

Fig. 23
Schematic drawing of the arteries of the right arm, showing the retention of developmental conditions: Persistence of a superficial brachial artery, which continues below the elbow as the radial artery, and persistence of a median artery.

teristics of these five stages of development are illustrated schematically.

Stage I. In this earliest stage of development, the lateral branch of the left and right sixth (seventh) cervical intersegmental artery becomes enlarged and elongated to form the axial artery of the upper limb. In the arm this axial artery extends to the wrist, where it terminates by dividing up into a capillary plexus from which the digital branches later arise. The proximal part of this artery becomes the brachial artery and its distal portion can be recognized as the interosseous artery of the adult.

Stage II is characterized by the development of the median artery from the interosseous artery while the interosseous artery itself subsequently undergoes atrophy. During this process the median artery fuses with the lower portion of the interosseous artery and ultimately forms the main channel for the digital branches, thus becoming the principal artery of the forearm.

Stage III. In embryos of about 18 mm the ulnar artery arises from the brachial artery and unites distally with the median artery to form the superficial carpal arch. The digital branches arise from this arch.

Stage IV. In embryos 21 mm long the superficial brachial artery develops in the axillary region and traverses the medial surface of the arm, running diagonally from the ulnar to the radial side of the forearm to the posterior surface of the wrist. There it divides over the carpus into branches for the dorsum of the thumb and index finger.

Finally in stage V, when the embryo reaches a length of about 23 mm, three changes occur. First the median artery undergoes degeneration, becoming a small, slender structure.

The superficial brachial artery gives off a distal branch which anastomoses with the superficial volar arch, which at that time is already present. At the level of the elbow, an anastomotic branch between the brachial artery and the distal portion of the superficial brachial artery hypertrophies and becomes the radial artery. The proximal portion of the superficial brachial artery undergoes a corresponding atrophy.

This is the normal embryological development of the arteries of the arm.

As far as the aetiology of the congenital anomalies of the arteries of the upper extremity is concerned, two theories should be mentioned. Singer believed that arterial anomalies could be explained embryologically. In 1933 in his article 'Embryological anomalies of the upper extremity of the arm' he concluded that congenital anomalies of the upper extremity arteries represent an inhibition of the development of the vessels at different stages of the embryonic period (Fig. 23). The other theory was established by Manners-Smith in 1910, who made a comparative study of the arteries of the limb in different groups of primates. After completion of his study he came to the conclusion that many of the variations in the upper extremity arteries which occur in man represent a retention or reappearance of primitive patterns which normally are found in the gorilla, chimpanzee, orangutan, gibbon, macacus rhesus and other primates.

REFERENCES

Congdon, E.D.: Transformation of the Aortic-arch System during the Development of the Human Embryo. *Contr. Embryol. Carneg. Inst., 68: 14-48, 1922.*

Manners-Smith, T.: The Limb Arteries of Primates. *J. Anat. Physiol., 45: 23-64, 1910.*

Moffat, D. B.: The Embryology of the Arteries. *Ann. Roy. Coll. Surg. Engl., 30: 368-882, 1962.*

Piersol, G. A.: Cited by E. Singer (1933).

Senior, H. D.: A note on the development of the radial artery. *Anat. Rec., vol. 32, p. 220, 1926.*

Singer, E.: Embryological Pattern Persisting in the Arteries of the Arm. *Anat. Rec., 55: 403-409, 1933.*

Chapter 6

ANATOMY OF THE ARTERIAL SYSTEM OF THE UPPER EXTREMITIES

Analysis Of Our Case Material

This chapter reviews the normal roentgenological anatomy and common congenital anomalies of the major branches of the aortic arch and the arteries of the upper extremities.

For each subject a short survey of relevant recent literature is followed by an extensive anatomical description and an analysis of the angiographic material.

The study includes 592 aortic arch angiograms and 750 selective subclavian and brachial arteriograms obtained between 1970 and 1980. The venous structures of the upper extremity are not included.

6.1 Aortic Arch (Arcus Aortae)

The first part of this chapter will deal with the congenital anomalies of the origin of the brachiocephalic vessels. Since these rare anomalies of the aortic arch are known in the literature, but were not encountered in our material, they are only described here. The double aortic arch, which may occur together with either a left or a right descending aorta, has been noted in the world literature in 136 instances (Klinkhamer, 1969). In 1943 Herbut described this aortic arch as a very rare anomaly, with an incidence of one in 5,000 to 10,000 necropsies. A less frequent anomaly is the so-called *cervical* aortic arch, which is situated in the neck. Twenty-five cases of this anomalous type have been reported in the literature: nine situated on the left side of the neck and sixteen on the right (Klinkhamer, 1969; Shuford *et al.*, 1972; Haughton, 1975). The aberrant right subclavian artery (*arteria lusoria*) with a coexistent bicarotid trunk (Fig. 28) was encountered only twice in our material (0.6%). From the reports of the literature the incidence of this artery has been estimated to be approximately 0.5 to 2.0 percent (Raider, 1967). Coarctation of the isthmus, patent ductus arteriosus, aortopulmonary window, aneurysm of the aortic sinuses and congenital kinking, the so-called pseudo-coarctation of the aorta, are not considered in this chapter. Other vascular rings associated with aortic arch anomalies are also not discussed.

6.1.1 Different Types of Aortic Arch

The material for this study was selected from 592 thoracic aortograms taken in our department. In order to determine the branching pattern of the brachiocephalic vessels only arteriograms which visualized their origin at the aorta were evaluated. The aortograms of the aortic arch of 323 patients were considered suitable for this purpose. The pa-

TABLE IV

Different Types of Aortic Arch.

Type	*Number*	*Percent*
I	235	72.8
II	45	13.9
III	18	5.6
IV	14	4.3
V	3	0.9
VI	1	0.3
VII	5	1.6
VIII	2	0.6
Total	323	100

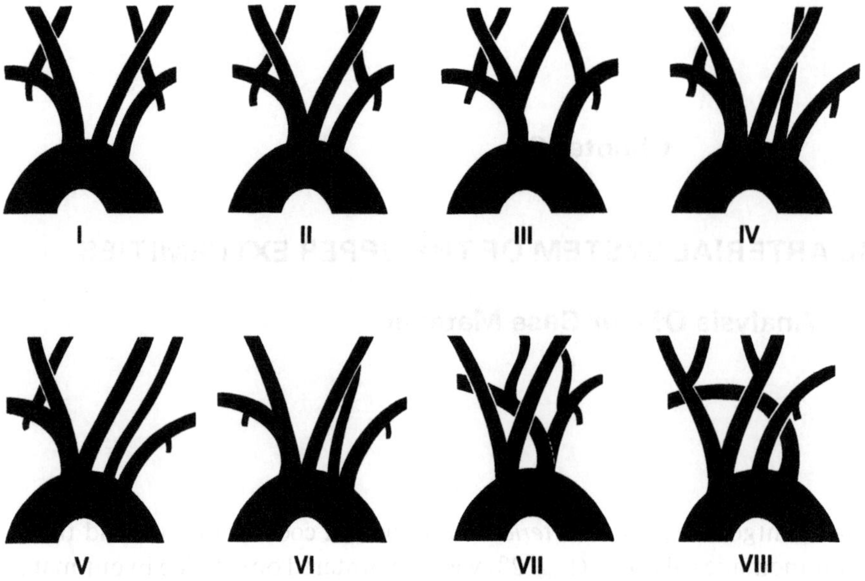

Fig. 24
Schematic representation of different types of aortic arch.

tients were of both sexes: 179 males and 144 females, varying in age from 15 to 80 years. The results of our study are shown in Table IV, together with the results of comparative studies by other

TABLE V

Comparison with the Results of Other Authors.

Type	*Present series*	*Lie 1968*	*Bosniak 1964*
I	72.8%	65-70%	69%
II	13.9%	16%	16%
III	5.6%	8%	8%
IV	4.3%	6%	6%

authors (Table V). For descriptive purposes the variations in the aortic arch have been divided into several types. The anatomy of the different arches is illustrated in Figures 24 and 25, where the structures are viewed in the anteroposterior projection. The aortic arch branches are marked in the order of origin from right to left.

In the present series eight different types of branching of the aortic/brachiocephalic tree could be distinguished:

Type I:
The innominate artery, the left common carotid artery and the left subclavian artery each have a separate origin from the aortic arch; both vertebral arteries originate from the subclavian arteries. This aortic arch, as illustrated in Figure 24, has a normal pattern of branching and is also called the *typical arch.* The type I branching pattern was the most commonly observed variant in the current series. Out of the 323 aortic arches in our material, this typical arch was present in 235 cases (73%) (Table IV). The branches given off from this aortic arch arise from the highest part of the arch, usually at unequal distances from one another. In elongated arches the brachiocephalic vessels may spring from the upper part of the ascending aorta (Fig. 2).

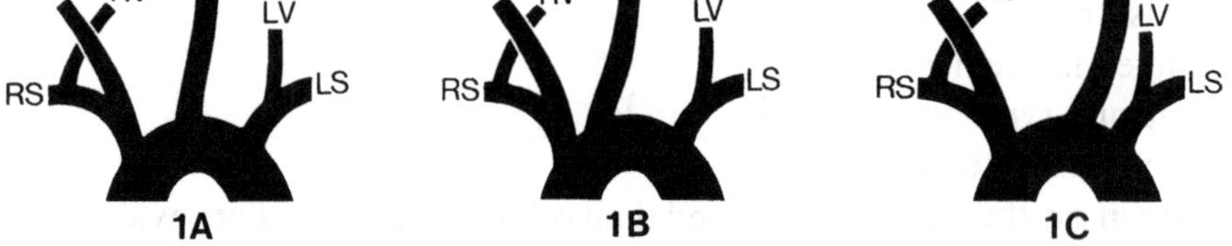

Fig. 25
Three subtypes of aortic arch I.

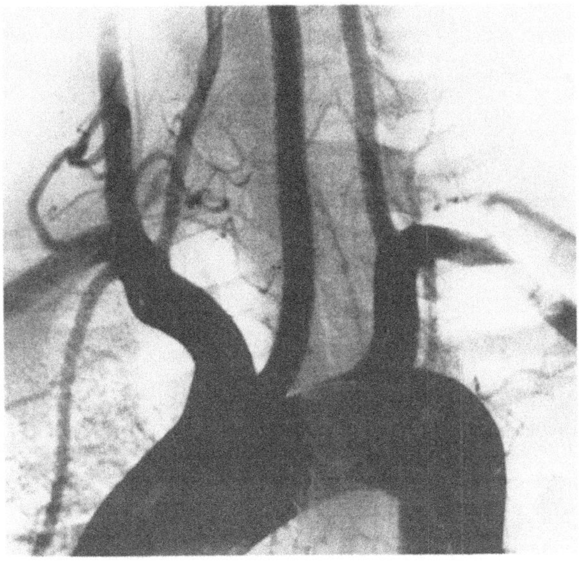

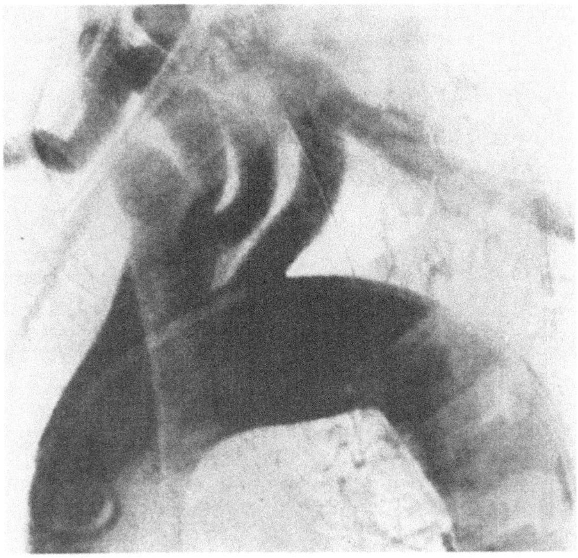

a b

Fig. 26
Two different types of aortic arch.
A. Aortic arch type II, the left common carotid artery and innominate artery have a common origin at the aorta.
B. The left common carotid artery originates directly from the innominate artery (Aortic arch type III).

The distance between the brachiocephalic vessels at their origin may be increased or diminished.

The location of the origin of the left common carotid artery between the innominate artery and the left subclavian artery can be close to the innominate artery, close to the subclavian artery or approximately halfway between these two vessels. On the basis of the distance of the origin of the left common carotid from the origins of the innominate and the left subclavian arteries, respectively, another subdivision into three types of aortic arches is made. These three types are indicated as IA, IB and IC (Fig. 25). If the origins of the three aortic branches are equidistant from one another, category IA is used. When the left common carotid arises close to the innominate artery, the arch is called type IB and when the left common carotid artery arises closer to the left subclavian artery, the arch is indicated as type IC.

TABLE VI

Different Types of Typical Aortic Arch.

Type	*Number*	*Percent*
IA	88	37.4
IB	115	48.9
IC	32	13.7
Total	235	100

The most frequent occurrence in this respect was the closer proximity of the left common carotid origin to the origin of the innominate artery (IB), which was observed in 48.9% of the cases. Types IA and IC occurred in 37.4% and 13.7%, respectively, of the 235 cases investigated in the current series (Table VI).

Type II (Fig. 26A):
In the type II branching pattern, the innominate artery and the left common carotid artery have a common origin which implies that bifurcation of the innominate artery and the carotid artery lies somewhat cranial to their common origin at the aorta. This branching pattern was observed in 13.9% of the cases.

Type III (Fig. 26B):
The left common carotid artery may also originate from the innominate artery and subsequently cross the midline. This variant occurred in 5.6% of our series.

Type IV:
The left vertebral artery has its origin at the aortic arch between the left common carotid and the left subclavian artery. The location of the origin of the left carotid artery may vary, as in IA, IB and IC. This variation was seen in 4.3% of our cases.

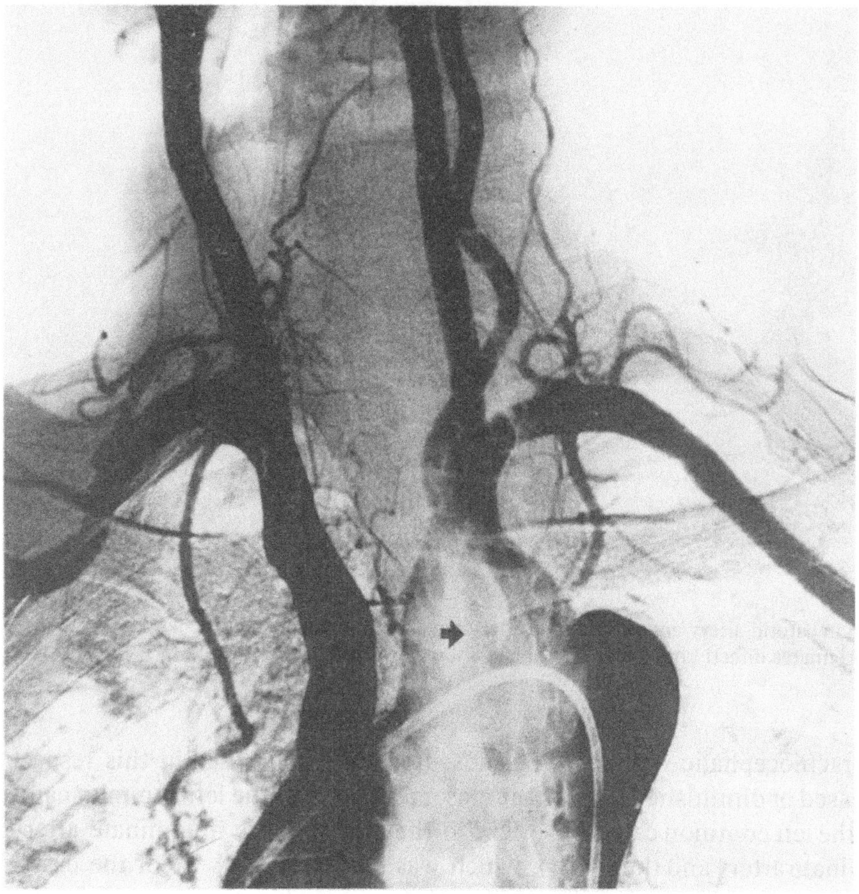

Fig. 27
Aortic arch type VI.
Large left vertebral artery (arrow) arising directly from the aortic arch between the origins of the left common carotid and the left subclavian artery. The right vertebral artery is absent.

Type V:
A common origin of the innominate and the left common carotid arteries at the aorta (see type II) in combination with a left vertebral artery originating from the aorta (see type IV) was observed on 0.9% of the aortic arch arteriograms in this series.

Type VI:
This type is a variation of the type IV branching pattern. It is associated with an aplasia of the right vertebral artery while the left vertebral artery, which is usually highly hypertrophic, arises from the aorta between the left carotid artery and the subclavian artery. This variation was observed only once (0.3%) (see Fig. 27).

Type VII:
In 4 cases a variation of the branches of the aortic arch was found which is called the bicarotid trunk: the two common carotid arteries have the same origin at the aorta and the left and right subclavian arteries have a separate origin at the aorta. The so-called bicarotid trunk arises at the original location of the brachiocephalic trunk at the aorta; medialwards and farther back are 2 separate subclavian arteries. The vertebral arteries arise from the subclavian arteries. This variation was observed in five cases (1.6%).

Type VIII (Fig. 28):
This variation comprises a bicarotid trunk and a left subclavian artery with an origin at the normal location. The right subclavian artery originates caudal to the left subclavian artery and is the most distal artery of the aortic arch. This aberrant right subclavian artery passes upward behind the left

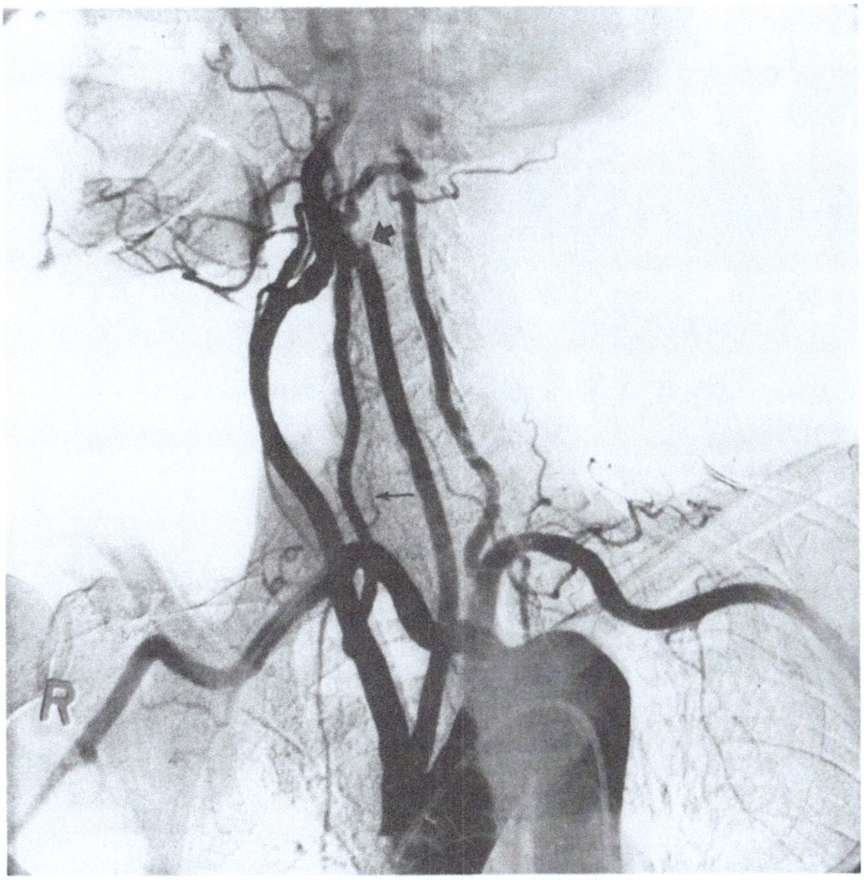

Fig. 28
Aortic Arch Type VIII.
The right subclavian artery originates distal to the left subclavian artery on the left side of the arch. It runs behind the left subclavian artery and both common carotid arteries, which originate from a common trunk. The right vertebral artery and the right internal mammary artery arise from the right common carotid artery. The ascending cervical artery (small arrow) originates from the right vertebral artery.
Note also the complete occlusion of the left internal carotid artery at its origin (large arrow).

subclavian artery, the oesophagus and the left and right common carotid arteries towards the right upper extremity. It has been stated that in very rare cases this artery may pass between the oesophagus and the trachea. Frequently the artery shows a dilatation at its origin which is known as the diverticulum of Kommerell, but this is not a constant finding.

There are considerable variations in the point of origin and size of the aberrant right subclavian artery. Usually it originates between the levels of the second and fourth thoracic vertebrae, although the level and length of the vessel varies from individual to individual. The impression of the aberrant right subclavian artery in the posterior wall of the oesophagus imparts characteristic roentgenological features, which may be observed during fluoroscopic examination of the oesophagus. In AP projection the most frequent sign is a compression of the left contour of the oesophagus (left notch) or a band-like oblique defect in the barium column created by the vessel as it passes upward from left to right. On lateral projection a compression is visible in the posterior wall of the oesophagus which varies from an almost imperceptible identation to almost complete occlusion of the barium column, depending upon the size of the vessel and its point of origin. Sometimes the pulsations of the vessel are visible.

The anomalous (retro-oesophageal) right sub-

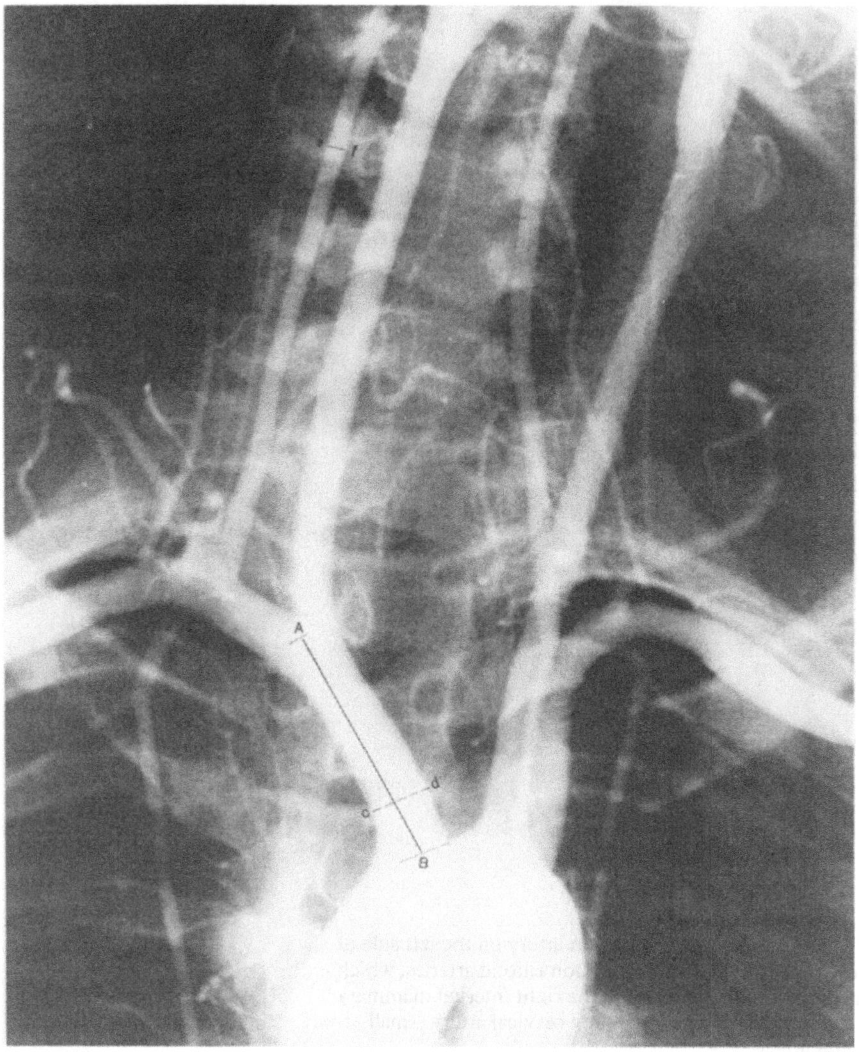

Fig. 29
Aortic arch aortography, RAO position, the innominate artery is suitably projected in its total length.

clavian artery may in some cases have clinical significance. In approximately 10% of patients, because of the compression of the oesophagus, it causes symptoms of *Dysphagia lusoria*. Therefore, the vessel is also called *arteria lusoria*, a term which was recommended by Arkin (1926). Usually this aberrant vessel represents a single anomaly of the aortic arch; however, it may be combined with coarctation, complete interruption of the aortic arch or a right-sided aortic arch (Abbott, 1928; Richter *et al.*, 1966; van Praagh *et al.*, 1970; Fishman *et al.*, 1976). Recent investigations have shown a predominance of the anomaly in females (Molz, 1976 and 1978).

This artery was found in our material in two cases (0.6%). In both cases the right vertebral artery arose from the right carotid artery and the remaining cervical arteries did not have their origin at the right subclavian artery (see Fig. 28). Both subjects were females. They had no other accompanying anomalies of the arch.

The eight brachiocephalic branching patterns described are depicted schematically in Figure 24. Although the aortic arches of types IV, V and VI show insignificant anatomical differences, they have been classified in three distinctive groups since they play an important role in the selective catheterization of the brachiocephalic vessels.

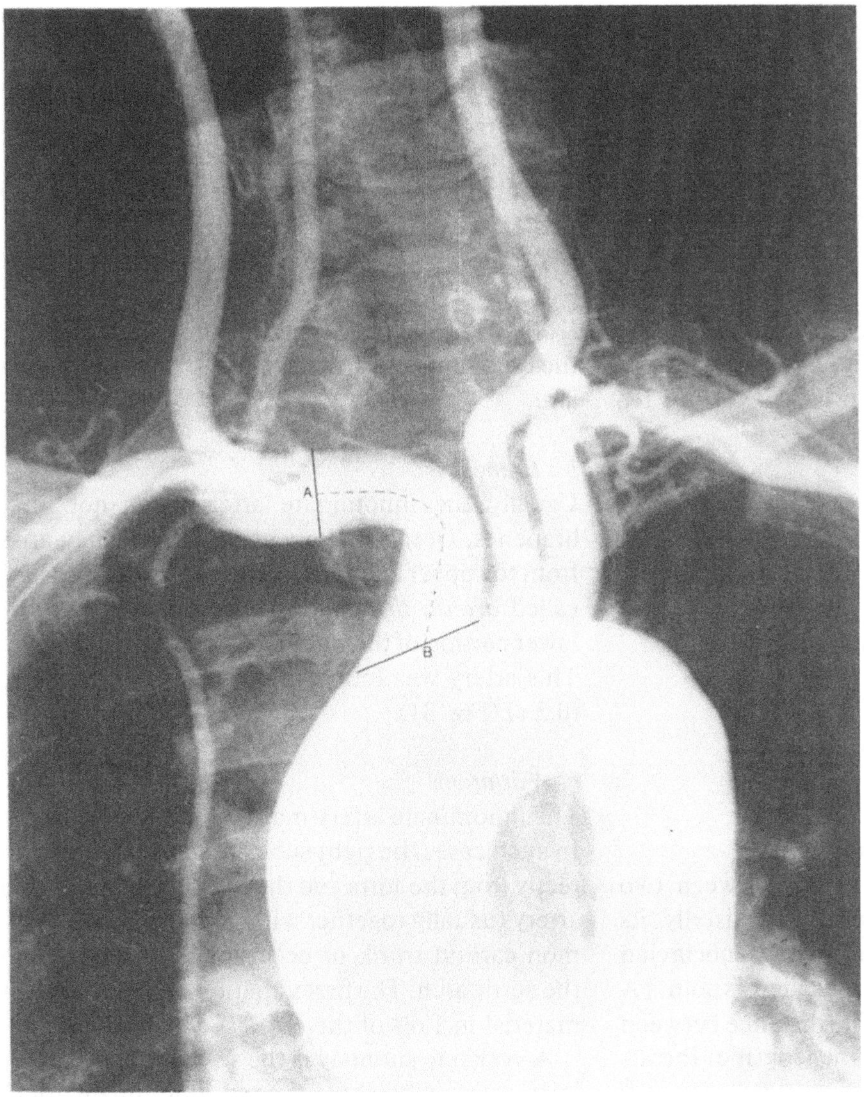

Fig. 30
Aortic arch aortography of a hypertensive patient with slight dilatation and tortuosity of the brachiocephalic vessels.

6.2 The Arteries of the Upper Extremities on the Aortograms

The upper extremity is supplied by one arterial trunk which originates at the aorta and continues as a single artery down to the elbow. Different portions of this trunk have received different names, according to the regions through which they pass. Thus we can recognize the innominate, subclavian, axillary and brachial arteries. Below the elbow, the brachial artery divides into two branches, the radial and the ulnar arteries.

In cases of obstruction, the arterial supply to the upper extremity is characterized by numerous collateral pathways. Each anatomical segment of the main arterial axis offers important collateral branches. In general, the more proximal the obstruction of the main stem, the more abundant and larger are the collateral vessels. The collateral pathways will be described more specifically for each anatomical area.

6.2.1 The Innominate Artery
(A. anonyma, truncus brachiocephalicus)

The innominate artery is usually the first branch originating from the aortic arch; it is also the largest vessel arising from the aortic arch. Since the dimensions and variations in this artery are important for the selective catheterization of the right subclavian and right carotid and vertebral arteries an analysis has been made of 323 thoracic aortograms on which the innominate artery was suitably projected. Only the aortograms which visualized the origin and the total length of the vessel were evaluated (Fig. 29).

Elongation, dilatation and tortuosity of the vessel in hypertensive and arteriosclerotic patients are also included in this study (Fig. 30). The results of the measurements are given in Tables VII en VIII.

TABLE VII

Length of the Innominate Artery.

cm	*Number*	*Percent*
0 -1		
1.1-2	2	0.6
2.1-3	13	4.2
3.1-4	90	28.8
4.1-5	142	45.6
5.1-6	52	16.7
6.1-7	11	3.5
7.1-8	2	0.6
Total	312	100

a. Dimensions of the Innominate Artery

The total length of the artery lies between two fixed points: proximally, its origin and distally, its bifurcation into the right carotid and subclavian arteries. These two points are indicated as points A and B in Figures 29 and 30. The distance between them was used to determine the length of the artery.

The diameter of the innominate artery is the distance between points C and D (Fig. 29) measured one centimeter distal to its origin (point B).

The average length of 312 innominate arteries was 4.54 cm, the shortest being 1.3 cm while the longest measured 8 cm. In 45.6% of the cases investigated the innominate artery measured between 4.1 and 5 cm in length (Table VII).

In 39% of the cases the diameter of the innominate artery was between 1.3 and 1.5 cm (Table VIII). The largest diameter measured was 3 cm, the smallest being 1.0 cm. The average diameter was 1.58 cm.

Of the most frequently occurring branching patterns of the brachiocephalic trunk (*i.e.* types I, II and III) it appeared that the innominate artery of the type I and III variants tends to have a large calibre.

b. Branches

Usually the innominate artery does not have branches. Occasionally a small branch may arise from the upper circumference of the artery, the so-called *arteria thyreoidea ima* which supplies the lower portion of the right lobe of the thyroid gland. This artery was found in our material only once (0.3%) (Fig. 31).

c. Variations

The innominate artery may sometimes be absent. In such cases the right subclavian artery arises directly from the aorta and the right common carotid artery (usually together with the left) from a common carotid trunk or occasionally directly from the aortic arch. The first variation was found in our material in 1.6% of the cases (Table IV).

A very rare anomaly is the so-called left innominate artery whereby a second innominate artery persists on the left side of the arch. The left common carotid and the left subclavian arteries stem from the left innominate artery; therefore such an aortic arch has only two branches and is called a bi-innominate arch. This variation was not found in our case material.

TABLE VIII

Diameter of Innominate Artery.

cm	*Nr.*	*%*	*Type of the aortic arch*			
			I	*II*	*III*	*Other*
1.0-1.2	37	12.3				
1.3-1.5	117	39.0				
1.6-1.8	101	33.7				
1.9-2.1	32	10.7	23 (72%)	5 (15.6%)	12 (39.3%)	1 (3%)
2.2-2.4	8	2.7	2 (25%)	2 (25%)	4 (50%)	
2.5-2.8	4	1.3	1 (25%)	0	3 (75%)	
2.9-3.1	1	0.3			1	
Total	300	100				

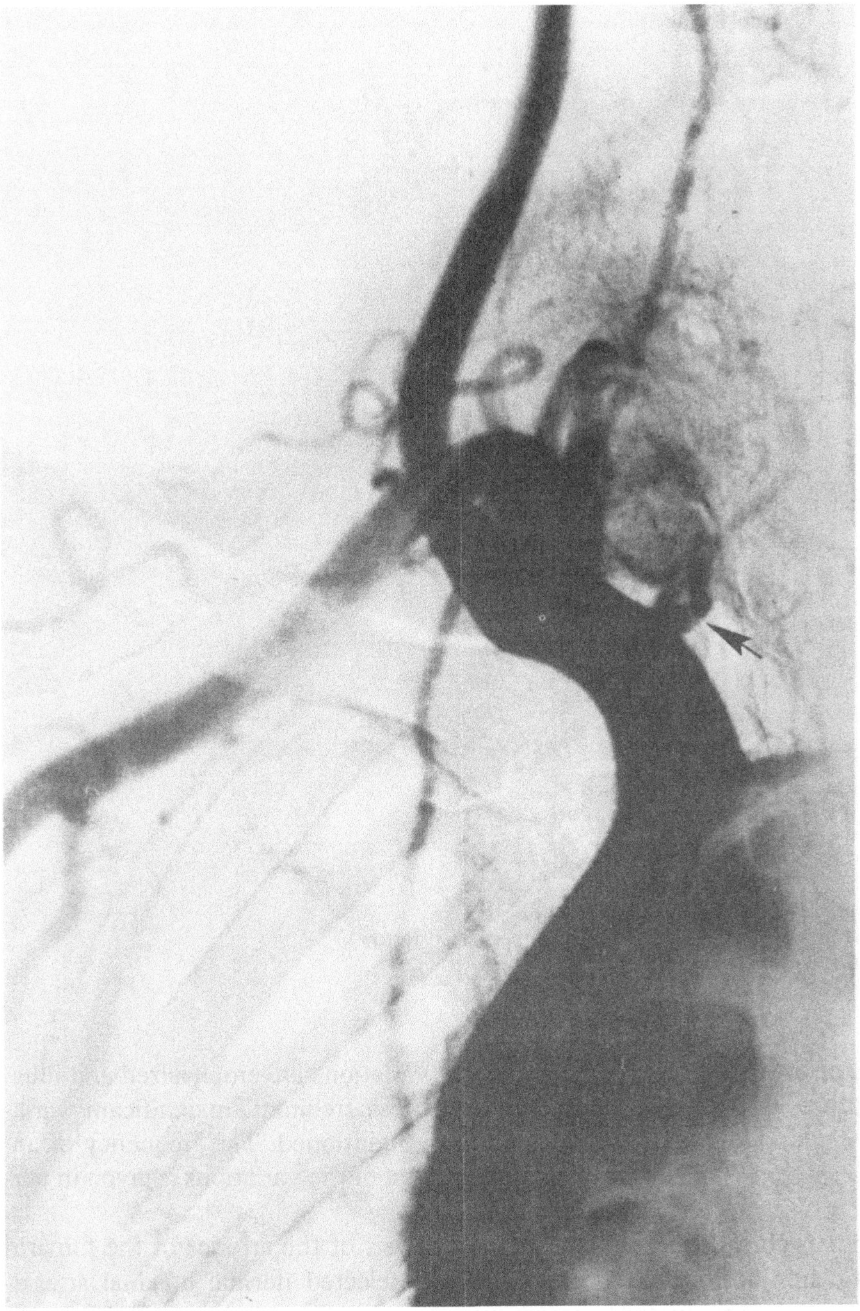

Fig. 31
Arteria thyreoidea ima (arrow).
The artery arises from the upper circumference of the innominate artery and supplies the lower part of a hypertrophic right lobe of the thyroid gland.

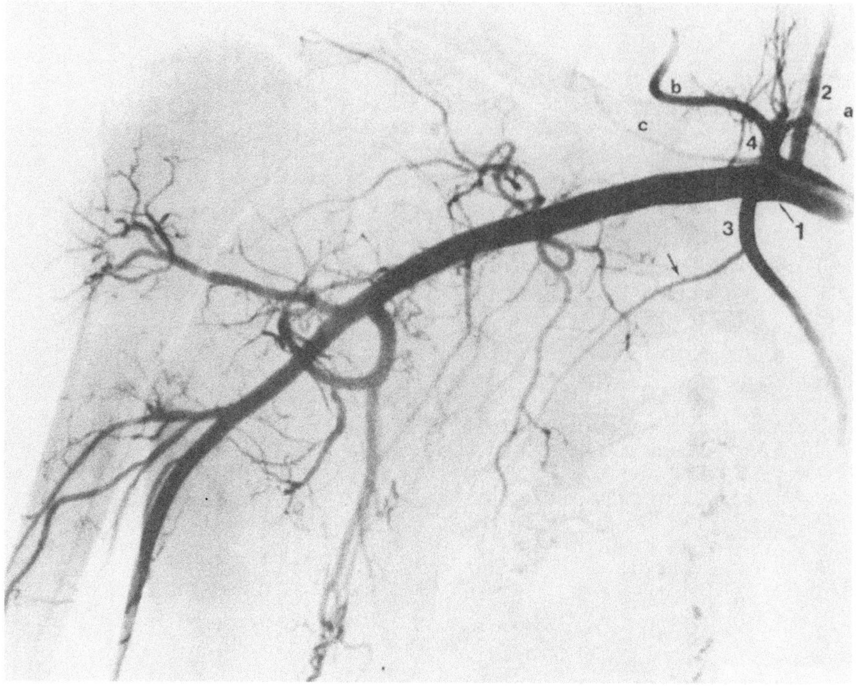

Fig. 32
1. Right Subclavian Artery
2. Vertebral Artery
3. Internal Mammary Artery
4. Thyrocervical Trunk
   a. Inferior Thyroid Artery
   b. Suprascapular Artery (Transverse Scapular Artery)
   c. Transverse Cervical Artery

The costocervical trunk is not present.
Note the small branch arising from the proximal part of the internal mammary artery (arrow), the ramus costalis lateralis; this branch is usually absent.

6.3 The Arteries of the Upper Extremities on Selective Arteriograms

Materials and Methods
Except the innominate and vertebral arteries, which were analysed on aortic arch aortograms, the other arteries of the upper limb were evaluated using 250 selective subclavian and 500 brachial arteriograms.

The results of the study of the arteries of the upper arm are based on an analysis of 250 selected normal subclavian arteriograms, which showed optimal visualization of all branches of the subclavian, axillary and brachial arteries. The study includes arteriograms of young patients of both sexes. The left and the right subclavian arteries were represented equally, each with 125 arteriograms.

Important variations are emphasized and illustrated. Other less frequent, insignificant variations are only mentioned. The frequency of appearance of most of the variations is given in percentages.

For the analysis of the arteries of the forearm and hand 500 selected normal brachial arteriograms were used. All arteriograms of this study were obtained by means of the transfemoral catheterization technique of Seldinger, as described in 3.4.

6.3.1 The Subclavian Artery (A. subclavia) (Figs. 32 and 36)

The subclavian artery is divided into three parts. The first portion extends from the origin of the vessel to the medial border of the anterior scalene muscle, the second lies immediately behind this

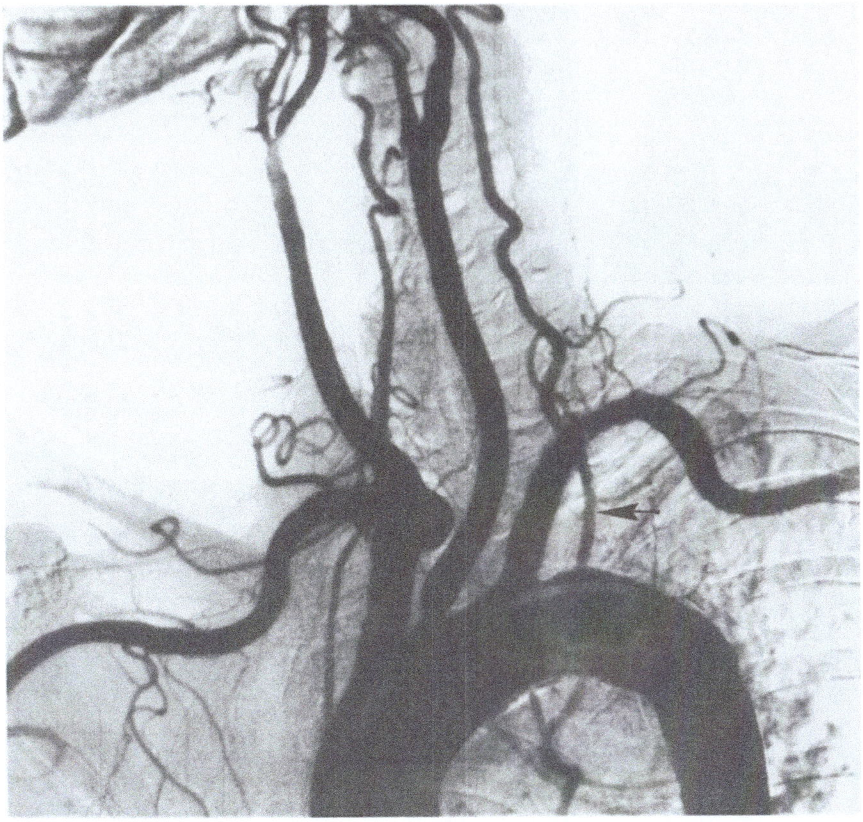

Fig. 33
Aortic arch arteriogram in AP projection demonstrates an anomalous origin of the left vertebral artery arising directly from the arch distal to the origin of the left subclavian artery (arrow).

muscle; the third extends from the lateral margin of the anterior scalene muscle to the outer border of the first rib, where it becomes the axillary artery. Since the left subclavian artery arises directly from the aortic arch and the right from the innominate artery, the first portion of the two vessels differs in length and direction. The origin and the proximal part of each subclavian artery lies in the thorax and is called the intrathoracic part.

6.3.2 The Vertebral Artery

The first branch of the subclavian artery, the vertebral artery, arises from the upper and posterior part of the first portion of the vessel at different distances from the aortic arch on the left and right side. The origin of this artery may vary. A direct origin of the left vertebral artery from the aortic arch between the left common carotid and left subclavian arteries (aortic arch types IV, V and VI) (Fig. 24) was found in our angiographic material in 5.5% of the cases. Less frequently this artery may originate from the aortic arch distal to the left subclavian artery (Fig. 33). In exceedingly rare cases the right vertebral artery will arise directly from the aortic arch. Occasionally this artery may even be absent. In our angiographic studies this was observed only once. The left vertebral artery in that case was very large with a diameter of 7.5 mm. The right vertebral artery may originate from the right common carotid artery. Apparently in all instances of such an origin, an aberrant right subclavian artery is also present (Fig. 28). On assessment of the literature, this anomaly appears to be very rare, but in our angiographic case material there were two such cases.

A so-called bifid origin of the vertebral artery with duplication of the proximal portion of the vessel was seen only twice (0.6%).

In both cases the anomaly was on the left side (Fig. 34).

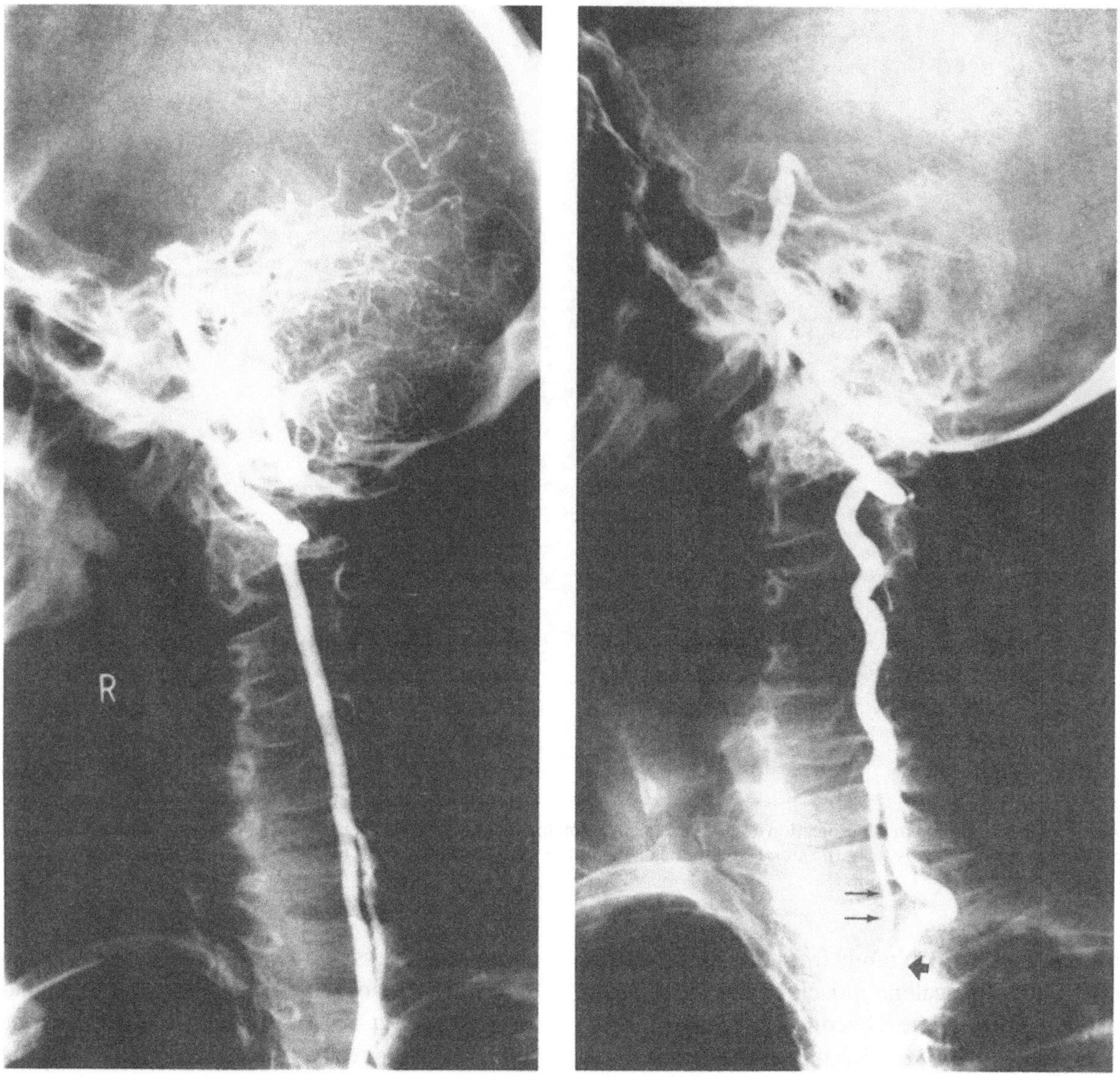

Fig. 34 a b

Bifid origin of the left vertebral artery.

A. The left vertebral artery originates directly from the aortic arch between the left common carotid and left subclavian arteries. A second left vertebral artery arises from the left subclavian artery, ascends to the foramen transversarium of the sixth cervical vertebra and unites with the first one.

B. The left vertebral artery (large arrow) arises from the left subclavian artery in the normal position and enters the foramen transversarium of the sixth cervical vertebra. A second anomalous left vertebral artery (double arrows) arises from the aortic arch (verified on aortic arch aortography) and ascends to enter the foramen transversarium of the sixth cervical vertebra. The two vertebral arteries unite at the level of the sixth cervical vertebra.

a. Calibre of the Vertebral Artery

Table IX summarizes the values found for the vertebral artery. A comparison was made between the sizes of the left and right vertebral arteries; these results are summarized in Table X.

The vertebral arteries were measured at the level of the sixth cervical vertebra.

The left vertebral artery appeared to have a larger calibre in 43.7% of the cases. The vertebral arteries had the same calibre in 28.3% of the cases. In 40.6% of the cases the diameter of the left vertebral artery was between 4.5 and 5.5 mm. The largest diameter of the left vertebral artery measured 7.6 mm; in this case the right vertebral artery was totally aplastic. In nine other cases (3.0%) the diameter was between 1.5 and 2.5 mm. In 38.8 percent of

TABLE IX

Diameter of the Vertebral Arteries.

mm	*Nr. L*	*% L*	*Nr. R*	*% R*
0 -1.5			1	0.3
1.5-2.5	9	3.0	12	4.0
2.5-3.5	31	10.4	51	16.8
3.5-4.5	80	26.8	118	38.8
4.5-5.5	121	40.6	89	29.3
5.5-6.5	51	17.1	25	8.2
6.5-7.5	5	1.7	6	2.0
> 7.5	1	0.4	2	0.6
Total	298	100	303	100

the cases the diameter of the right vertebral artery was between 3.5 and 4.5 mm. The largest diameter of the right vertebral artery was 8 mm, the smallest being 0.5 mm.

The average diameter was 4.5 mm for the left vertebral artery and 4.1 mm for the right vertebral artery. The standard deviations were 1.06 mm for the left side and 1.08 mm for the right. The most frequently found diameters of the right and the left vertebral arteries were 4 and 5 mm, respectively, and the difference between these two vessels was often found to be 1 or 2 mm (Table X).

6.3.3 The Internal Mammary Artery (A. mammaria interna)

This artery arises from the inferior surface of the first portion of the subclavian artery, usually opposite the origin of the thyrocervical trunk. The proximal part runs caudalwards and slightly medialwards to enter the chest behind the clavicle and the cartilage of the first rib. After descending laterally to the sternum it usually ends in the sixth intercostal space by dividing into two branches.

The extrathoracic (cervical) portion of the internal mammary artery gives off no branches. The thoracic portion lies behind the cartilages of the six upper ribs; the branches on the medial side go to the mediastinum, thymus, pericardium and sternum. The lateral branches of the internal mammary artery are the first six anterior intercostal arteries: two for each of the six intercostal spaces. The anastomoses between these arteries and the branches of the lateral thoracic and subscapular arteries play an important role in the collateral circulation to the brachial artery in cases of occlusion of the second or third portion of the subclavian artery.

a. Variations

This artery does not show many variations. Sometimes a lateral costal branch (ramus costalis lateralis) arises from the upper thoracic portion, close to the first rib. This branch is usually small in calibre, but sometimes it is significantly larger, i.e. about the same as or even larger than the continuation of the internal mammary artery. It descends behind the ribs in the caudolateral direction and gives off some of the intercostal arteries (Fig. 35).

The lateral costal branch has been observed on 24 arteriograms or 9.6 per cent of our material.

Sometimes this branch does not originate from the proximal part of the internal mammary artery but from the middle portion, as was observed in one case. In another case two lateral branches were seen.

TABLE X

Comparison of the Left and the Right Vertebral Arteries.

R and L equal mm	*R = L Nr.*	*%*	*R and L difference mm*	*R > L Nr.*	*R > L %*	*L > R Nr.*	*L > R %*
2	1	0.03	0.5	22	7.5	15	5.0
2.5			1	28	9.5	44	14.9
3	7	2.4	1.5	4	1.3	18	6.1
3.5	1	0.3	2	18	6.0	25	8.5
4	35	11.8	2.5	2	0.7	8	2.8
4.5	7	2.4	3	8	2.7	15	5.1
5	27	9.1	3.5	1	0.3	1	0.3
5.5	1	0.3	4			2	0.7
6	5	1.7	4.5			1	0.3
Total	84	28.3		83	28.0	129	43.7

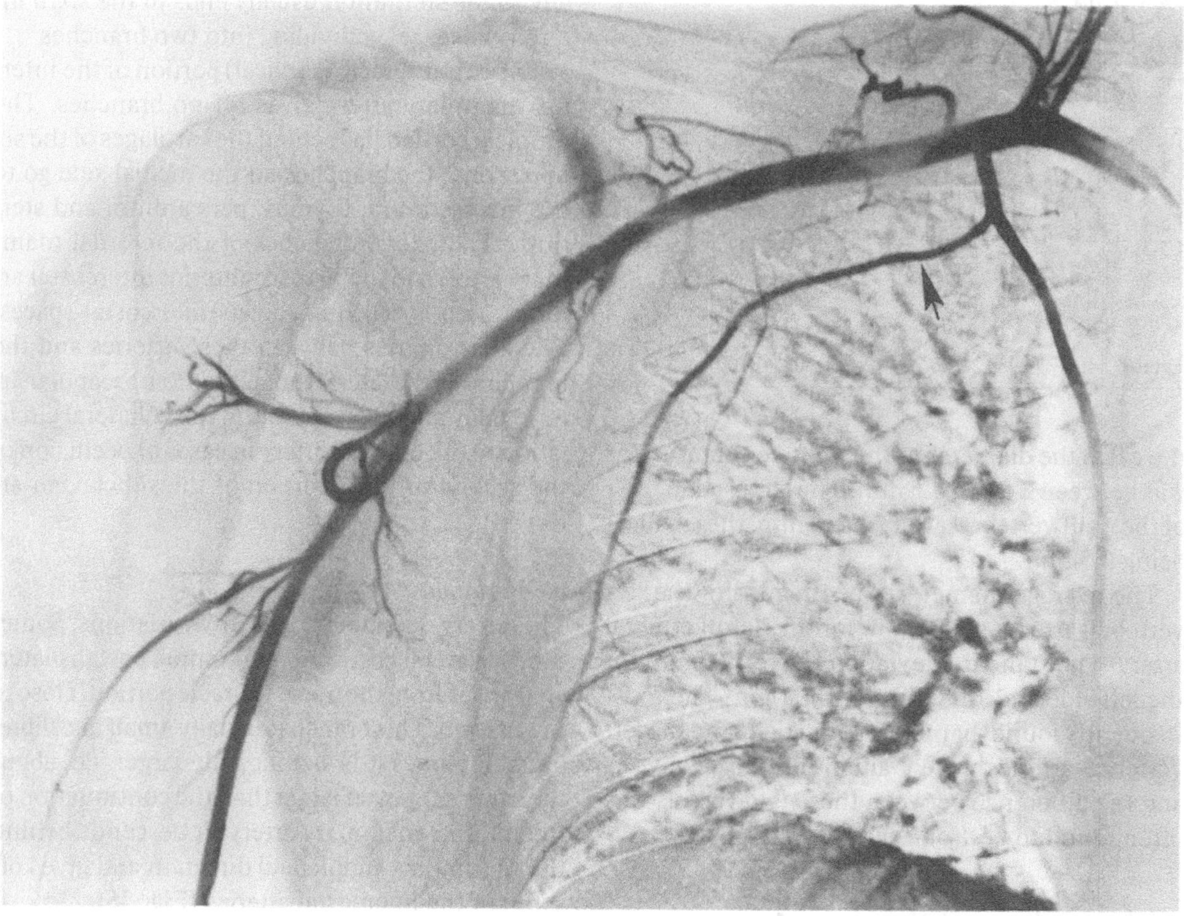

Fig. 35
Large lateral costal branch (arrow) of the internal mammary artery which gives off some of the intercostal arteries.

6.3.4 The Thyrocervical Trunk
(Truncus thyrocervicalis or thyroid axis) (Figs. 32 and 36)

The thyrocervical trunk is the shortest branch of the subclavian artery. It arises from the superior and anterior wall of the first portion of the subclavian artery. Usually it is a thick trunk which divides almost immediately into three branches: the inferior thyroid, the suprascapular (transverse scapular) and the transverse cervical arteries.

a. Variations

Since the thyrocervical trunk is sometimes subjected to selective catheterization in cases of thyroid gland pathology, the variations in this vessel may be relevant. All of the branches of the thyrocervical trunk or one of them may arise directly from the subclavian artery (Figs. 36B and 37). On very rare occasions the inferior thyroid artery can be absent; in such instances the superior thyroid artery usually supplies the territory normally nourished by the inferior thyroid artery.

The suprascapular artery anastomoses with the descending branch of the transverse cervical artery and the branches of the scapular circumflex artery.

The transverse cervical artery lies inferior to the suprascapular artery. It runs nearly parallel to the suprascapular artery and then divides into two branches: an ascending and a descending branch. The descending branch anastomoses with the suprascapular and scapular circumflex arteries as well as the posterior branches of some intercostal arteries. In cases of occlusion of the third portion of the subclavian artery, the collateral circulation for the arm is established mainly via anastomoses of the suprascapular and transverse cervical arteries with the scapular circumflex artery.

The second collateral pathway is through the in-

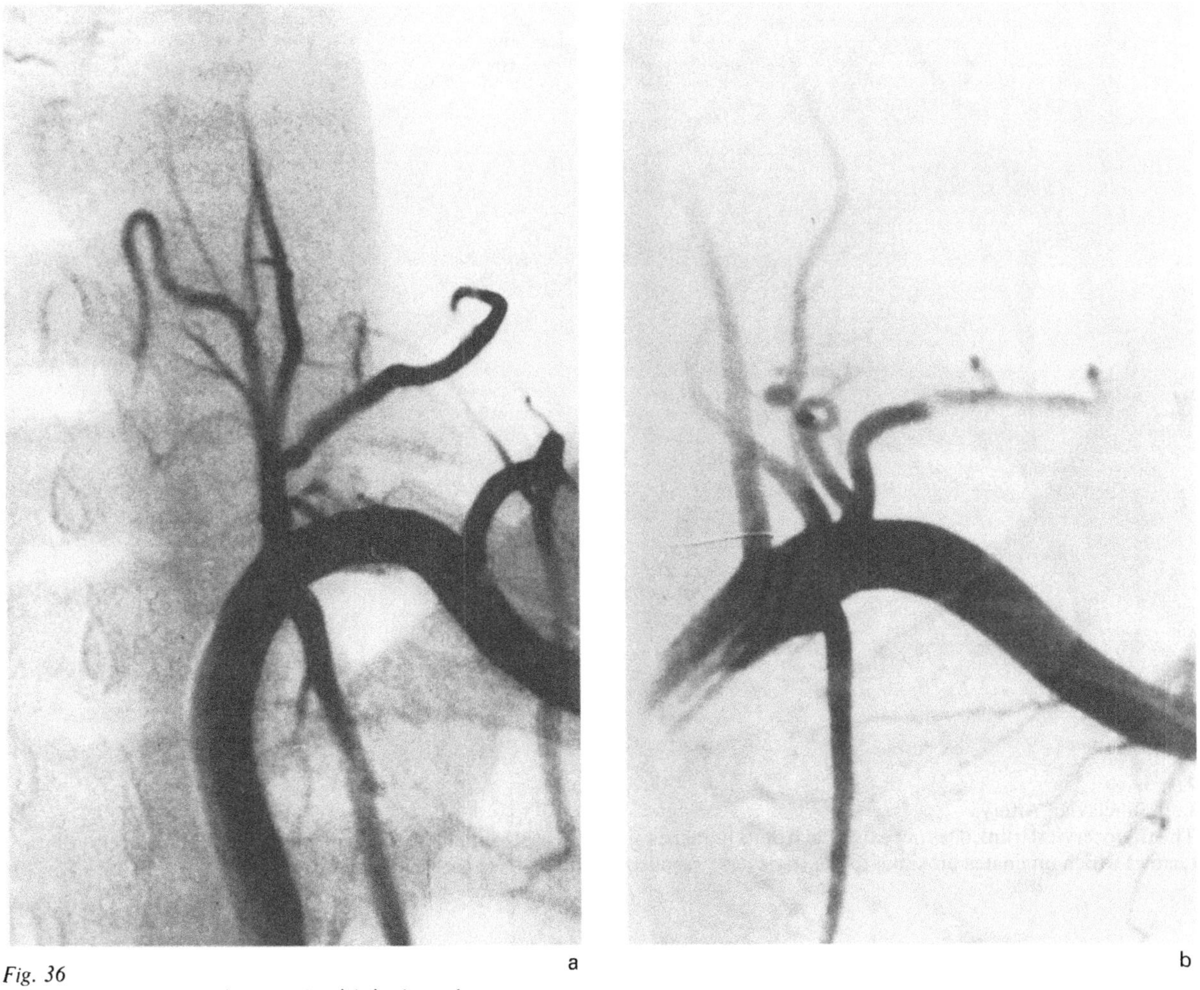

Fig. 36
A. Persistent thyrocervical trunk with its branches.
B. Bifid origin of the thyrocervical vessels. The inferior thyroid artery arises separately from the subclavian artery. The suprascapular and ascending cervical arteries have a common origin.

ternal mammary and intercostal arteries to the subscapular and lateral thoracic arteries.

A single thyrocervical trunk with its branches (Fig. 36A) was visualized in 131 cases (52.4%). Independent origin of all thyrocervical branches from the subclavian artery (Fig. 36B) with absence of the trunk was seen 78 times (31.2%).

In all other cases (16.4%) one of the branches originated independently from the subclavian artery and the remaining branches from the trunk. The transverse cervical artery arose from the subclavian artery as a single vessel 19 times (7.6%) and together with the suprascapular artery in 5 cases (2.0%); in the latter case the ascending cervical artery and the inferior thyroid artery branched off from the thyroid trunk.

The suprascapular artery arose directly from the subclavian artery as a single vessel in 4.0 percent of the cases. The remaining arteries in such cases originate as branches of the trunk. In the event that the ascending branch of the transverse cervical artery is small in calibre or totally absent it may be replaced by an artery originating directly from the thyrocervical trunk which usually runs upwards and lateralwards in the neck. This artery is called *the superficial cervical artery*; it supplies the same area as the ascending branch of the transverse cervical artery. Occasionally the descending branch of the same artery may originate from the third or, more rarely, from the second part of the subclavian artery. The first variation, that of the superficial cervical artery, was found in 22 percent of our cases.

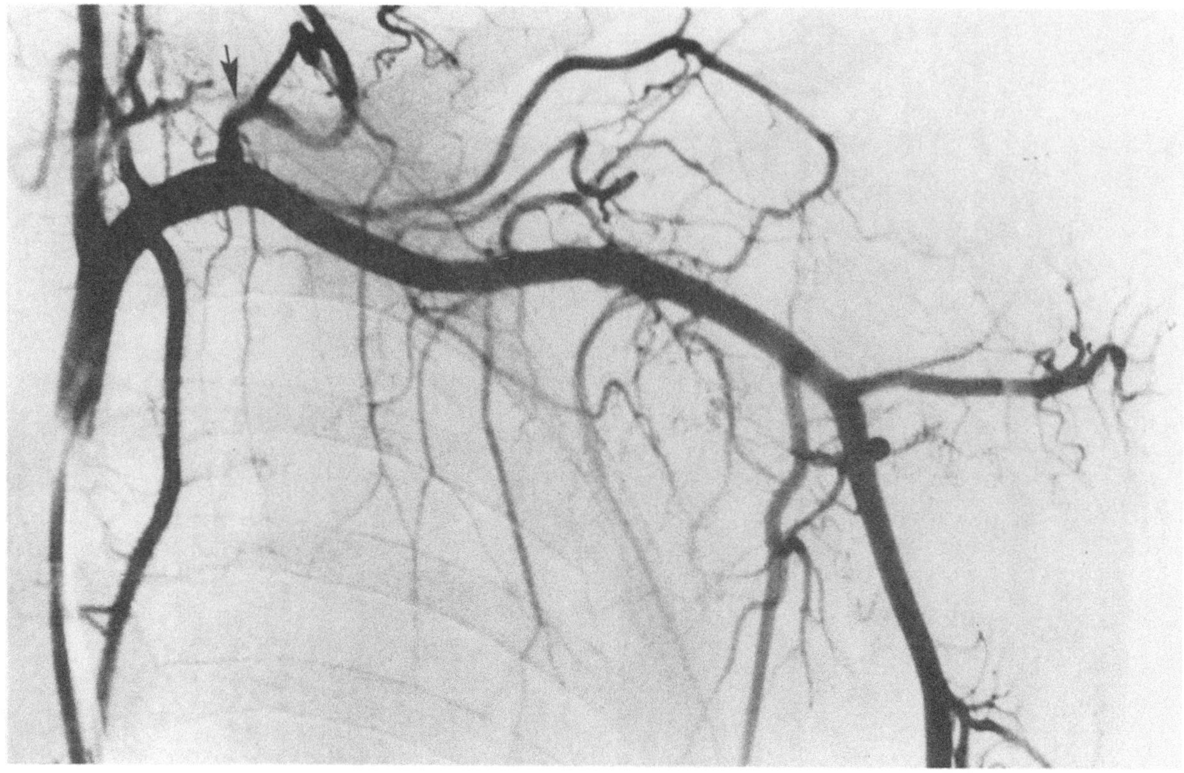

Fig. 37
Left Subclavian Artery.
The thyrocervical trunk does not exist. Each of its branches arises directly from the subclavian artery. Normal costocervical trunk (arrow) which originates proximal to the transverse scapular and transverse cervical arteries.

6.3.5 The Costocervical Trunk (Truncus costocervicalis) (Fig. 37)

This is a short stem that usually arises from the posterior aspect of the second portion of the subclavian artery. It is the most distal branch of the subclavian artery. Beyond this point, the subclavian artery continues as the axillary artery. This trunk is not always present. In our case material it was visualized on 221 arteriograms (88.4%).

a. Branches
The branches of the costocervical trunk are the superior intercostal artery and the deep cervical artery.

Variations of the branches of the costocervical trunk were not noted.

6.3.6 The Axillary Artery (A. axillaris) (Fig. 38)

The axillary artery is the direct continuation of the subclavian artery which passes through the axillary fossa. It begins at the lateral border of the first rib and ends at the lower border of the tendon of the greater pectoral muscle where it continues as the brachial artery. For descriptive purposes the main trunk of the axillary artery has been divided into three segments: the first segment lies medial to the smaller pectoral muscle, the second behind and the third below and lateral to this muscle. Each portion of the artery gives off a number of branches.

a. Branches (Fig. 38)
A. From the first portion:
1. the highest thoracic artery.

B. From the second part:
2. lateral thoracic artery
3. thoracoacromial artery

C. From the third part:
4. subscapular artery
5. humeral circumflex artery

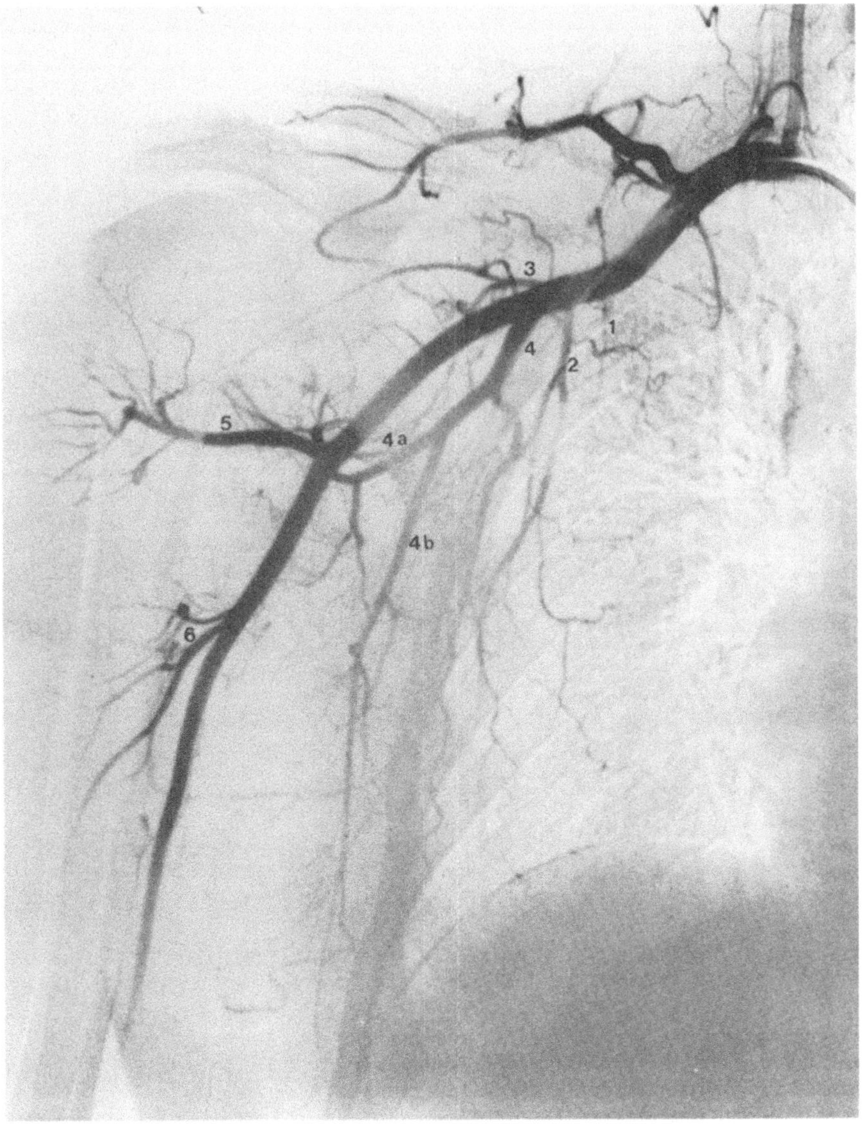

Fig. 38
Axillary Artery (normal pattern).
1. Highest Thoracic Artery (A. thoracica suprema)
2. Lateral Thoracic Artery (A. thoracica lateralis)
3. Thoracoacromial Artery (A. thoracoacromialis)
4. Subscapular Artery (A. subscapularis)
   4a. Scapular circumflex artery (A. circumflexa scapulae)
   4b. Thoracodorsal Artery (A. thoracodorsalis)
5. Humeral Circumflex Artery (A. circumflexa humeri)
6. Deep Brachial Artery (A. profunda brachii).

In case of occlusion of the axillary artery, the collateral circulation will be supplied by the same branches that take over after occlusion of the third part of the subclavian artery.

b. Variations

The branches of the axillary artery show many variations, but they are almost never subjected to superselective catheterization. They may play a role during the selective catheterization of the brachial artery, especially the large branches which sometimes cannot be avoided during catheterization.

One important variant which plays a significant

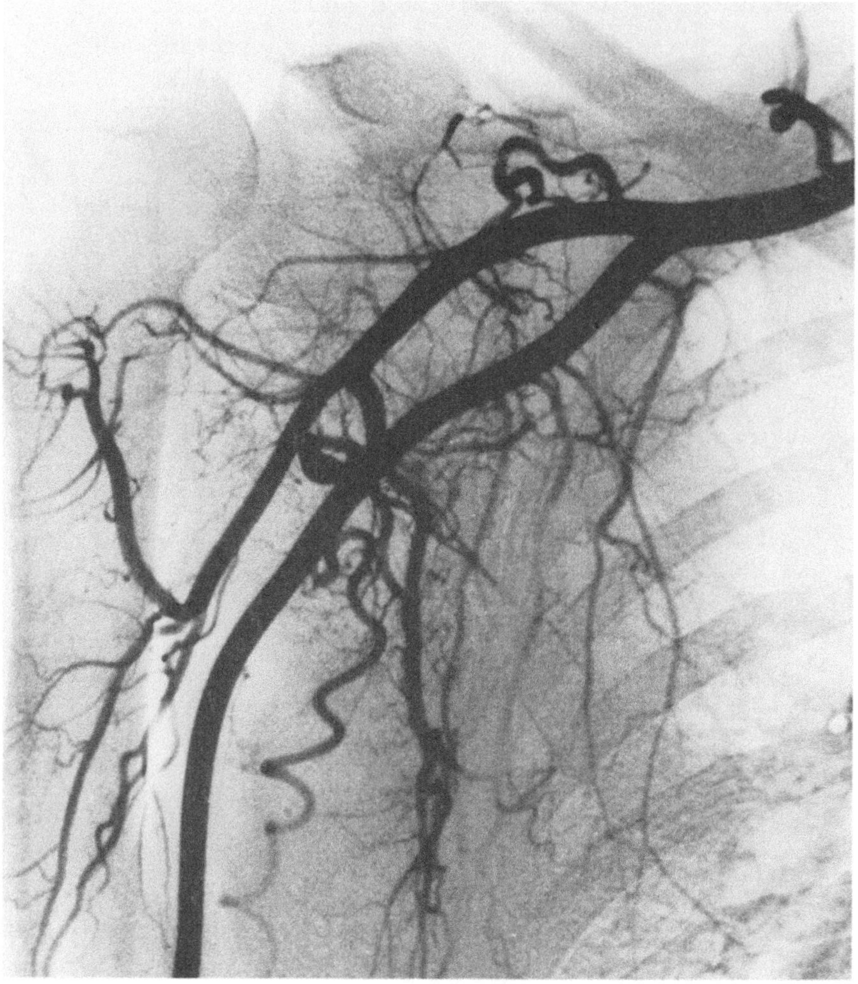

Fig. 39
A large common trunk for several branches which normally arise from the axillary and brachial arteries. The calibre of this vessel is approximately the same as that of the axillary artery. Since it follows the same course it can play an important role during the selective catheterization of the brachial artery, because it is difficult to avoid.

role in the selective catheterization of the brachial artery is shown in Figure 39. It is the large vessel which arises from the first part of the axillary artery and extends cranialwards and almost parallel to the axillary artery. This branch may have the same calibre as the axillary artery and during catheterization of the brachial artery it is sometimes difficult to keep the catheter from entering this vessel. This branch gives off several arteries which normally arise from the axillary and brachial arteries. In the proximal part it gives off the thoracoacromial and thoracodorsal arteries and when it reaches the level of the lower border of the teres major muscle it divides into the anterior and posterior humeral circumflex arteries and the deep brachial artery, which normally arise from the proximal part of the brachial artery. The highest thoracic, the lateral thoracic and the scapular circumflex arteries are in this case the branches of the axillary artery. These variations are apparently not very frequent, since they were seen on ten arteriograms (4.0%): six times on the left side and four on the right.

Another important variant which may play a role during catheterization of the brachial artery is demonstrated in Figure 40. It is a common trunk for the humeral circumflex and the subscapular arteries, usually separate branches of the axillary artery. This vessel may be quite large and usually runs caudal to the axillary artery. This common

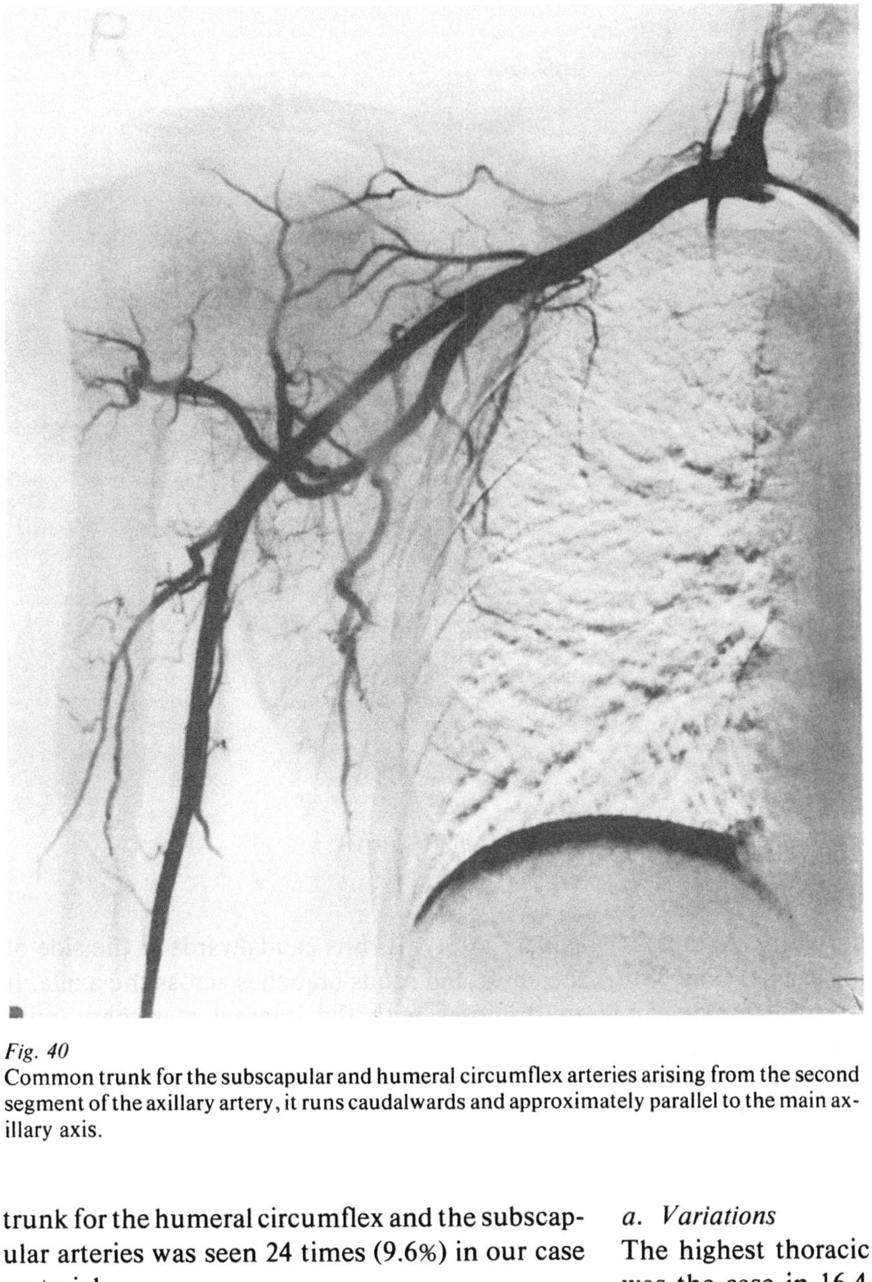

Fig. 40
Common trunk for the subscapular and humeral circumflex arteries arising from the second segment of the axillary artery, it runs caudalwards and approximately parallel to the main axillary axis.

trunk for the humeral circumflex and the subscapular arteries was seen 24 times (9.6%) in our case material.

6.3.7 The Highest Thoracic Artery
(A. thoracica suprema; A. thoracica superior) (Fig. 38)

This artery is a small vessel which arises in the first portion of the axillary artery. It is the most proximal branch of the axillary axis and supplies the medial part of the anterior thoracic wall. The peripheral branches of the artery anastomose with the terminal branches of the internal mammary and intercostal arteries.

a. Variations
The highest thoracic artery may be absent; this was the case in 16.4 percent of our material. In such instances the medial branch of the lateral thoracic artery vascularized the territory of the highest thoracic artery.

We have observed on our arteriograms that this artery may be double (3.6%) or even triple (0.4%). In all of these cases the arteries were very tiny. We have also seen that this artery may be a branch of the thoracoacromial artery, or it may arise together with the latter (3.6%). A single highest thoracic artery arising independently from the axillary artery was present on 190 arteriograms or 76 percent of our series.

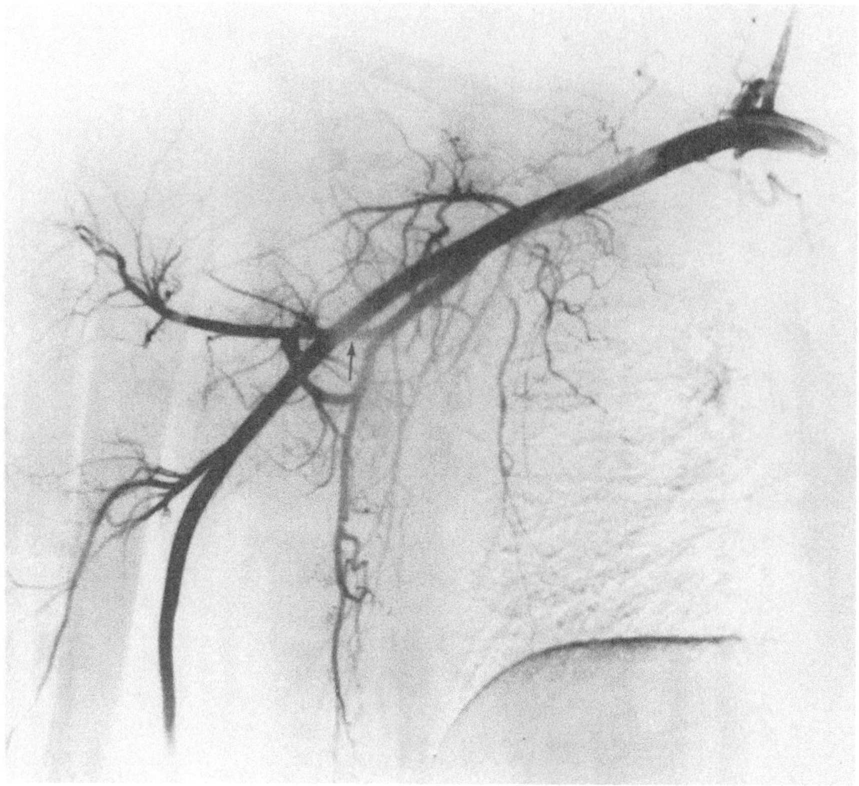

Fig. 41
Arteriogram of the right upper arm shows a different origin of the humeral circumflex artery. It arises from the subscapular artery (arrow).

6.3.8 The Thoracoacromial Artery (A. thoracoacromialis; syn. thoracic axis) (Fig. 38)

This artery arises from the second part of the axillary artery behind the medial edge of the minor pectoral muscle. It is a short vessel which usually divides into two branches immediately after its origin a descending branch which anastomoses with the branches of the lateral thoracic and internal mammary arteries and an ascending branch which runs lateralwards and terminates in several small branches, which anastomose with the terminal branches of the humeral circumflex arteries. Marked variations of this artery were not seen in our case material. Sometimes it may replace the lateral thoracic artery, or the latter may be a branch of the thoracoacromial artery.

6.3.9 The Lateral Thoracic Artery (A. thoracica lateralis, syn: external mammary artery; long thoracic artery) (Fig. 38)

This artery arises from the second segment of the axillary artery. It runs caudalwards to the side of the chest and sends branches across the axilla. It anastomoses with the internal mammary, subscapular, thoracoacromial and intercostal arteries. In females it supplies a part of the mamma.

a. Variations

The origin, course and distribution of the lateral thoracic artery vary greatly. Usually it stems directly from the axillary artery. This was the case on 64.4 percent of our arteriograms. We saw a different origin of this artery 89 times (35.6%).

It originated together with the thoracoacromial in 71 cases (28.4%), and it was a branch of the subscapular artery in 18 cases (7.2% or our series).

The lateral thoracic artery is usually a single vessel (38.4%), but it may be represented by two, three or multiple vessels. In our series we observed a double lateral thoracic artery on 56 arteriograms (22.4%). A triple vessel was seen 8 times (3.2%); once (0.4%) the artery was represented by multiple tiny vessels, all of which originated directly from the axillary artery.

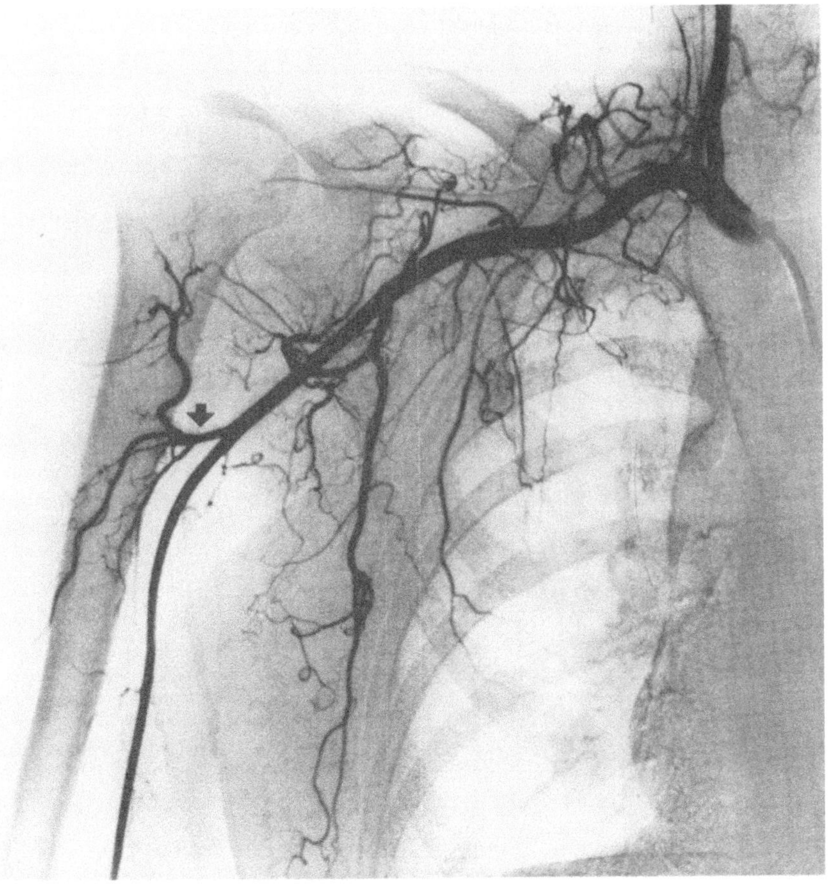

Fig. 42
Arteriogram of the right upper arm demonstrates a common arterial stem (arrow) which arises from the proximal brachial artery and divides into the humeral circumflex and deep brachial arteries.

6.3.10 The Subscapular Artery
(A. subscapularis) (Fig. 38)

This is the largest branch of the axillary artery, arising from the inferior wall of the third portion of the axillary artery. It runs caudalwards almost parallel to the thoracic wall and the lateral border of the scapula which it follows up to the inferior angle of the scapula. The terminal branches of this artery anastomose with the lateral thoracic and intercostal arteries. The subscapular artery also anastomoses with the descending branch of the transverse cervical artery.

The main branches of the subscapular artery are the scapular circumflex artery, which usually arises 4 cm from the origin of the subscapular artery, and the thoracodorsal artery, which parallels the course of the subscapular artery as far as the angle of the scapula where it anastomoses with the intercostal arteries and the branches of the lateral thoracic artery.

a. Variations

The subscapular artery may arise from the second part of the axillary artery. It usually runs lateral and caudal to the main axillary trunk. The proximal portion gives off the lateral thoracic branch and then divides into the scapular circumflex and thoracodorsal arteries. This variation was found on our arteriograms 18 times (7.2%).

Very often the subscapular artery originates with the humeral circumflex artery from a common trunk (Fig. 40). This variation was seen on 24 arteriograms or 9.6 percent of our series. Occasionally the scapular circumflex and thoracodorsal arteries arise directly from the axillary artery; this was observed six times (2.4%). In 3 cases (1.2%) we observed a common trunk arising from the third

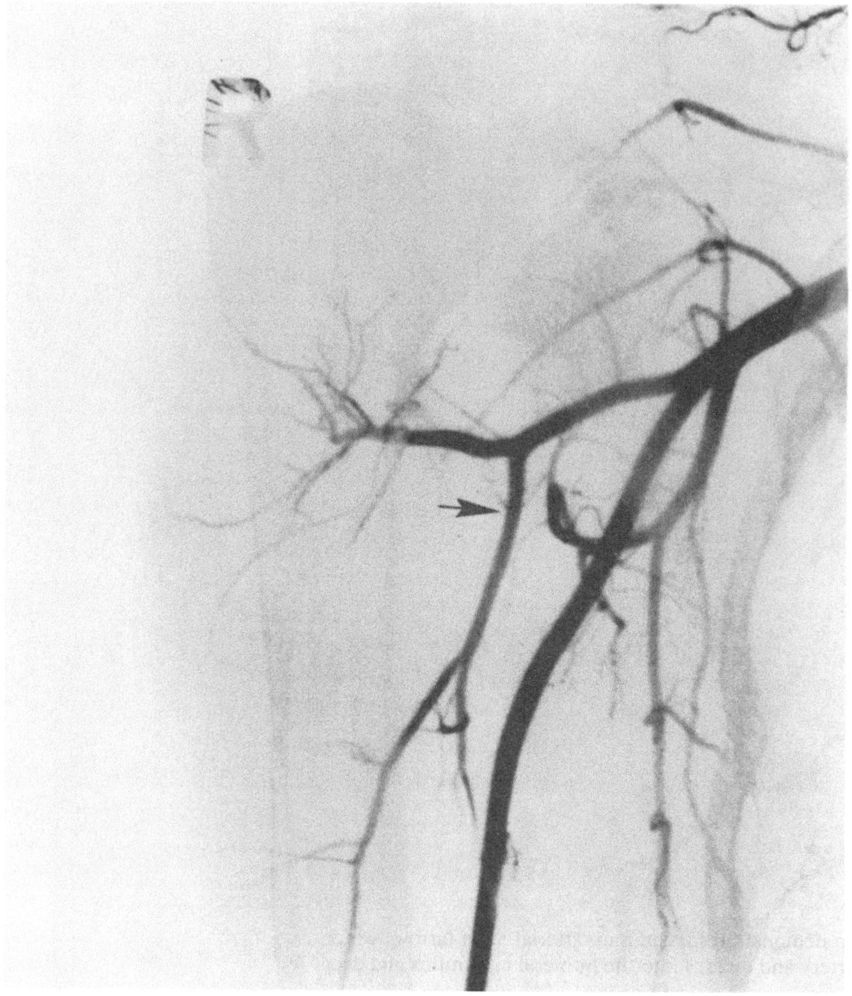

Fig. 43
The same variation as in Fig. 42. A long deep brachial artery arises from the stem of the humeral circumflex artery (arrow).

portion of the axillary artery which gave rise to the subscapular, humeral circumflex and deep brachial arteries.

6.3.11 The Scapular Circumflex Artery
(A. circumflexa scapulae; syn: A. dorsalis scapulae) (Fig. 38)

This is the largest branch of the subscapular artery, even larger than the continuation of the subscapular artery. It curves around the lateral border of the scapula, runs dorsal to the scapula in the infraspinous fossa and terminates by dividing into two branches which anastomose with the transverse scapular artery and the descending branch of the transverse cervical artery.

a. Variations
This artery may arise directly from the axillary artery; in such cases the subscapular artery is small in calibre. A direct origin of the scapular circumflex artery was observed on 6 arteriograms (2.4%). Other variations of this artery were not noted.

6.3.12 The Humeral Circumflex Artery
(A. circumflexa humeri) (Fig. 38)

It originates from the axillary artery. According to the course and distribution of the main branches of this artery two distinct vessels can be recognized: the anterior and the posterior humeral circumflex arteries.

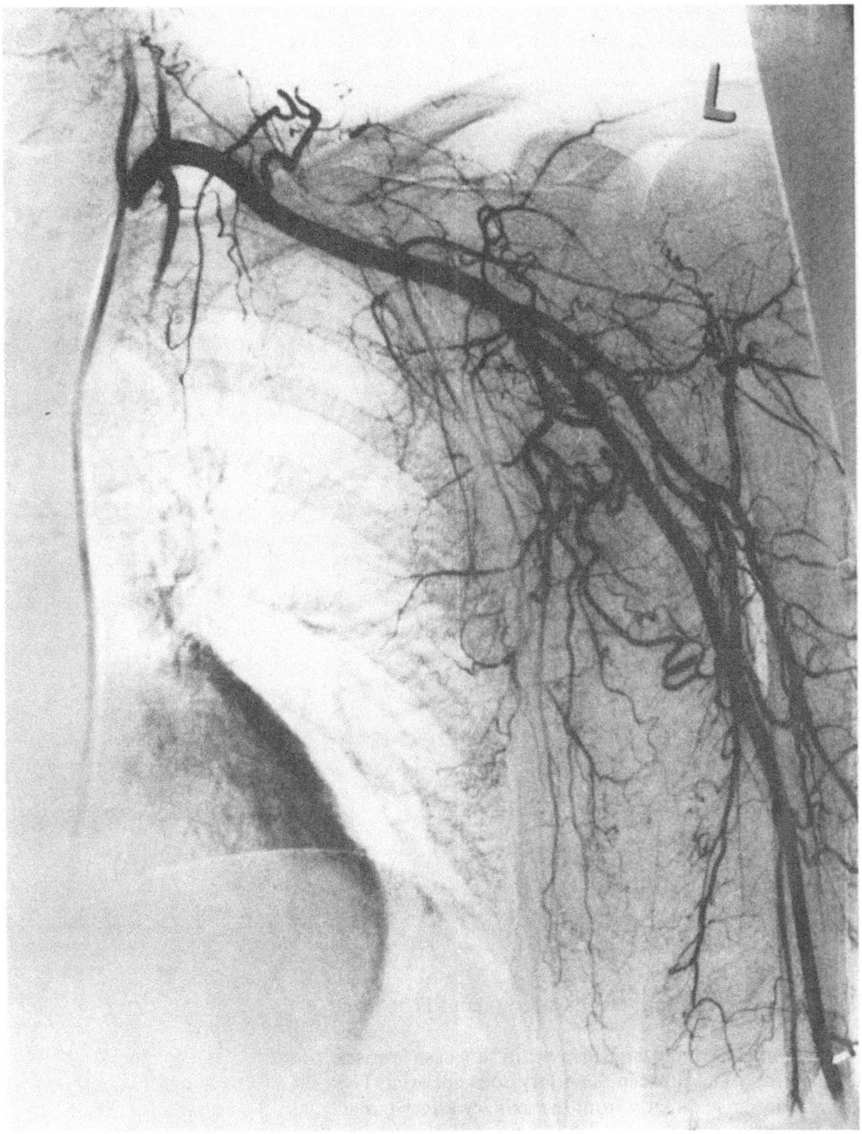

Fig. 44
A long arterial trunk which arises from the third portion of the left axillary artery giving rise to the humeral circumflex artery, the deep brachial artery and some branches of the thoracodorsal artery.

a. The Posterior Humeral Circumflex Artery (A. circumflexa humeri posterior; A. circumflexa posterior)
This artery is the most distal branch of the axillary artery; it runs posteriorwards until it curves around the posterior surface of the neck of humerus and ends with small branches to the deltoideus region and shoulder joint which anastomose with the branches of the anterior humeral circumflex artery and the deep brachial artery.

b. The Anterior Humeral Circumflex Artery (A. circumflexa humeri anterior; A. circumflexa anterior)
This originates on the lateral side of the distal part of the axillary artery, just beyond the origin of the posterior humeral circumflex artery. It is usually smaller in calibre than the posterior humeral circumflex artery. It extends in the horizontal direction in front of the neck of humerus, terminating in small branches which anastomose with

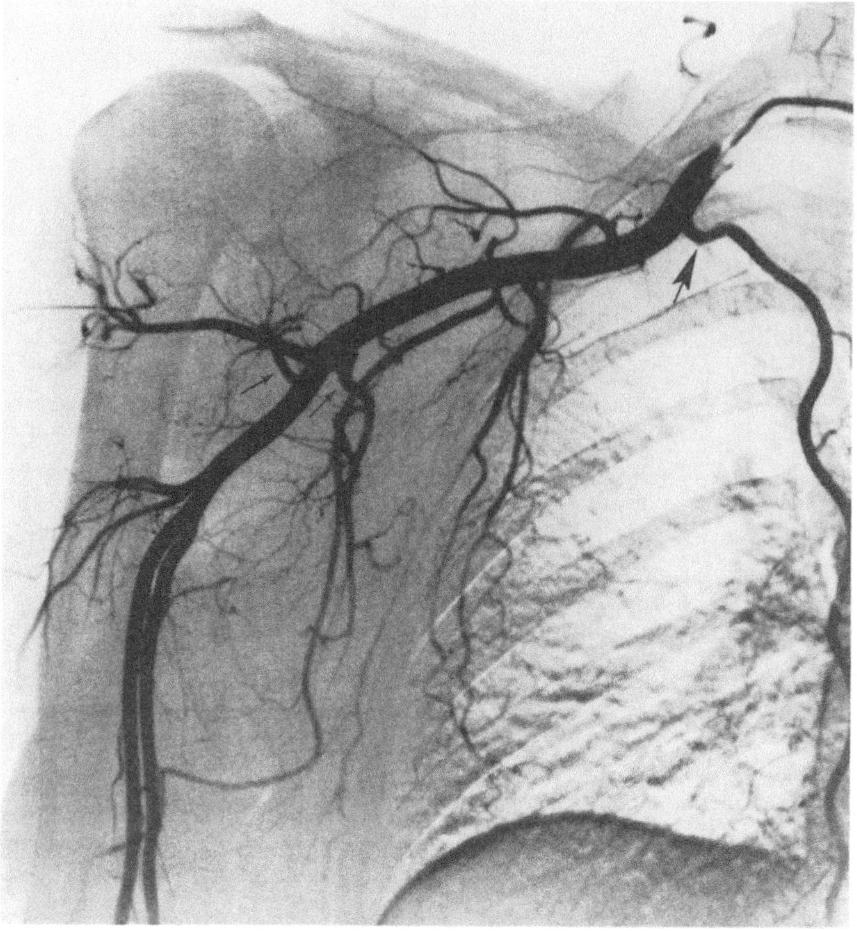

Fig. 45
Right subclavian arteriogram shows high bifurcation of the brachial artery, about 1 cm distal to the origin of the deep brachial artery.
Note the unusual origin of the internal mammary artery (large arrow); in this case it arises from the second section of the subclavian artery. The subscapular artery does not exist. The scapular circumflex and thoracodorsal arteries arise directly from the axillary artery (small arrows).

the branches of the posterior humeral circumflex artery and the branches of the deep brachial artery.

c. Variations

The anterior and posterior humeral circumflex arteries may originate from a common arterial trunk, which usually is short but may also be a few centimeters long (Fig. 38). This common arterial trunk of the humeral circumflex arteries was seen in our angiographic material more frequently than the separate origin of these two vessels. The common arterial trunk was observed on 175 arteriograms (70%). On the other hand, a separate origin of the humeral circumflex arteries was observed on only 6 arteriograms (2.4%). The humeral circumflex artery may originate in common with the deep brachial artery. This variation was found 30 times or in 12 percent of the cases. The common trunk of the humeral circumflex and deep brachial arteries is usually a short vessel, which originates from the proximal brachial artery (Fig. 42). On rare occasions it may arise from the axillary artery and be quite long (Fig. 44).

A common origin of this artery with the subscapular artery is sometimes present and was found on 24 arteriograms (9.6%) (Fig. 40). In 10 cases (4.0%) the humeral circumflex artery arose from a larger common trunk together with the subscapular, thoracoacromial and deep brachial arteries (Fig. 39). On very rare occasions both humeral circumflex arteries may be represented by

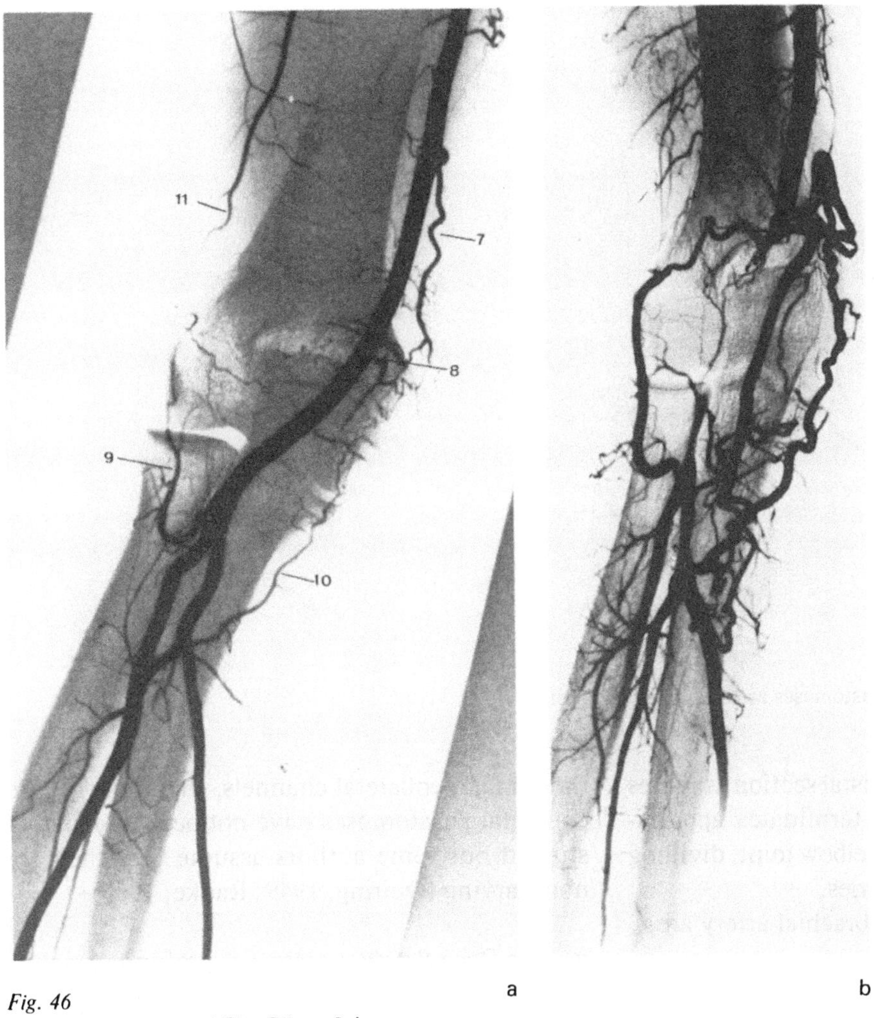

Fig. 46
Anastomoses Around The Elbow Joint.
A. Normal pattern.
7. Superior ulnar collateral (A. collateralis ulnaris superior)
8. Inferior ulnar collateral (A. collateralis ulnaris inferior)
9. Radial recurrent (A. recurrens radialis)
10. Ulnar recurrent (A. recurrens ulnaris)
11. Anterior branch of deep brachial artery.
B. Large elbow collaterals due to occlusion of the distal brachial artery.

three or four very small branches. This variation was observed in 5 cases (2.0%). On extremely rare occasions the axillary artery may divide into the radial and ulnar arteries; in such cases there is no brachial artery. A more common variation is a short brachial artery with a high bifurcation (Fig. 45). This high bifurcation of the brachial artery and similar variations of the axillary artery are of importance when angiography is attempted by means of direct brachial or axillary puncture or by transfemoral catheterization of the brachial artery, as described and illustrated in 3.5.1.

6.3.13 The Brachial Artery
(A. brachialis) (Figs.38 and 46A)

At the lower border of the teres major muscle, which lies at the level of the anatomical neck of humerus, the axillary artery continues distalwards as the brachial artery. Since the course of this vessel along the medial aspect of the arm is quite superficial, it is easily palpated throughout its length or compressed against the humerus over the proximal section, as shown and illustrated in 9.9.

The proximal section of the brachial artery lies

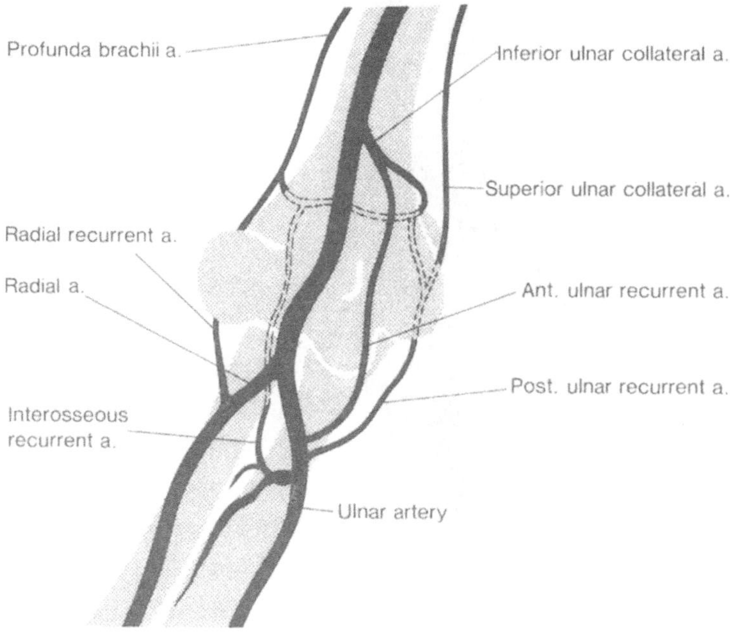

Fig. 47
Schematic representation of the anastomoses around the elbow joint.

medial to the humerus; the distal section assumes a more anterior position. It terminates approximately 2 to 3 cm distal to the elbow joint, dividing into the radial and ulnar arteries.

The chief branches of the brachial artery are:
1. The deep brachial artery
2. Superior ulnar collateral
3. Inferior ulnar collateral
4. Several small, muscular and nutrient, unnamed branches, arising usually from the lateral side of the artery.

6.3.14 Anastomoses around the Elbow Joint (Figs. 46 and 47)

When the brachial artery is occluded at the elbow, two anterior and two posterior collateral pathways are available to maintain distal flow (Fig. 47). The two anastomoses located posterior to the elbow joint are the superior ulnar collateral artery, which joins with the posterior ulnar recurrent artery, and the middle branch of the deep brachial artery, which joins with the interosseous recurrent artery. The anterior anastomoses are formed by the inferior ulnar collateral artery with the anterior ulnar recurrent artery and the lateral branch of the deep brachial artery with the radial recurrent artery. Several small anastomoses may also interconnect these major collateral channels. Variants of these collateral anastomoses have not been adequately studied but some authors assume that they are non-varying (Quiring, 1949; Radke, 1969).

a. The Deep Brachial Artery (A. profunda brachii; syn: superior profunda artery) (Fig. 38)
This is the most proximal and largest branch of the brachial artery. In addition to several muscular branches, it also gives off the middle and radial collateral arteries.

The middle collateral branch descends behind the humerus to the elbow and anastomoses on the dorsal side of the humerus with the interosseous recurrent artery and the inferior ulnar collateral artery. The radial collateral branch runs ventral to the humerus as a continuation of the deep brachial artery. Ventral to the lateral epicondyle of the humerus it anastomoses with the radial recurrent artery (Fig. 47).

b. The Superior Ulnar Collateral Artery (A. collateralis ulnaris superior) (Figs. 46A and 47)
This is a small-sized vessel which arises from the brachial artery, usually a little below the middle of the humerus, but it may also originate from the upper part of the deep brachial artery. Behind the medial epicondyle of the humerus it anasto-

moses with the posterior ulnar recurrent artery (Fig.47).

c. *The Inferior Ulnar Collateral Artery* (A. collateralis ulnaris inferior; syn: supratrochlear artery) (Fig. 47).

This artery usually originates about 5 cm above the elbow joint. It runs medialwards and divides almost immediately into two branches which anastomose with the anterior ulnar recurrent artery in front of the medial epicondyle and with the superior ulnar collateral behind the medial epicondyle of the humerus.

The anastomoses around the elbow joint are significant collateral pathways to the forearm in cases of complete occlusion of the brachial artery at the level of the elbow (Fig. 46B).

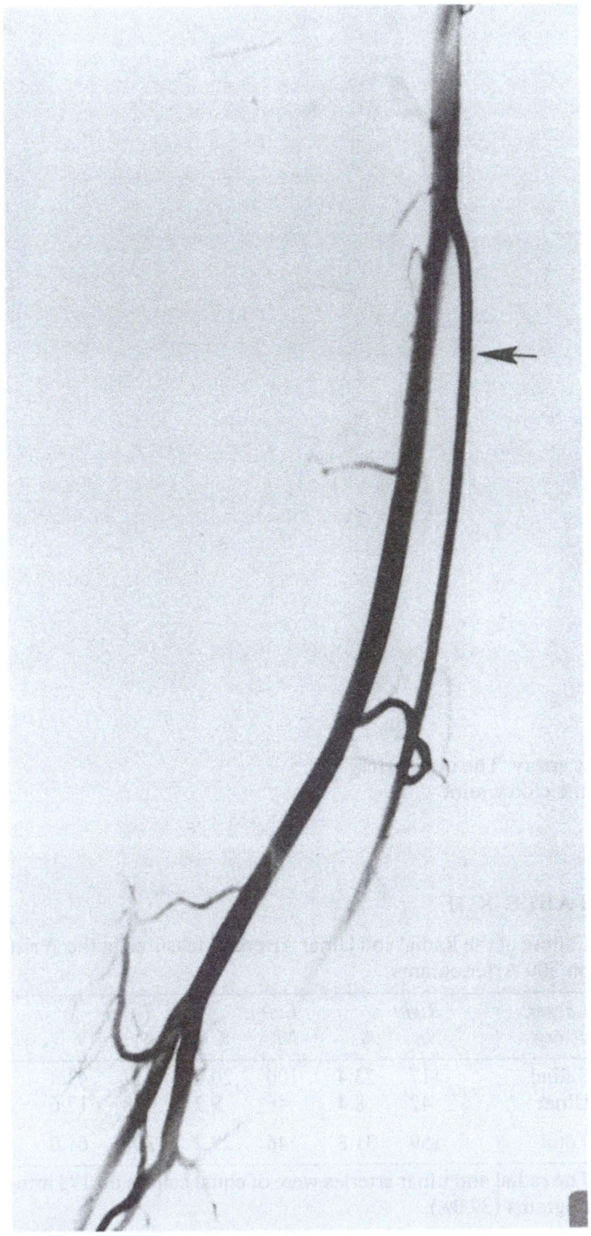

Fig. 48
Superficial Brachial Artery (arrow).

d. *Variations*

A common variation is the *superficial brachial artery* (Fig. 48) which arises below the origin of the deep brachial artery. It follows a typical course along the medial aspect of the arm and usually rejoins the brachial artery at its distal end (Fig. 55A). It may continue into the forearm to form the radial artery (Fig. 23); occasionally it remains as a separate vessel, the so-called superficial antebrachial artery. This artery was seen on six arteriograms (2.4%).

Frequently the division of the brachial artery occurs at a higher level; in such cases the radial artery usually branches off first. The other trunk of the bifurcation consists of the ulnar and interosseous arteries and this usually divides below the elbow joint. The radial artery can arise from the axillary artery (Fig. 49) or from the upper or lower part of the brachial artery (Figs. 50 and 51; see Table XI). Occasionally the ulnar artery will branch off at a higher level; in extremely rare cases the common interosseous artery will arise higher up.

Since the level of bifurcation of the brachial artery is important in selective catheterization of the brachial artery or when arteriography is carried out via direct puncture of the brachial or axillary artery, as discussed and illustrated in 3.5.1, an analysis of our series of 250 normal brachial arteriograms was carried out. The results of this study are presented in Table XII. The most frequent variation was found to be a bifurcation of the brachial artery in the middle of its course (see Table XII).

TABLE XI

Incidence of Axillary Origin of the Radial Artery on 250 Arteriograms.

	Number	*Percent*
Right	6	2.4
Left	7	2.8
Total	13	5.2

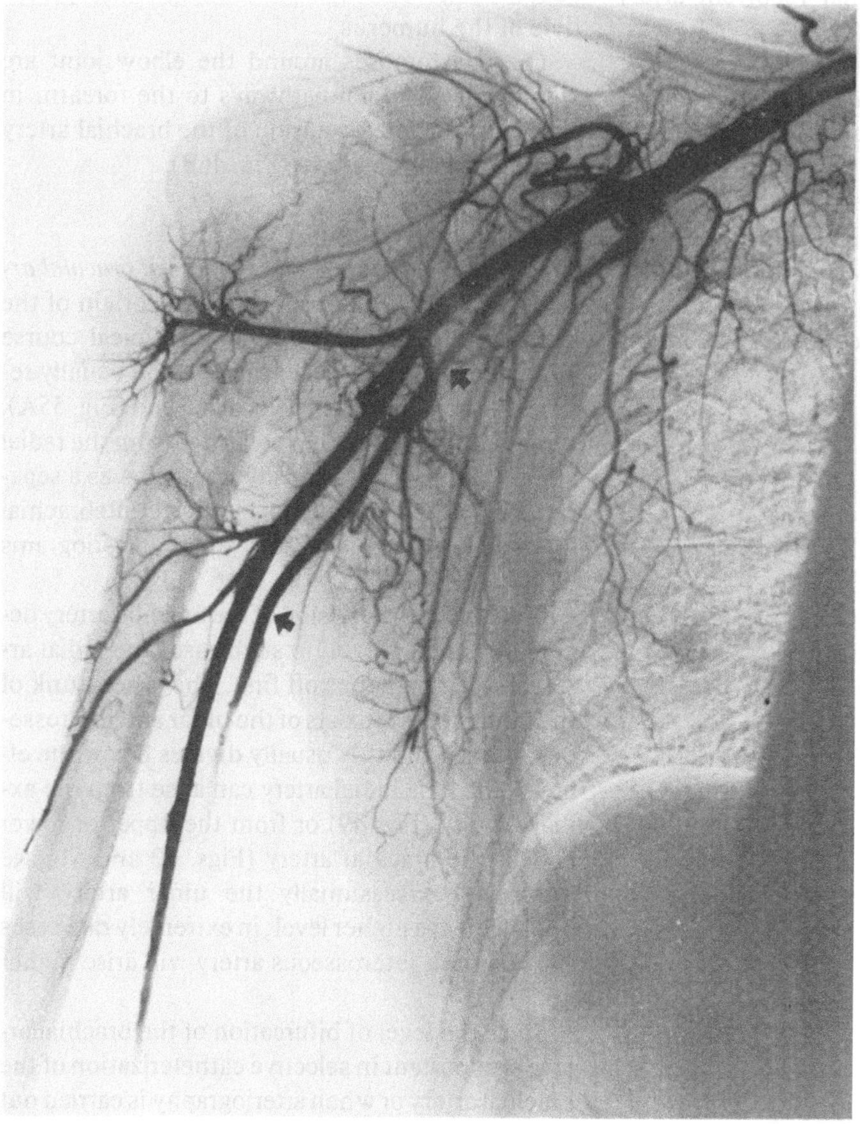

Fig. 49
The radial artery (arrows) arises from the second part of the axillary artery. The ulnar artery in this particular case gives rise to the interosseous artery below the elbow joint.

TABLE XII

Incidence of High Bifurcation of the Brachial Artery on 250 Arteriograms.

	Right Nr.	%	*Left* Nr.	%	*Total* Nr.	%
Proximal third	9	3.6	10	4.0	19	7.6
Middle third	19	7.6	5	2.0	24	9.6
Distal third	3	1.2	2	0.8	5	2.0
Total	31	12.4	17	6.8	48	19.2

TABLE XIII

Calibre of the Radial and Ulnar Arteries Measured at the Wrist on 500 Arteriograms.

Larger artery	*Right* Nr.	%	*Left* Nr.	%	*Total* Nr.	%
Radial	117	23.4	100	20.0	217	43.4
Ulnar	42	8.4	46	9.2	88	17.6
Total	159	31.8	146	29.2	305	61.0

The radial and ulnar arteries were of equal calibre on 195 arteriograms (39.0%).

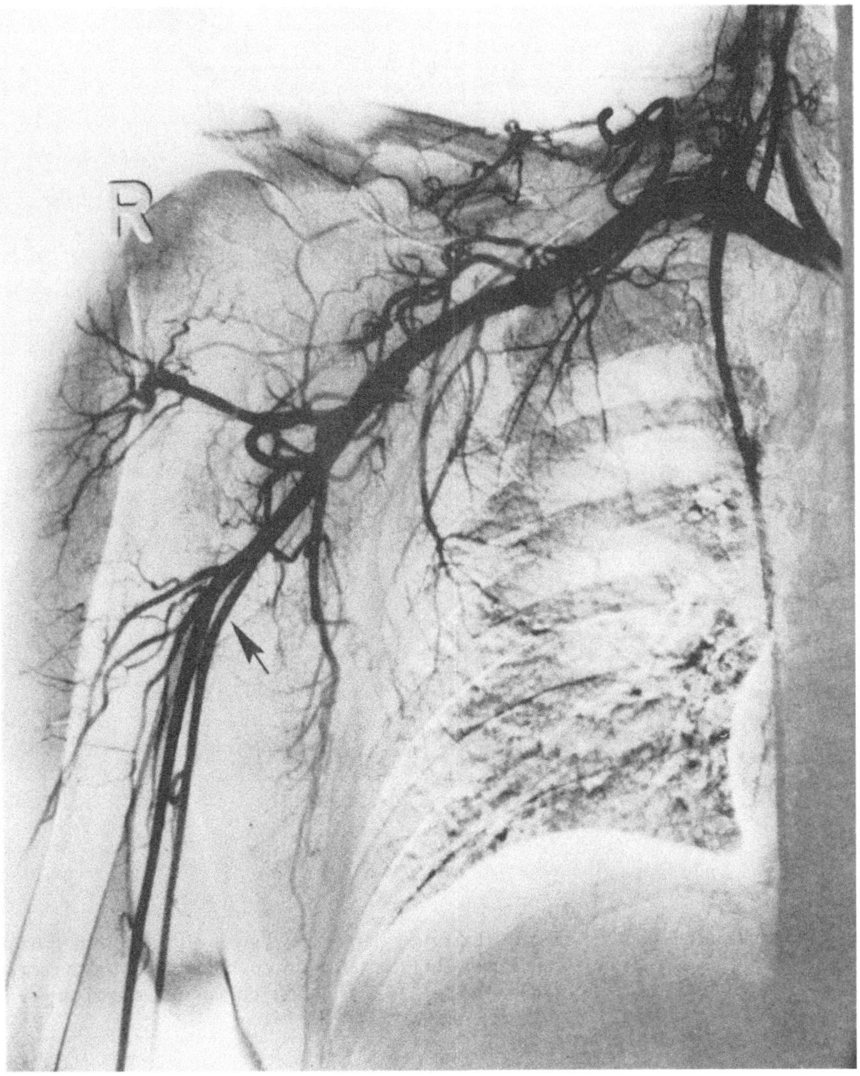

Fig. 50
Right subclavian arteriogram shows a high origin of the radial artery (arrow). It arises from the brachial artery proximal to the origin of the deep brachial artery.

Altogether high bifurcation of the brachial artery occurred in 19.2 percent of the cases (Table XII). Manifestation in the right arm is more frequent (12.4%).

6.4 The Arteries of the Forearm

The brachial artery divides into the radial and ulnar arteries 2-3 centimeters below the elbow joint. Further distalwards the ulnar artery gives off the interosseous artery.

6.4.1 The Radial Artery (A. radialis)

This artery follows the same course as the brachial artery and appears as its continuation. It passes along the radial side of the forearm to the wrist where it winds backwards, ventral to the lateral side of the carpus, and turns medialwards into the palm to take part in the formation of the deep volar arch. The calibre of the radial artery is, according to anatomical literature, smaller than that of the ulnar artery. On our arteriograms this was the rule only when a median artery was present. Our measurements at the level of the wrist show that in the

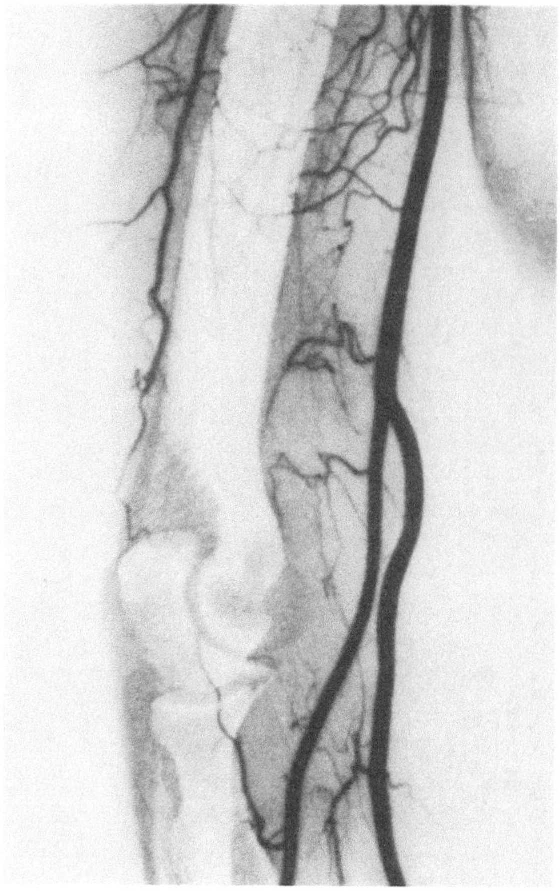

Fig. 51
The right brachial artery divides just proximal to the elbow joint into the radial and ulnar arteries.

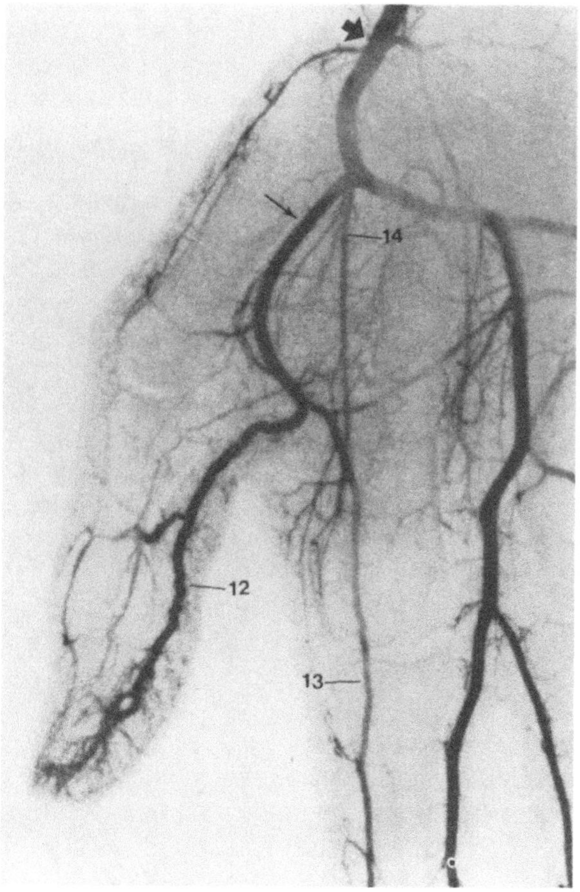

Fig. 52
Distal radial artery (large arrow) gives off the common trunk (small arrow) of the arteria princeps pollicis (12) and the arteria radialis indicis (13). The first dorsal metacarpal artery is numbered 14.

majority of cases the radial artery was the larger of the two (43.4%) (see Table XIII). The ulnar artery was larger in only 17.6 percent of the cases. In 39 percent of the cases the two arteries were of the same calibre (Table XIII).

The important branches in the hand are: (Figs. 52 and 61)

1. princeps pollicis
2. radialis indicis
3. first dorsal metacarpal
4. volar metacarpal arteries.

a. Variations

The variations in the origin and the calibre of this artery have already been discussed.

A total aplasia of the radial artery was encountered only once in our case material. It was observed on a left arm arteriogram of a female patient. In this particular case almost the entire palm and all fingers were supplied by the ulnar artery. The deep volar arch was formed by the deep branch of the ulnar artery and the termination of the volar interosseous artery (Fig. 54).

A large median artery may replace the radial artery in the formation of the superficial volar arch as described and illustrated in 6.8.1 (complete superficial arch, type V).

6.4.2 The Ulnar Artery (A. ulnaris)

The proximal portion of the ulnar artery is usually the larger of the two terminal branches of the brachial artery. It runs obliquely downwards and medialwards, crosses the ulna and reaches the medial

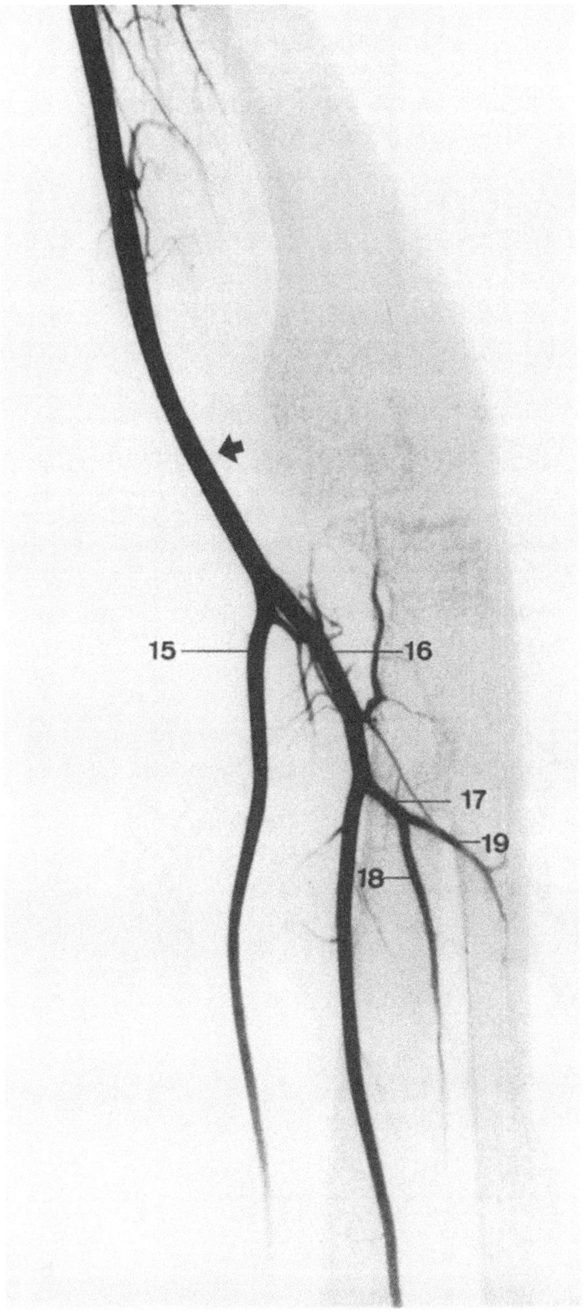

Fig. 53
The branches of the brachial artery (arrow) to the forearm:
15. The radial artery (A. radialis)
16. The ulnar artery (A. ulnaris)
17. The common interosseous artery (A. interossea communis)
18. The anterior interosseous artery (A. interossea volaris)
19. The posterior interosseous artery (A. interossea dorsalis).

side of the forearm at a point about midway between the elbow and the wrist. Lateral to the pisiform bone it divides into two branches: the deep branch which participates in the formation of the deep volar arch, and the superficial branch which continues across the palm as the superficial palmar arch.

a. Branches
In the forearm the most important branch is the common interosseous artery. Distal to the branching off of this artery, the ulnar artery may be smaller in calibre than the radial artery (Table XIII, Fig. 53).

b. Variations
The ulnar artery may originate high up in the upper arm, as described in 6.3.14d, but it may also arise about 5 to 7 cm below the elbow joint. This variation was observed several times on our arteriograms. On one of our arteriograms the ulnar artery was completely absent (aplastic) (Fig. 55). The territory of the ulnar artery in this particular case was supplied by hypertrophic branches of the anterior and posterior interosseous arteries.

The ulnar artery may give off the median artery, which normally arises from the common interosseous artery.

6.4.3 The Common Interosseous Artery
(A. interossea communis)

This is the largest branch of the ulnar artery. As measured on our arteriograms, it is about 1 cm long; it then divides into two branches: the anterior interosseous artery and the posterior interosseous artery.

a. Variations
Some anomalies of the terminal branches of the anterior interosseous artery may be found. In one type, reinforcing vessels are given off from the terminal part of the anterior interosseous artery. According to Manners-Smith (1910) this variation resembles the normal arrangement in gibbons, in whom the radial artery is highly attenuated at the wrist and the anterior interosseous artery either ends in a crossbranch connecting the ulnar with the radial artery or gives off a branch which joins with one of the two.

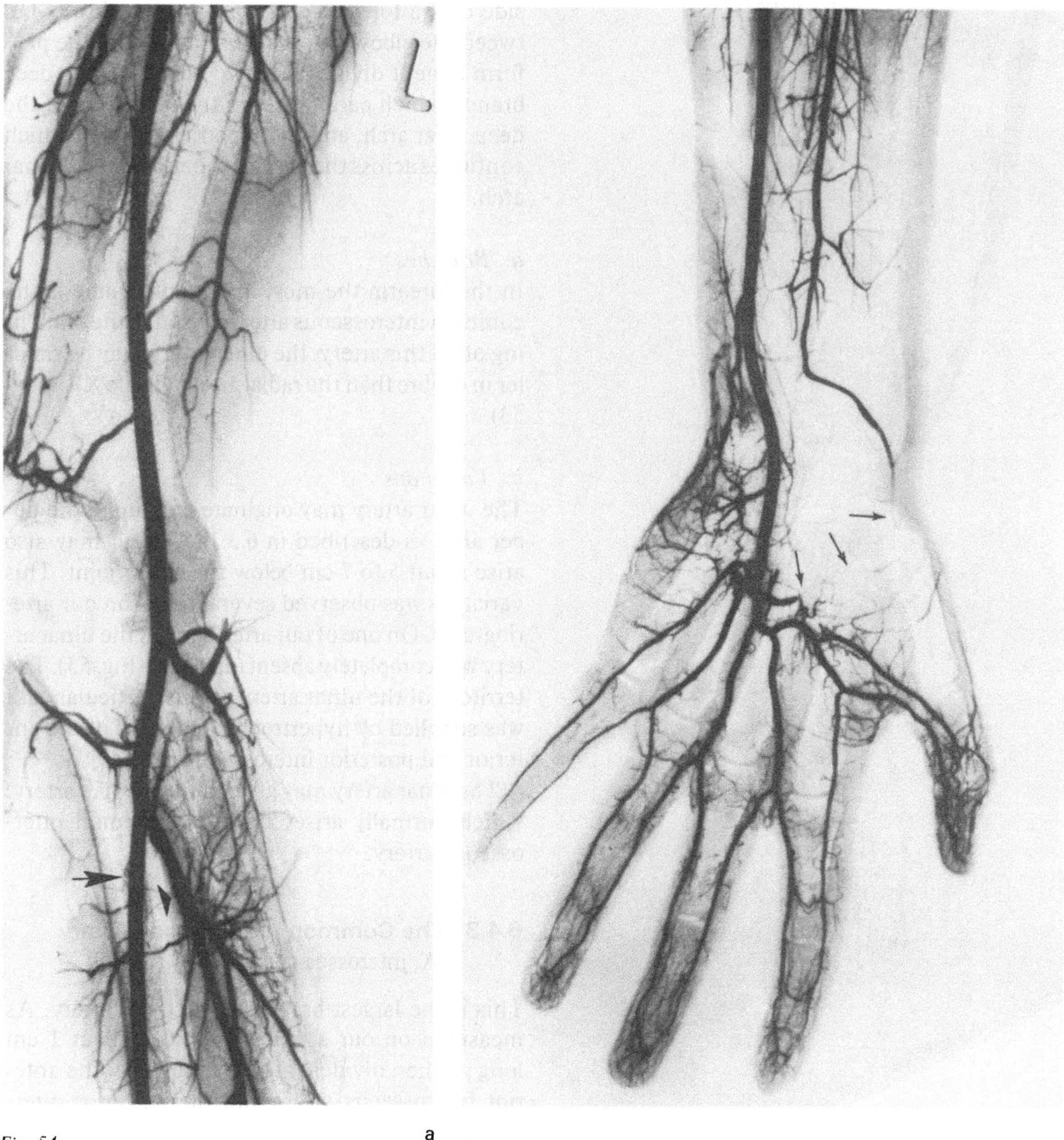

Fig. 54
Arteriograms of the left arm of a patient with total aplasia of the radial artery.
A. There is a division of the brachial artery into the ulnar artery (large arrow) and common interosseous artery (arrow head).
B. A large ulnar artery supplies the entire hand. The radial artery is absent (aplastic). The termination of the anterior interosseous artery runs through the palm and joins the deep volar arch (arrows).

We found the same arrangement on the arteriograms of the right arm of two female patients. In the first case the anterior interosseous artery connects a medium-sized radial artery with a short transverse branch at the wrist (Fig. 56; arrow). In the second case it terminates as a transverse branch joining the radial artery at the wrist (Fig. 57). In this particular case the radial artery arose higher up along the brachial artery. We also observed that one of the branches of the anterior interosseous artery may cross the carpal bones and either terminate in the hypothenar (Fig. 58) or join one of the palmar arches (Fig. 54).

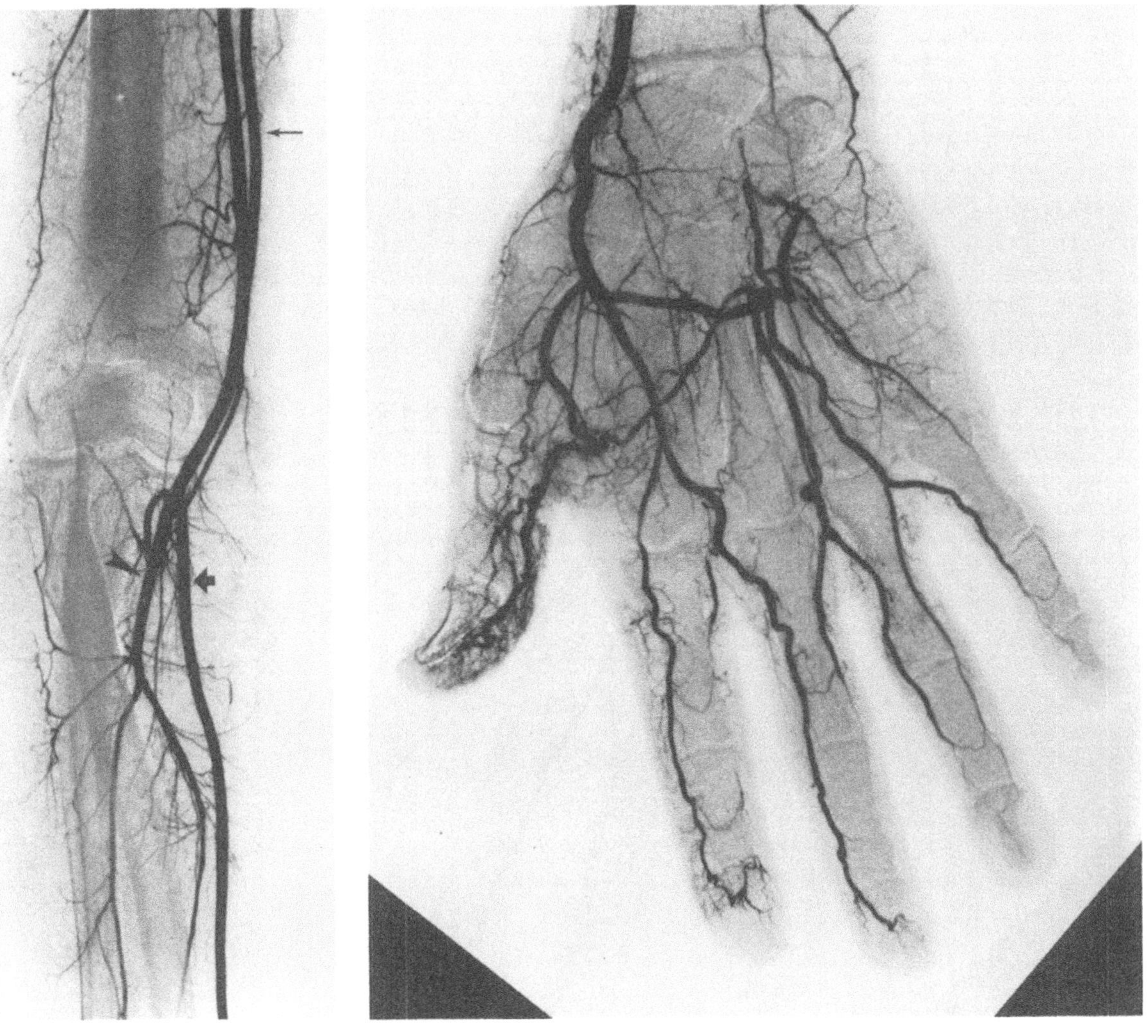

a b

Fig. 55
Absent (aplastic) Ulnar Artery.
A. Duplication of the distal brachial artery due to presence of a superficial brachial artery (arrow), which rejoins the brachial artery above the elbow joint. Just distal to the elbow the brachial artery divides into the radial artery (large arrow) and common interosseous artery (arrow head).
B. Hand arteriogram of the same patient.

6.4.4 Persistent Median Artery

A median artery was found in our angiographic material in 2.2 percent of the cases. It is usually a slender vessel that arises from the proximal part of the anterior interosseous artery. We have observed in our material that the median artery may originate from the common interosseous artery and that it can be large (Fig. 59). Sometimes it may contribute to the formation of the complete superficial volar arch, as described and illustrated in 6.8.1a.

6.5 The Arteries of the Hand

6.5.1 Introduction

The degree of peripheral ischaemia is not only determined by the state of the afferent arteries but also by the anatomical characteristics of the palmar arches.

It might be assumed that incomplete palmar arches play a certain role in ischaemic disease and may even contribute to digital ischaemia.

It is well known that injury of the ulnar artery or superficial palmar arch may compromise the arte-

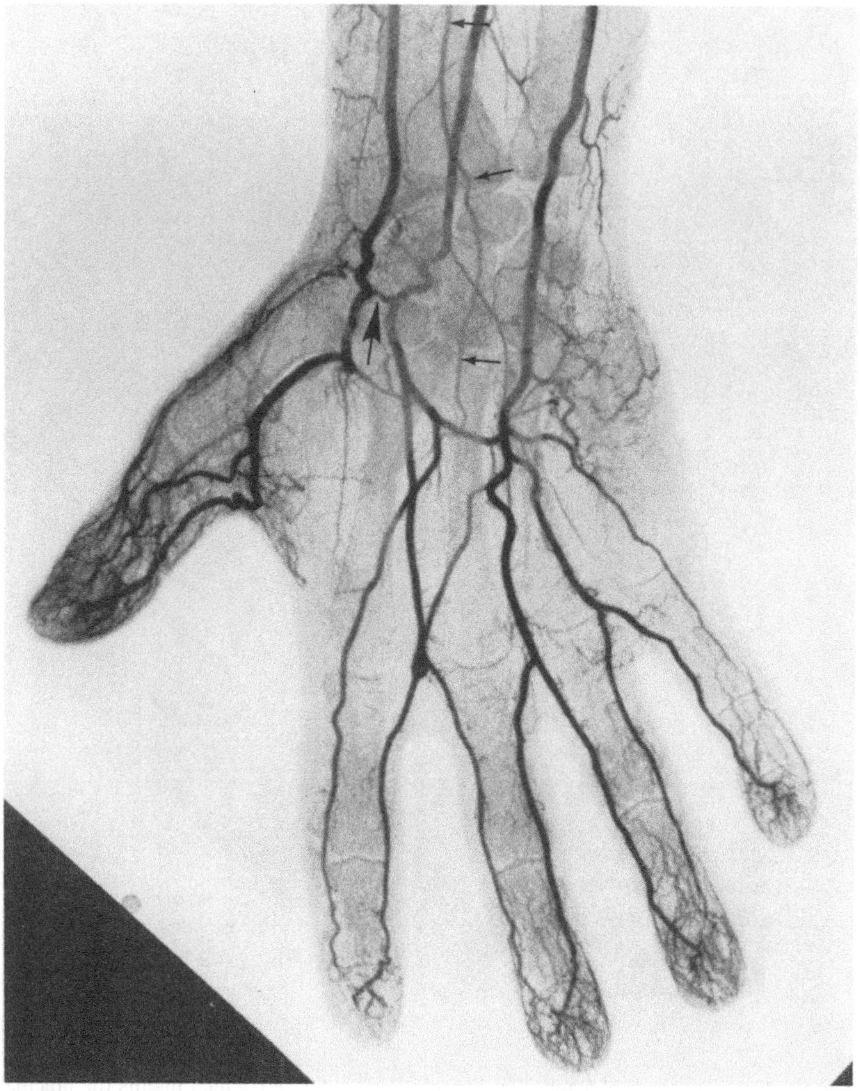

Fig. 56
The anterior interosseous artery reinforces a medium-sized radial artery with a short transverse branch at the level of the wrist (arrow); moreover it takes part in the formation of the superficial volar arch. In addition a slender median artery persists (small arrows) which terminates in the thenar of the palm.

rial supply to the fingers if there is a poor anastomosis between the superficial and deep volar arches.

On the other hand an optimal anatomical arrangement with two complete palmar arches provides a reserve in blood supply in case of occlusion of one of the arches or one of the major afferent arteries to the hand, as shown in Figure 60.

For this reason a thorough knowledge of the anatomy of these vessels is required to understand and interpret an arteriogram.

Many arteries do not conform to a single anatomical pattern and for this reason the interpretation of arteriograms of the hand can be difficult. Complicated anatomical texts and sketches may be confusing; therefore for the understanding of angiographic findings a schematic drawing of the arteries and their common variations in relation to the osseous structures may be very helpful.

The arteries of the hand show considerable variations in their distribution, which are described in anatomical literature. Very limited material has been published so far concerning the angiographic anatomy of these vessels. The majority of radiological publications deal with the use of angiography for the detection of pathology. An extensive

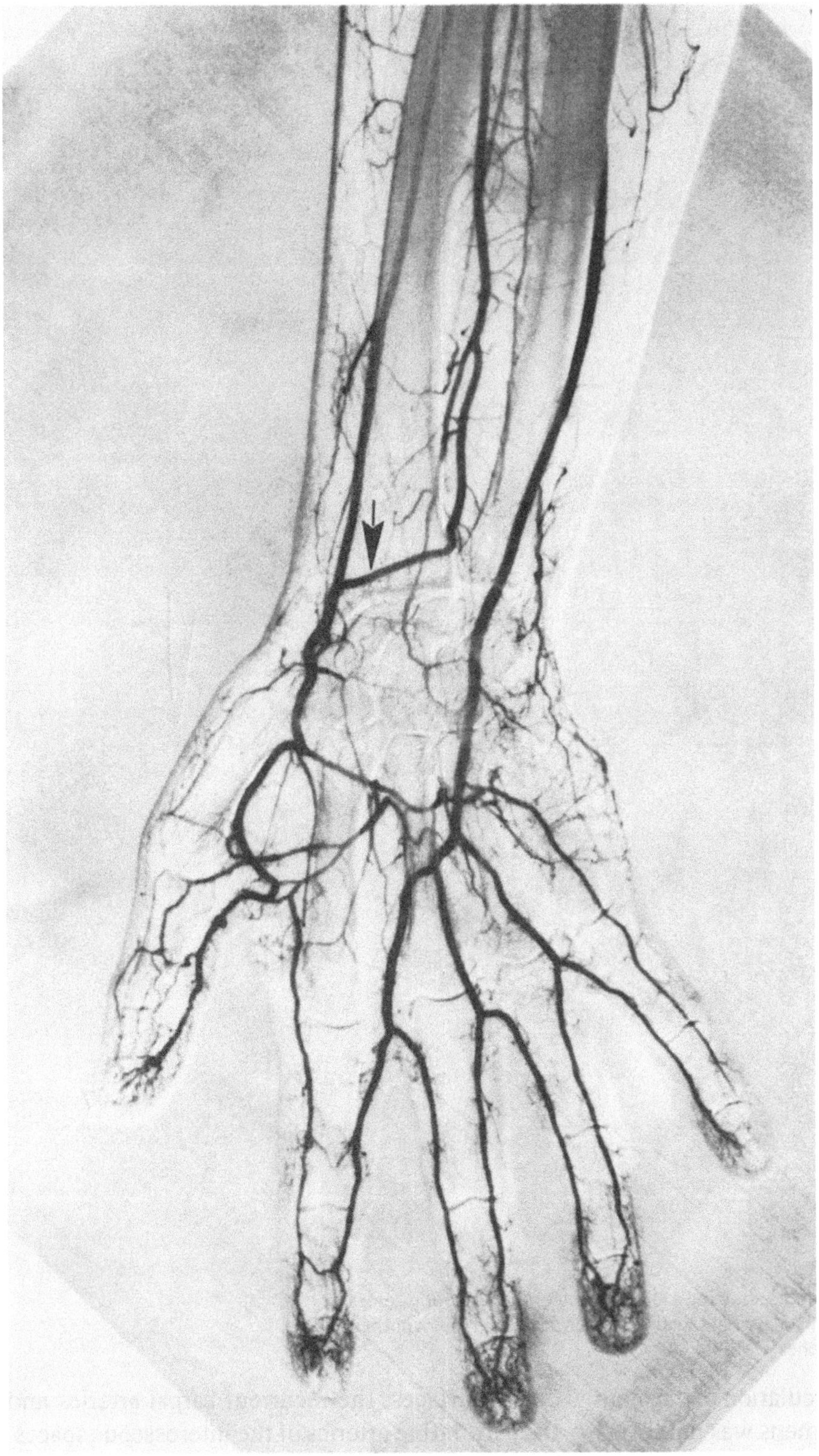

Fig. 57
A large anterior interosseous artery terminates as a transverse branch (arrow). It reinforces the radial artery by joining it at the wrist.

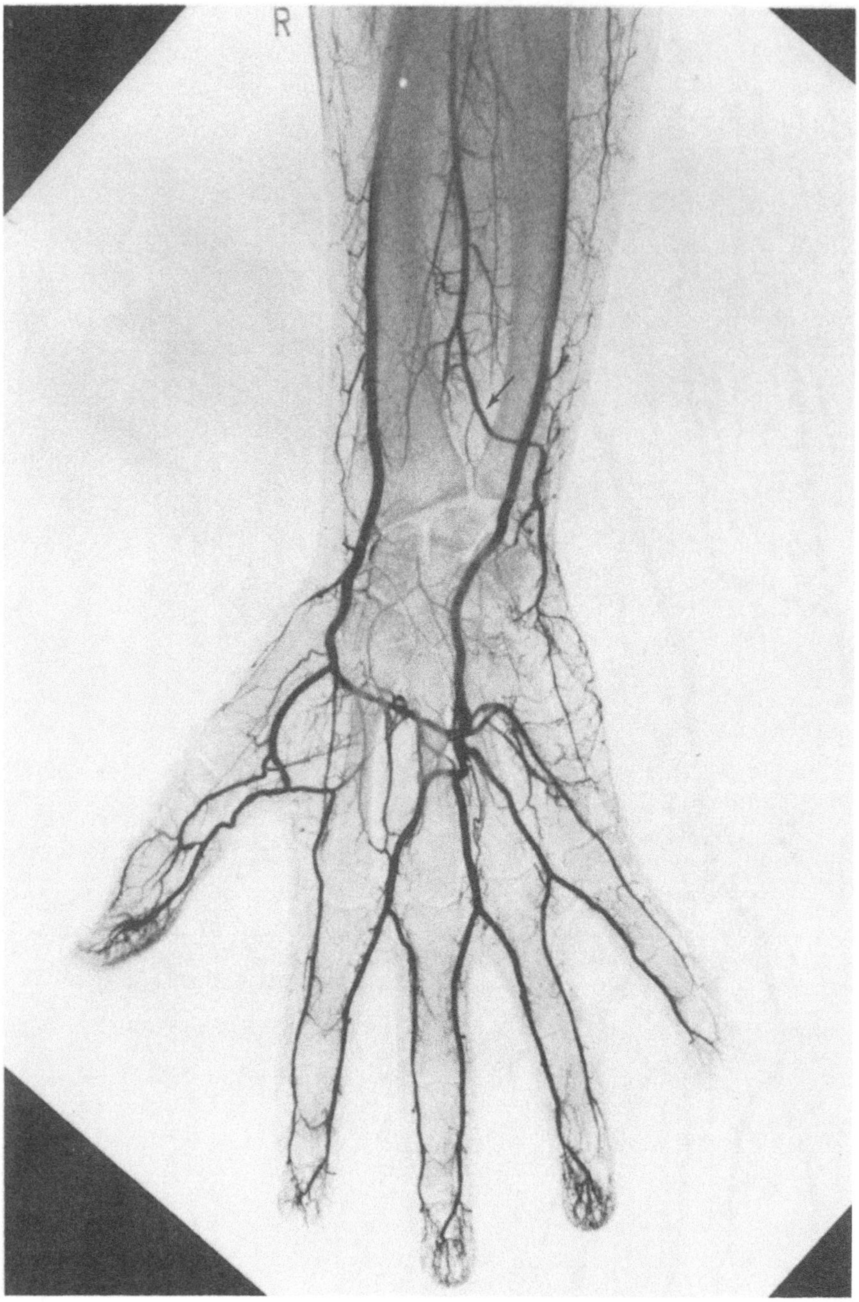

Fig. 58
Arteriogram of the right forearm and hand showing a large branch of the anterior interosseous artery (arrow) which crosses the distal part of the ulna and terminates in the hypothenar by dividing into multiple small branches.

study of the anatomy of the circulation of the hand based on analysis of 650 specimens was published by Coleman and Anson in 1961. They separated the different patterns of the vascular distribution into a few well-defined categories. Since their study included a large number of dissections they were able to carry out a complete analysis of all arteries of the hand, e.g. the arteries of the volar and dorsal surfaces, the recurrent carpal arteries and the perforating arteries of the interosseous spaces. This excellent anatomical study could never be surpassed by an angiographic investigation. In the following radiological analysis the main emphasis will be on the large arteries of the hand which are important for the interpretation of an arteriogram. The superficial and the deep volar arches with

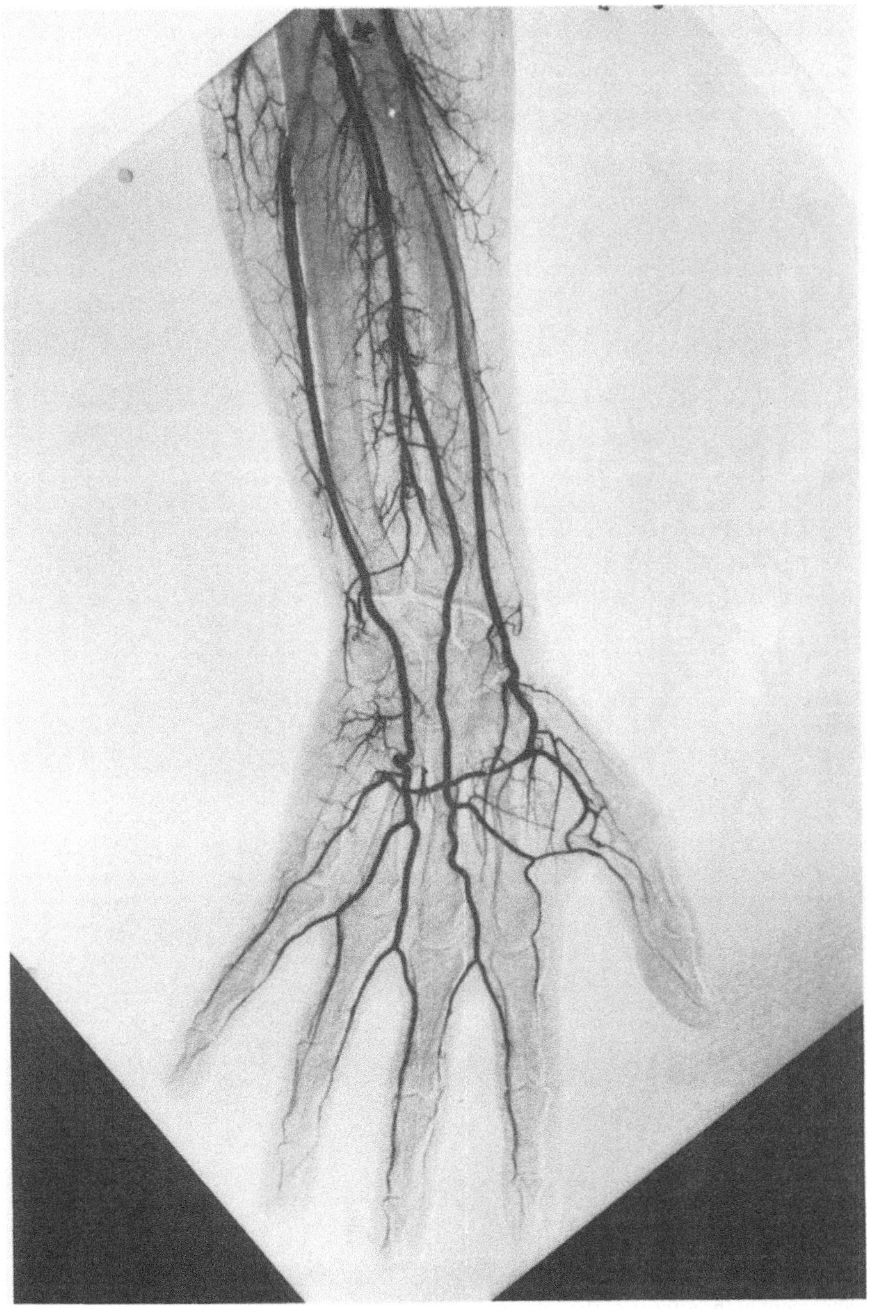

Fig. 59
Large median artery which arises from the common interosseous artery (arrow).

their major branches will be evaluated with regard to their variations and the frequency with which they occur. Since the digital arteries usually follow a standard pattern, they will be considered only briefly here.

The study is based on a series of 500 arteriograms of the hand. In the conclusion the results will be compared with those of other authors.

6.6 Arterial Patterns in the Hand: Based upon a Study of 500 Arteriograms

6.6.1 Materials and Methods

The material for the present study was obtained from 730 angiograms of the hand, obtained in our

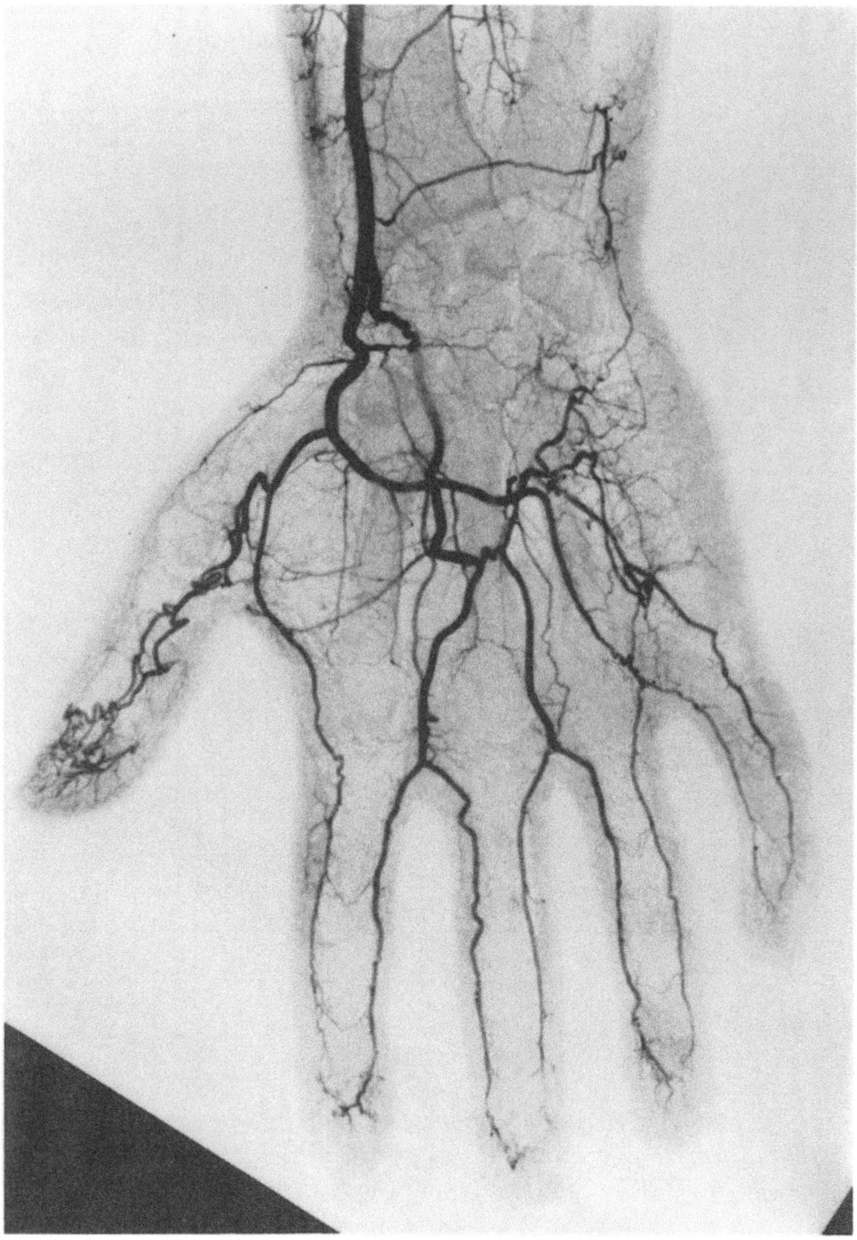

Fig. 60
Thanks to the optimal anatomical arrangement of the arteries of the palm and two complete volar arches, this patient had no symptoms of digital ischaemia despite total occlusion of the ulnar artery. This case demonstrates the importance of the completeness of the superficial and deep volar arches and the anastomoses between them.

department between 1970 and 1980. The study includes arteriograms of patients of both sexes, varying in age between sixteen and seventy years old. More than 70 percent of the patients included in this study were under 50 years of age. In order to determine the branching pattern of the deep and superficial volar arches only arteriograms which visualized these vessels completely were evaluated. Arteriograms which showed spasticity of the arteries or incomplete opacification due to pathological occlusion were excluded from the study.

Hence, although 500 hand arteriograms were studied, in some of the categories the number of arteriograms used for statistical analysis will be smaller than the total. For the same reason both extremities are not represented equally.

The arteries of the hand were classified into two main categories as follows:
1. The deep volar arch and its branches.
2. The superficial volar arch and its branches.

The variations of the arches, based on the way in which the contributing arteries join, are divided into two groups, i.e. Group I: complete arches and Group II: incomplete arches. Similarly, on the basis of the different branching patterns of the arches, each group is subdivided into several types. All detected arterial patterns are described and schematically reproduced, and their frequency has been established. The deep and the superficial volar arches are illustrated separately, as shown in Figure 88.

6.7 The Deep Volar (Palmar) Arch
(Arcus volaris profundus)

The deep volar arch (Fig. 61) is formed primarily by the terminal part of the radial artery, which is also called the deep volar branch of the radial artery. At the level of the wrist this vessel curves over the radial side of the carpus, slightly beyond and lateral to the styloid process of the radius, and runs behind the trapezium and the base of the first metacarpal bone. Passing between the first and the second metacarpal bones the artery arrives ventral to the second and third metacarpal bones to anastomose with the deep palmar branch of the ulnar artery at the lateral margin of the fourth metacarpal bone.

The variations of this arch may be divided into two large groups, *i.e.* Group I: complete arches and Group II: incomplete arches.

6.7.1 Group I: Complete Arch

A complete arch means a fusion of the deep volar branch of the radial artery with the deep palmar ramus of the ulnar artery to form an uninterrupted vessel at the base of the palm.

This arch is situated between the lateral border of the trapezium and the distal end of the hamate bone at the level of the base of the metacarpal bones. On radiographs it is always projected about 1 cm proximal to the superficial arch.

a. Different Types of Complete Deep Volar Arch
Group I, in which the deep volar arch is complete,

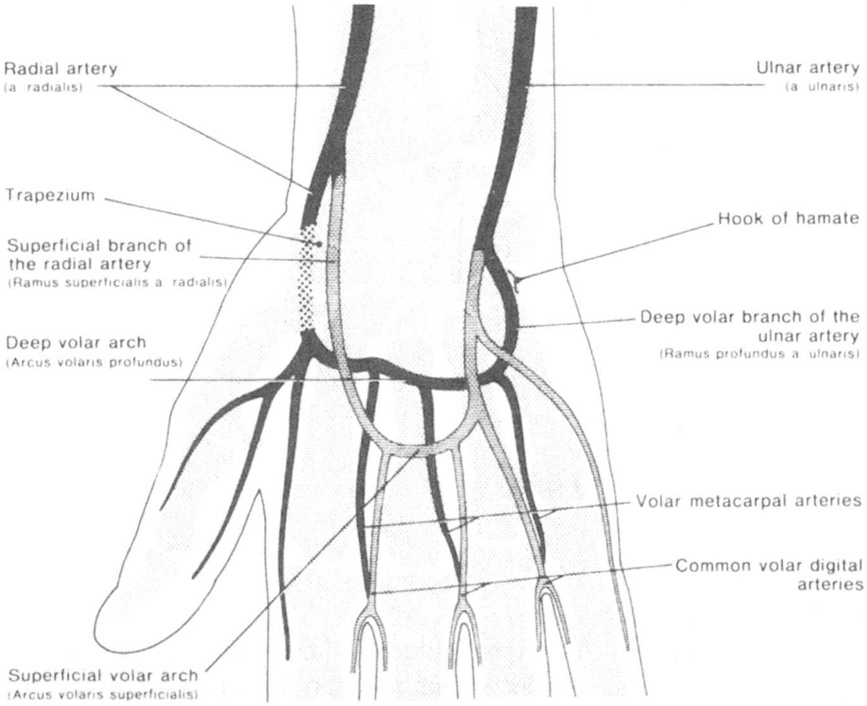

Fig. 61
Schematic representation of the superficial and the deep volar arches with their main branches on the volar side.

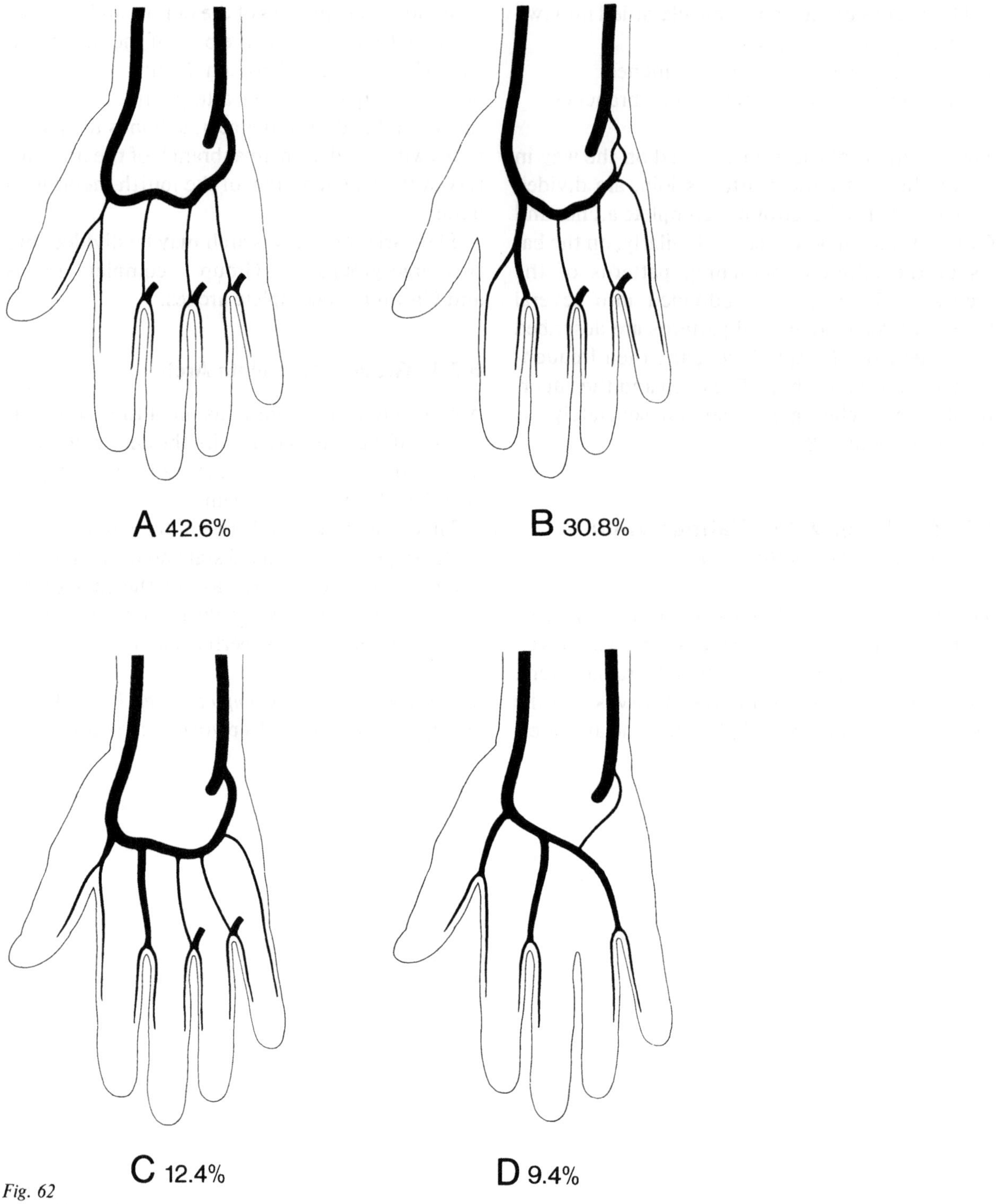

Fig. 62
Arcus Volaris Profundus.
Different types found on 500 arteriograms.

is by far the largest group. Of the 500 hands in this study, 476 or 95.2 percent possessed complete arches.

Within this group four main types can be distinguished (Fig. 62).

Type A:
This type includes all complete arches in which the deep volar branch of the radial artery anastomoses with the inferior or superior branch of the ulnar artery, or with both of them (Fig. 63). The main characteristic of these arches is that they give

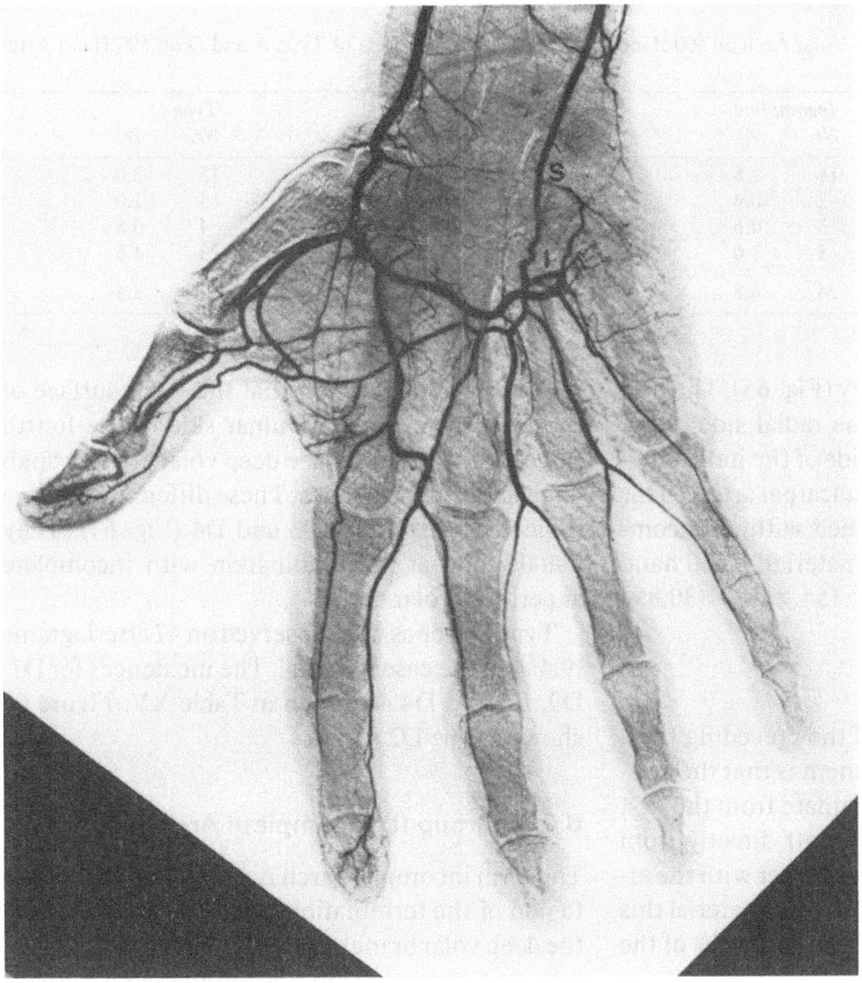

Fig. 63
Complete deep volar arch, in which the deep volar branch of the radial artery anastomoses with the superior and inferior deep volar branches of the ulnar artery indicated as S and I.

off branches from the convexity of the arch in an uniform manner. These branches are: the arteria princeps pollicis, the arteria radialis indicis which usually arises in common with the preceding vessel, and three volar metacarpal arteries which extend distalwards in the second, third and fourth interosseous spaces to terminate by anastomosing with the common digital arteries from the superficial arch.

Because the anastomosis of the deep volar branch of the radial artery on the ulnar side varies, a further subdivision of this arch into types A1, A2 and A3 is made.

When the deep volar branch of the radial artery anastomoses with the inferior branch of the ulnar artery, it is type A1; when it anastomoses with the superior branch it is type A2; and when the deep volar branch of the radial artery joins both branches of the ulnar artery, the arch is called A3 (Fig. 64). The incidence of type A arches in our series of 500 arteriograms was 213 or 42.6% (Table XIV). Type A1 was present in 32%, A2 in 8.6% and A3 in 2% (Table XV) of the cases.

Type B:

This type comprises those arches in which the deep volar branch of the radial artery anastomoses with small branches of the ulnar artery in the hypothenar to form a complete deep arch. The main characteristic of this type of arch is persistence of a large first metacarpal artery which supplies the index finger and radial side of the third finger. It is usually the only artery for this region. The arteria radialis indicis in this type of arch always arises

TABLE XIV

Incidence of Different Types of Deep Volar Arch on 500 Hand Arteriograms.

Types	*Complete* Nr.	*Complete* %	*Incomplete* Nr.	*Incomplete* %
A	213	42.6	14	2.8
B	154	30.8	2	0.4
C	62	12.4	3	0.6
D	47	9.4	5	1.0
Total	476	95.2	24	4.8

TABLE XV

Complete Deep Arches of Type A and D on 500 Hand Arteriograms.

Subtypes	*Type A* Nr.	*Type A* %	*Type D* Nr.	*Type D* %
1	160	32.0	15	3.0
2	43	8.6	5	1.0
3	10	2.0	4	0.8
4			23	4.6
Total	213	42.6	47	9.4

from the first metacarpal artery (Fig. 65). The proper volar digital arteries on the radial side of the third finger and on the ulnar side of the index finger are branches of the first metacarpal artery. This type of arch is usually combined with an incomplete superficial arch. In our material of 500 hand arteriograms it appeared in 154 cases (30.8%) (Table XIV).

Type C:
This arch is a modification of the preceding type. The only difference between them is that the arteria radialis indicis does not originate from the first metacarpal artery but branches off directly from the radial artery, separately or together with the arteria princeps pollicis (Fig. 66). In our material this type of arch was found in 62 hands or 12.4% of the cases (Table XIV).

Type D:
This arch is not a characteristic single type but comprises several rare types of complete volar arch which have in common that the volar surface of the fifth finger and the ulnar side of the fourth finger are supplied by the deep volar arch through large metacarpal arteries. These different types are indicated as D1, D2, D3 and D4 (Fig. 67). They usually appear in combination with incomplete superficial volar arches.

Type D arches were observed on 47 arteriograms (9.4%) of the case material. The incidences for D1, D2, D3 and D4 are given in Table XV. Figure 68 shows a type D2 arch.

6.7.2 Group II: Incomplete Arch

The term incomplete arch is used when there is no fusion of the termination of the radial artery with the deep volar branch of the ulnar artery. Both vessels end separately in the interosseous spaces. They usually anastomose with the perforating arteries, but these connections are not visible on the arteriograms.

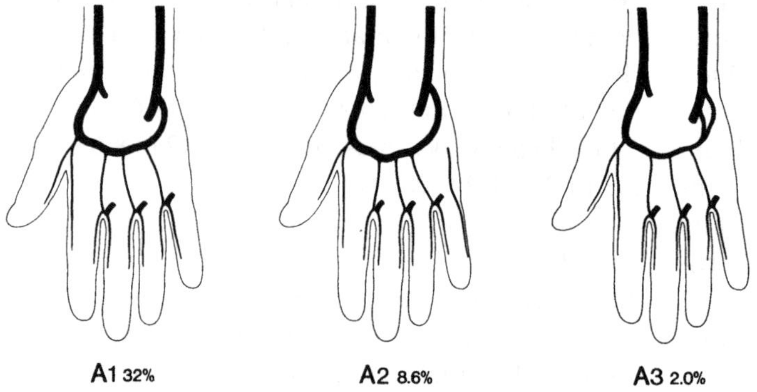

Fig. 64
Subtypes of Complete Deep Arch A.
A1. The deep volar branch of the radial artery joins the inferior volar ramus of the ulnar artery to form a complete deep volar arch.
A2. The deep volar arch is formed by the anastomosis between the deep volar branch of the radial artery and the superior deep volar ramus of the ulnar artery.
A3. The deep volar branch of the radial artery joins the superior and inferior deep volar branches of the ulnar artery.

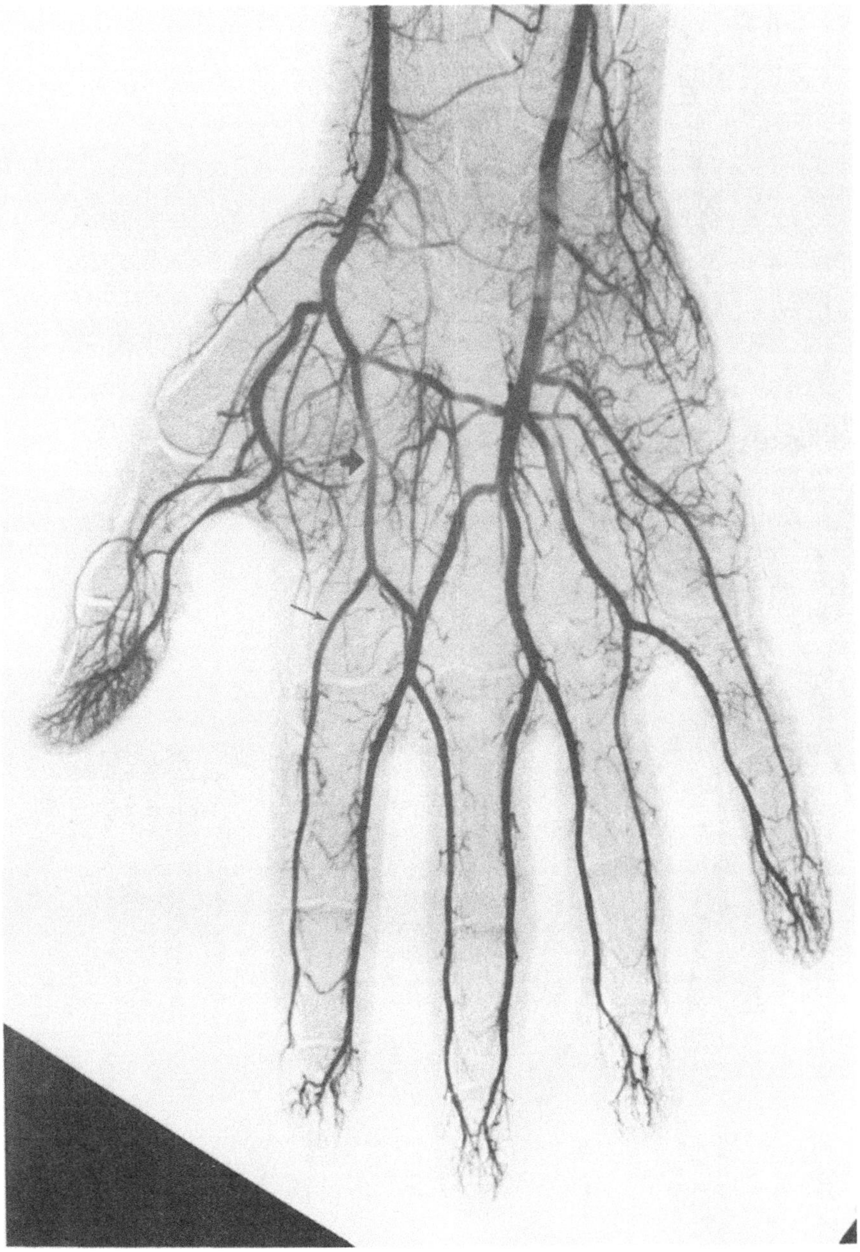

Fig. 65
Complete Deep Volar Arch of type B.
The arch has a large first metacarpal artery (large arrow) which gives off the arteria radialis indicis (small arrow). The deep volar branch of the radial artery anastomoses with small branches of the ulnar artery in the hypothenar.
Note a supplemental branch from the ulnar artery which joins the common trunk of the digital arteries of the second and third fingers.

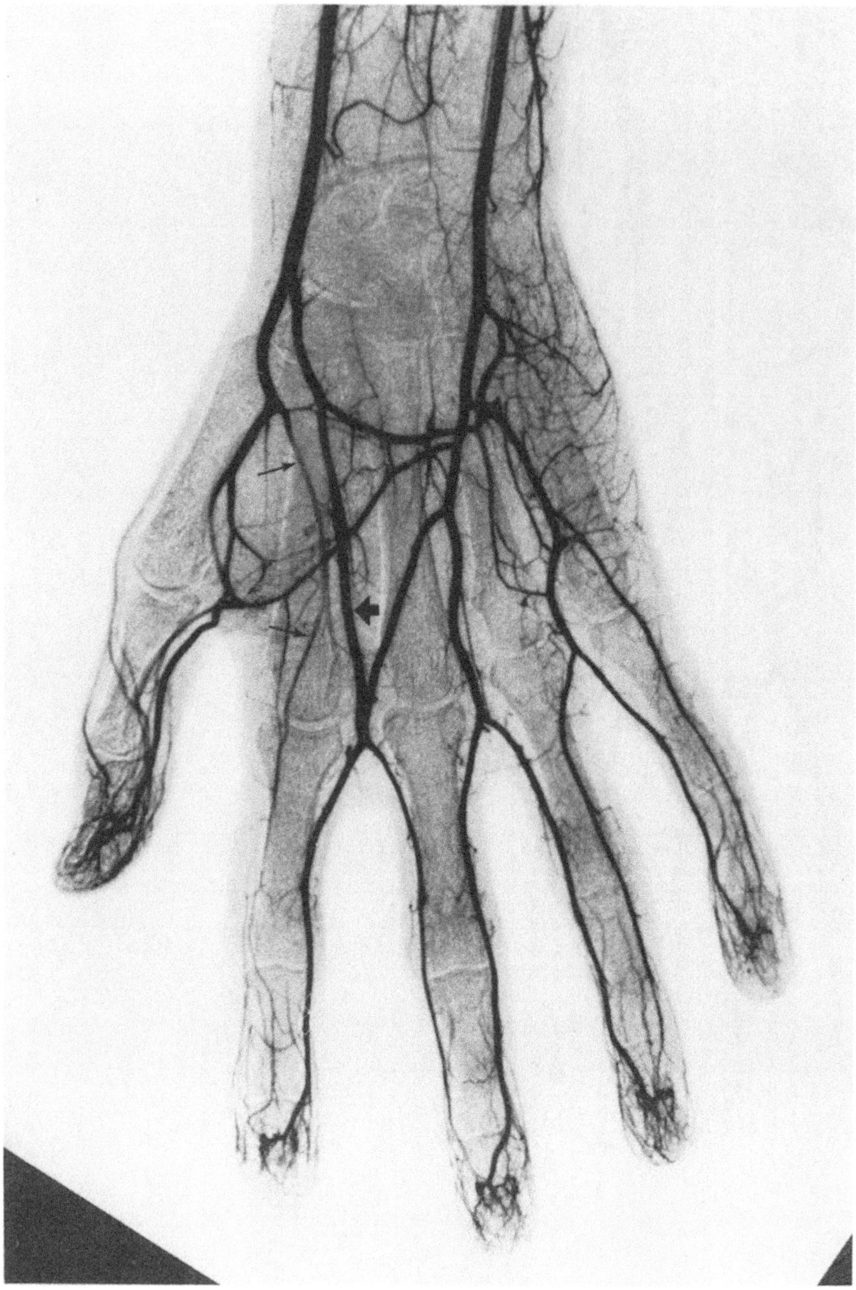

Fig. 66
Complete Deep Volar Arch of type C.
The deep arch possesses a large first metacarpal artery (large arrow). The arteria radialis indicis (small arrows) originates together with the arteria princeps pollicis from a common trunk of the radial artery.

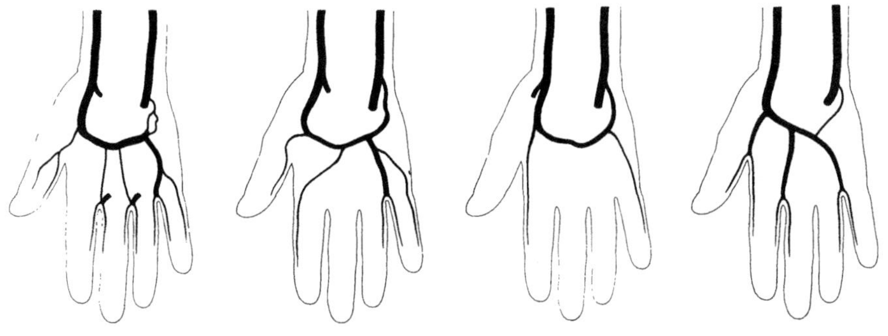

Fig. 67
Subtypes of Complete Deep Arch D.
D1. The volar surface of the fifth finger and the ulnar side of the fourth finger are totally supplied by the deep volar arch through a large metacarpal artery which gives off the proper digital arteries.
D2. The same as the preceding type. The only difference is that the arteria radialis indicis arises from the middle portion of the deep volar arch.
D3. The deep volar arch gives off the arteria radialis indicis and the fifth volar digital artery on the ulnar side.
D4. The deep volar arch gives off the arteria princeps pollicis and arteria radialis indicis and the proper digital arteries for the ulnar side of the index finger and the radial side of the middle finger, as well as the digital arteries on the ulnar side of the fourth and radial side of the fifth fingers via hypertrophic metacarpal arteries.

a. Different Types of Incomplete Deep Volar Arch
Group II consists of four different types of incomplete arch, indicated as types A, B, C and D in Figure 69.

Type A:
In this type of arch, the deep volar supply to the thumb and radial side of the index finger is derived from the deep volar branch of the radial artery which in turn terminates in the second interosseous space. The deep volar ramus of the ulnar artery ends in the third interosseous space. In our material this type of arch was found 14 times (2.8%) (Table XIV, Fig. 70).

Type B:
The deep volar supply to the thumb and the index finger is derived from the deep volar branch of the radial artery. The deep volar ramus of the ulnar artery terminates in the third interosseous space. In our material this type of arch was observed only twice (0.4%) (Table XIV).

Type C:
In this type of arch the arteries for the deep volar supply to the thumb, the ulnar side of the index finger and the radial side of the third finger as well as the appropriate arteries on the ulnar side of the fourth and the radial side of the fifth fingers originate from the deep branch of the radial artery. The deep volar branch of the ulnar artery is completely absent. This type of arch was seen on three hand arteriograms (0.6%) (Table XIV).

Type D:
The volar arterial supply to the thumb and the radial side of the index finger comes from the termination of the radial artery. The arch is incomplete since the deep branch of the ulnar artery terminates after giving off two metacarpal arteries in the second interosseous space. This arch appeared 5 times in our case material (1%) (Table XIV).

6.7.3 Other Observations and Discussion

6.7.4 The Arteria Princeps Pollicis (Principal artery of the thumb)

The arteria princeps pollicis arises from the radial artery after it has turned medialwards towards the palm. It extends distalwards on the ulnar side of the first metacarpal bone; proximal to the metacarpophalangeal joint it usually divides into two

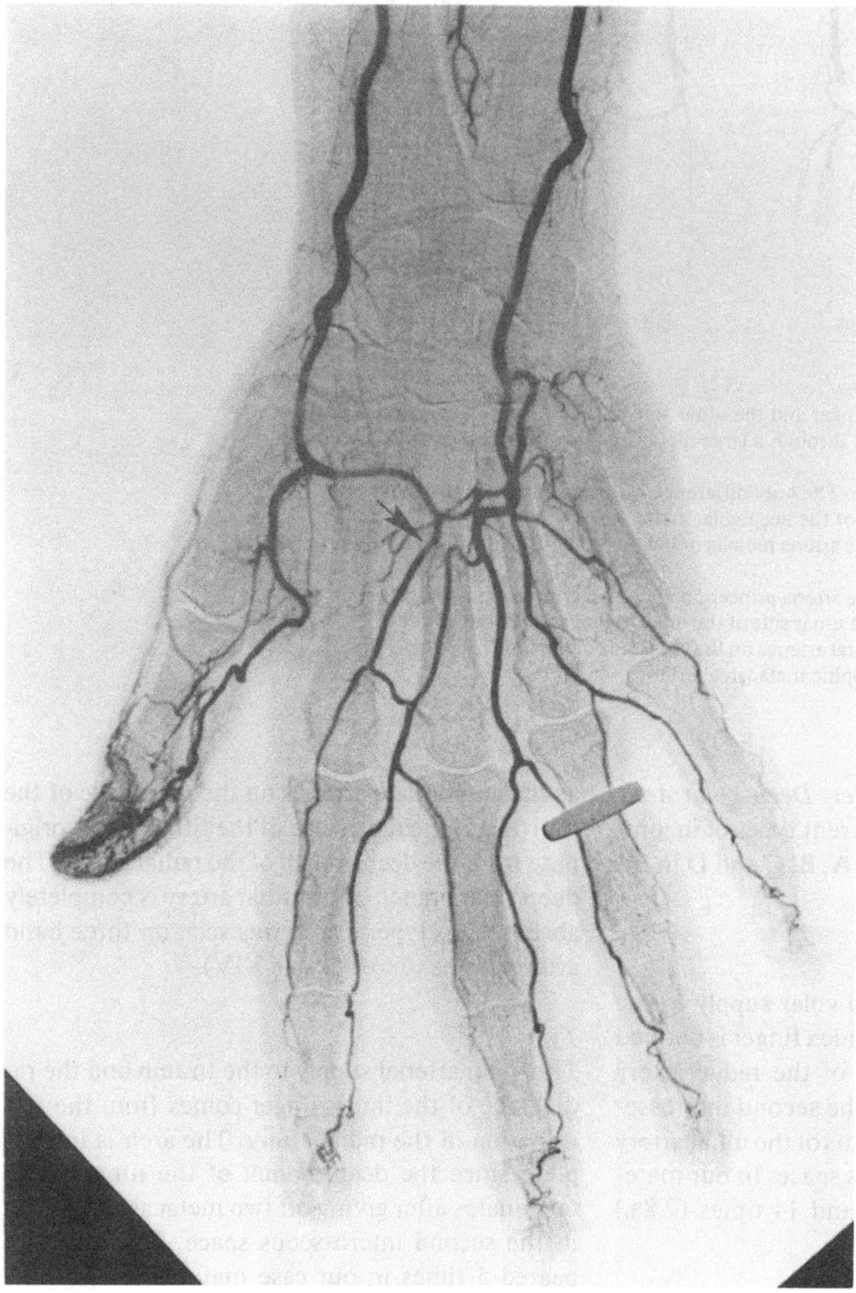

Fig. 68
Complete Deep Arch of type D2.
Arteria radialis indicis arises from the middle portion of the deep volar arch (arrow). It also gives off the last metacarpal artery with the corresponding proper digital arteries and the volar digital artery for the fifth finger on the ulnar side.

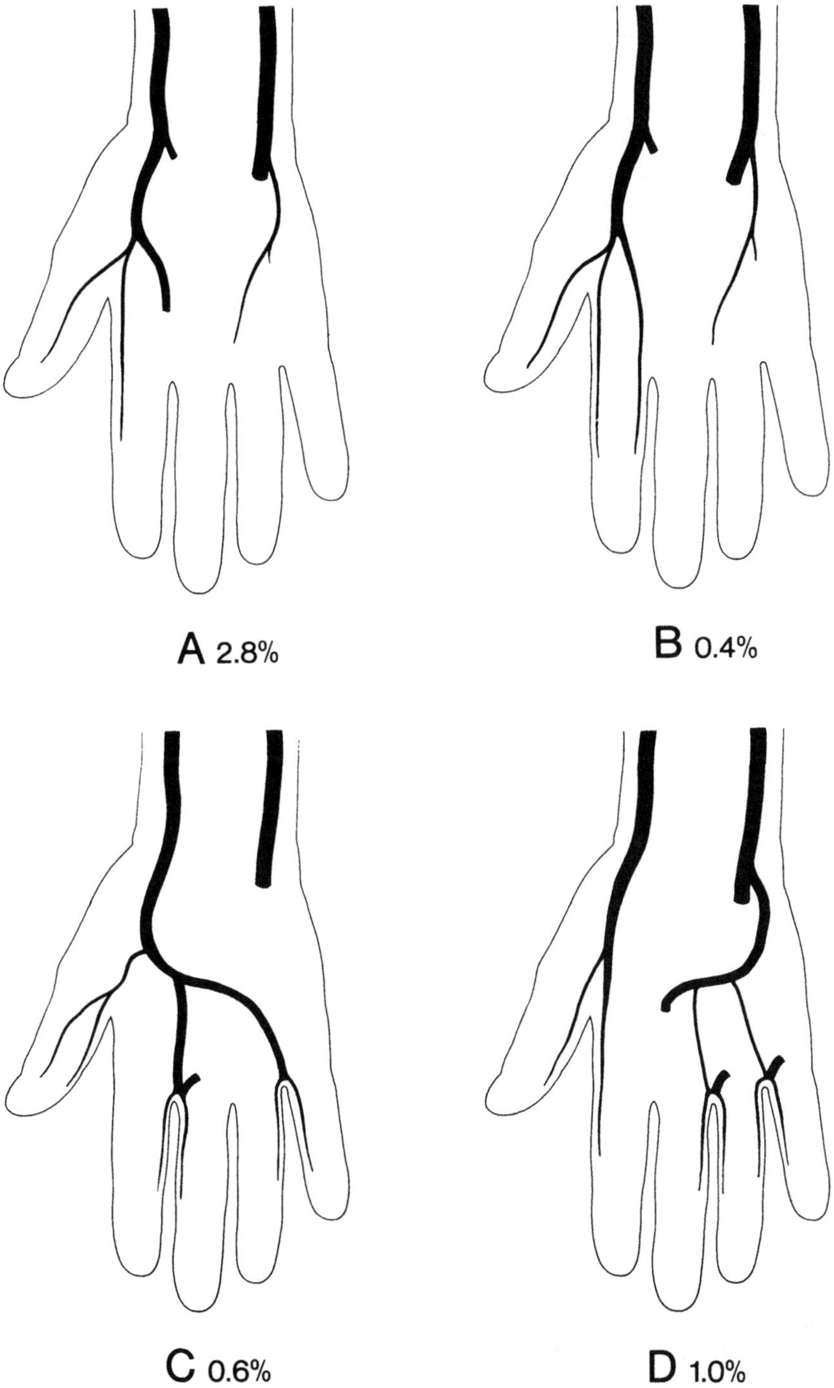

Fig. 69
Different types of incomplete arcus volaris profundus found on 500 hand arteriograms.

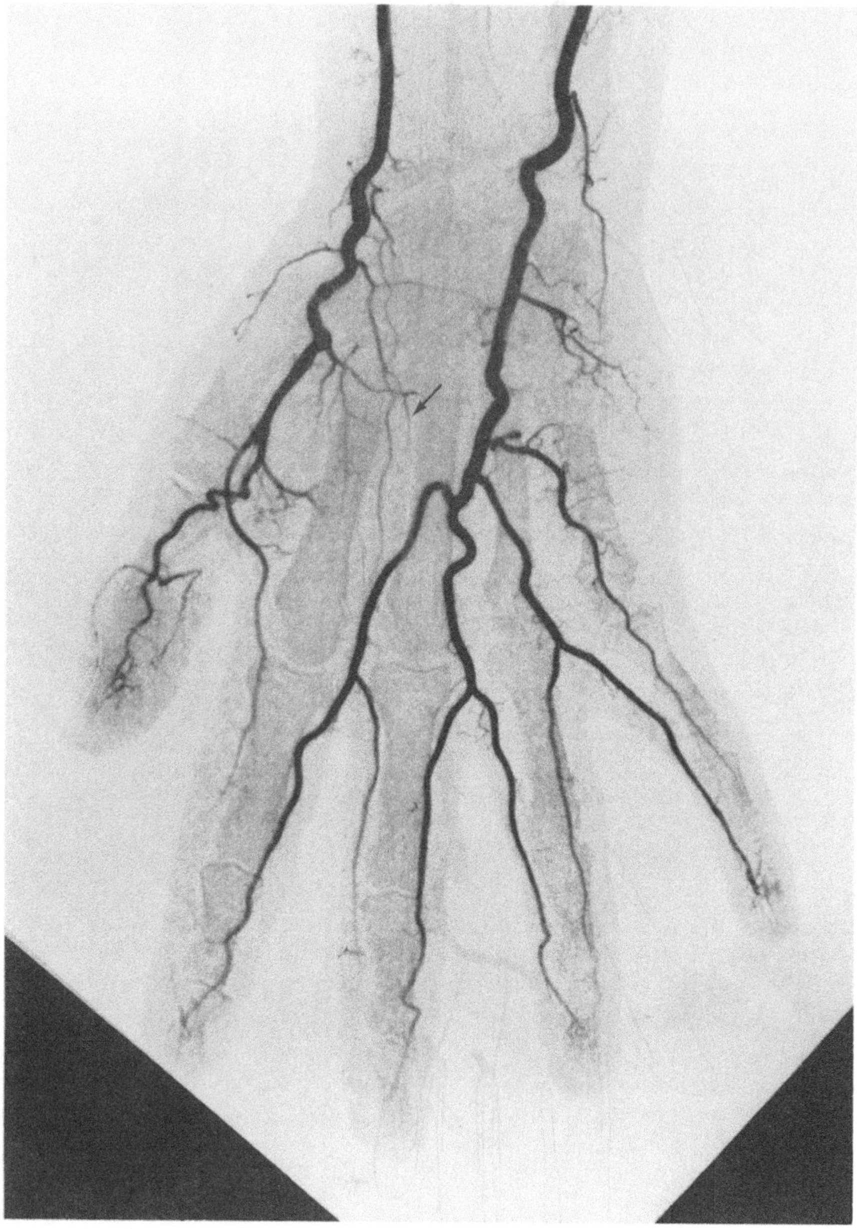

Fig. 70
Incomplete Deep Volar Arch of type A.
The deep volar branch of the radial artery after giving off the common trunk of the princeps pollicis and radialis indicis arteries, terminates in the second interosseous space (arrow).

branches; one to each side of the volar surface of the thumb. It may also run undivided to the end of the thumb as a single branch or it may divide into more branches (Fig. 71). These vessels anastomose with one another at the end of the thumb, like the other digital arteries.

Tandler (1897) proposed that the arteria princeps pollicis between the arch and its bifurcation should be called the first volar metacarpal artery.

a. Variations

The arteria princeps pollicis may arise in common with the arteria radialis indicis (Fig. 66). This common trunk of both arteries is usually very short but occasionally may be quite long (Fig. 72, arrows). In some anatomy books it is termed the first volar metacarpal artery. A common trunk for the arteria princeps pollicis and radialis indicis appeared in 48% of our cases. The principal artery of the thumb

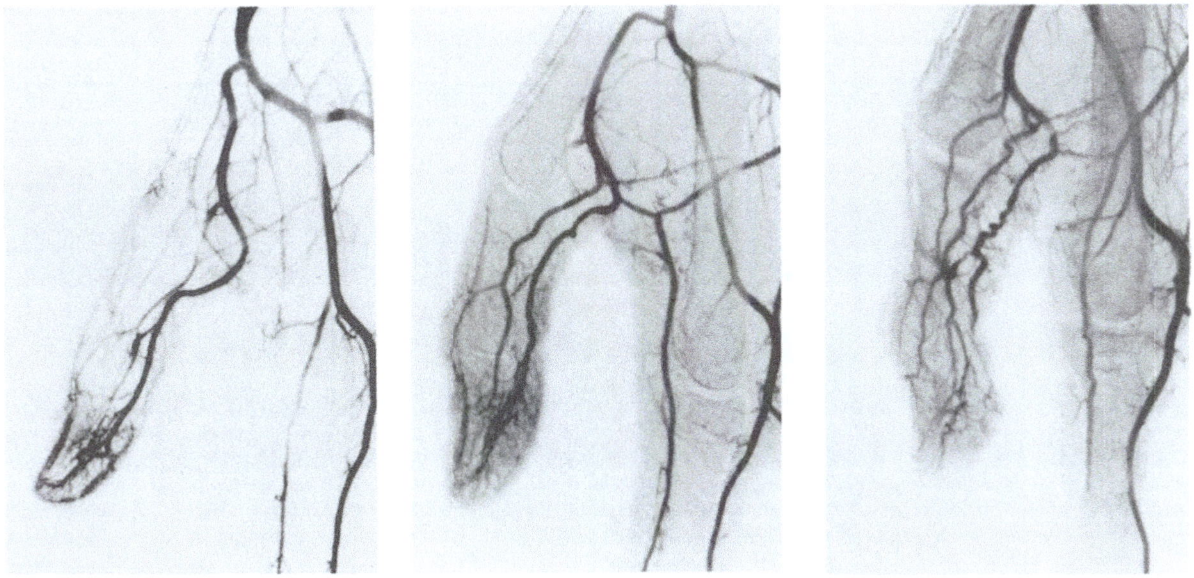

a b c

Fig. 71
Arteria princeps pollicis.
A. A single artery.
B. The artery divides into two branches (most common pattern).
C. The artery divides into three branches.

may be double or even triple. In such cases each of these arteries arises separately from the termination of the radial artery (Fig. 86); one of them can be the lateral branch of Tandler's artery (Fig. 99). On rare occasions both arteriae princeps pollicis may arise from the superficial arch (Fig. 76), or one may originate from the deep and the other from the superficial volar arch (Fig. 77).

A double arteria princeps pollicis was found in 52 percent of the cases; three principal arteries of the thumb were seen only twice (0.4%).

6.7.5 The Arteria Radialis Indicis (Radial artery of the index finger)

In 52 percent of the cases, this artery arises from a common trunk with the arteria princeps pollicis.

If this artery originates separately from the radial artery, then its origin lies somewhat beyond the origin of the arteria princeps pollicis (Fig. 79).

It descends distalwards along the lateral side of the index finger decreasing gradually in calibre towards the fingertip, where it anastomoses with the digital artery on the opposite side (similar to other digital arteries).

a. Variations

This artery may also originate from the metacarpal artery of the first interosseous space, as in the complete deep arches of type B (Fig. 65). This variable origin was found in 30.8% of our cases (Table XIV). In 1% of the cases it originated from the middle portion of the deep volar arch, as in complete deep arch type D2 (Fig. 68). In such cases the artery runs distal- and lateralwards, crossing the third and second metacarpal bones to reach the supply area on the radial side of the index finger. In rare instances this artery may arise from the superficial arch (Fig. 76) or may be totally absent. In the latter case, the final termination of the superficial branch of the ulnar artery in the palm is usually an artery which supplies the territory normally nourished by the radialis indicis (Fig. 100). The arteria radialis indicis may also originate from a branch of the median artery, as in incomplete superficial arch type L (Fig. 95) or from the volar interosseous artery when this vessel helps to supply the palm, as in incomplete superficial arch type N (Fig. 98). This is described and illustrated in 6.8.2d.

6.7.6 The Volar Metacarpal Arteries (Aa. metacarpeae volares) (Fig. 61)

They arise from the convexity of the deep volar arch, extend distalwards in the interosseous spaces and anastomose with the common digital

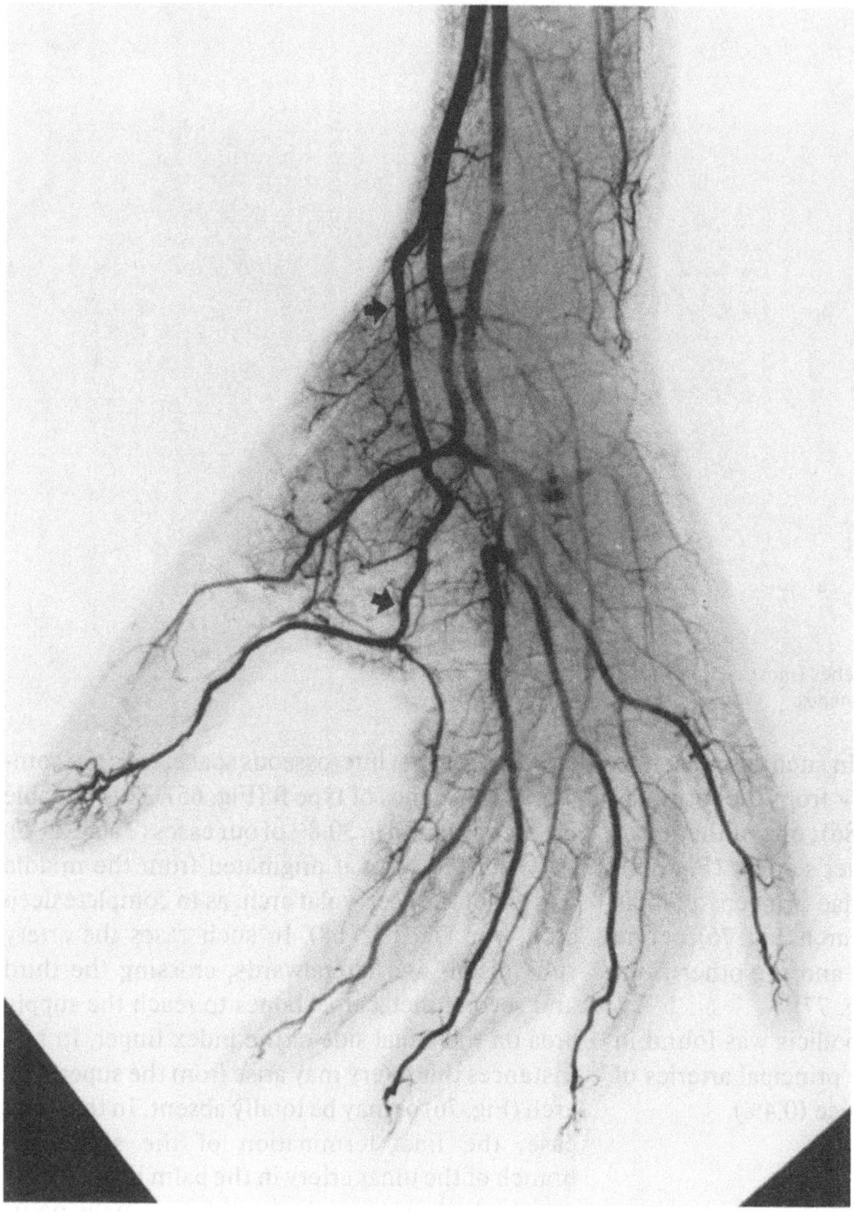

Fig. 72
A long common trunk of arteria princeps pollicis and arteria radialis indicis (arrows). This trunk is also called the first volar metacarpal artery, a term which is not generally accepted.

arteries of the superficial volar arch at or proximal to the bifurcation of the latter into the proper digital arteries. On an arteriogram a volar metacarpal artery can be identified as the artery which arises from the deep arch and runs distalwards at least as far as the metacarpophalangeal joint. These arteries were found to be highly variable as far as both number and distribution are concerned.

On a number of arteriograms identification of these vessels was not possible. Out of 500 selected hand arteriograms, all enhanced by subtraction, the volar metacarpal arteries were fully opacified in only 432 cases. The number, course and area of supply of these arteries vary considerably. Excluding the vessels to the thumb and index finger, the smallest number of metacarpal arteries found in any hand was 2; the largest number was 6. About 54 percent of the hands contained three metacarpal arteries, two and four metacarpal arteries were found in about 20 percent of the cases and six metacarpal arteries in less than 1 percent (Table XVI).

We observed several times that when a volar metacarpal artery is enlarged, the corresponding common volar digital artery from the superficial arch will usually be small in calibre. When a branch of the superficial arch is completely absent, the area of supply of the missing artery is nourished by a volar metacarpal artery, which in such instances is usually large (Fig. 83).

Like other investigators, we found that a volar metacarpal artery does not always join the corresponding common volar digital artery. In such cases it usually joins one of the adjacent arteries (Fig. 73). This variation was seen in about 7% of our cases. The relationship of these metacarpal arteries to the corresponding metacarpal bones and interosseous spaces varied. They cross the metacarpals and run partially through the next interosseous space before anastomosing with the common volar digital arteries of the superficial arch.

In 18 cases or 4% of our arteriograms two volar metacarpal arteries join the same common volar digital artery. In 12 percent of the cases we observed that one volar metacarpal artery divided into two branches which joined two adjacent common volar digital arteries (Fig. 74). A complete absence of one or more metacarpal arteries was also observed.

Finally, the small arteries which supply the dorsum of the hand, the recurrent carpal arteries and the perforating arteries which arise from the dorsal surface of the arch were not analysed in this study. In our opinion roentgenological evaluation of these vessels is not possible, even on good subtraction films.

TABLE XVI

Number of Volar Metacarpal Arteries Found on Arteriograms of 432 Hands.

Number of arteries	*Number of hand arteriograms*	*Percent*
Two	88	20.4
Three	236	54.6
Four	93	21.5
Five	11	2.6
Six	4	0.9
Total	432	100

6.8 The Superficial Volar (Palmar) Arch

(Arcus volaris superficialis; syn: arcus volaris sublimis)

The variations of the superficial volar arch can be divided into two main groups, *i.e.* Group I: complete arch and Group II: incomplete arch. There are six types of complete superficial volar arch subdivided according to the contributing arteries and the number of common volar digital arteries arising from it. Similarly, there are nineteen types of incomplete arch, divided according to the different branching patterns. All types of complete and incomplete superficial volar arch are schematically illustrated in Figures 75, 82, 89, 94 and 97.

6.8.1 Group I: Complete Arch

According to the arteries which contribute to the formation of a complete arch, three different arches can be distinguished:

a. *Radio-ulnar* arch, which is formed by the branches of the radial and ulnar arteries.
b. *Mediano-ulnar* arch, composed of the ulnar artery and an enlarged median artery.
c. *Radiomediano-ulnar* arch, in which three vessels join to form the arch (Fig. 75).

a. Different Types of Complete Superficial Volar Arch

There are four types of complete radio-ulnar arch (Fig. 75).

Type I:

The so-called normal, or classical, radio-ulnar arch (Figs. 61 and 76) is formed chiefly by the ulnar artery. When the ulnar artery enters the palm it divides into two branches, the superficial and the deep. The superficial branch is a direct continuation of the ulnar artery and is usually the larger of the two.

At the level of the carpal bones it runs medialwards to the hook of hamate, then descends over a short distance, turns toward the thumb, crosses the third and fourth metacarpal bones and combines with the superficial volar ramus of the radial artery. The superficial volar branch of the radial artery usually arises at the level of the styloid process of the radius, or a little beyond it (Figs. 61 and 77).

The complete superficial arch is always convex

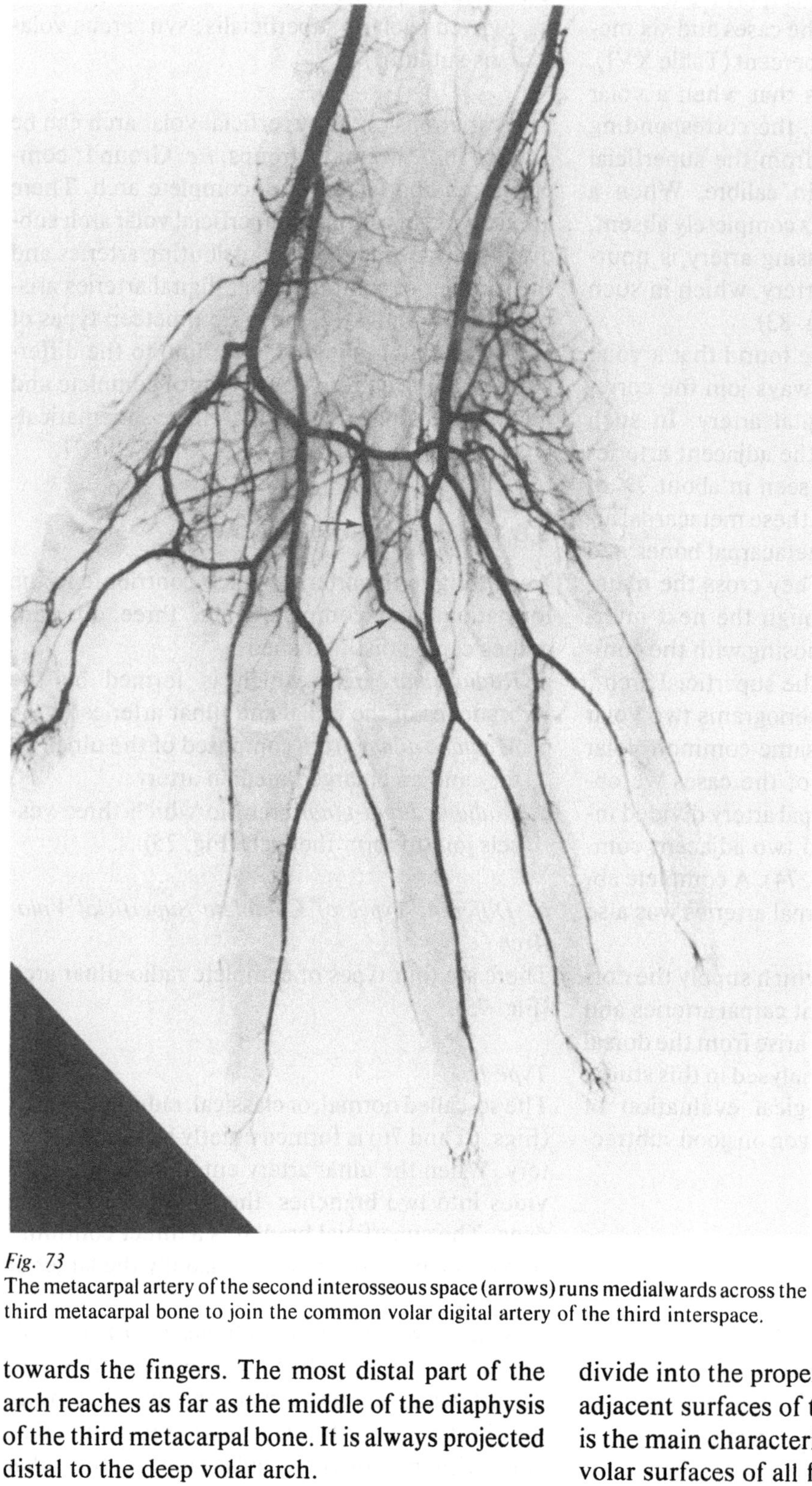

Fig. 73
The metacarpal artery of the second interosseous space (arrows) runs medialwards across the third metacarpal bone to join the common volar digital artery of the third interspace.

towards the fingers. The most distal part of the arch reaches as far as the middle of the diaphysis of the third metacarpal bone. It is always projected distal to the deep volar arch.

This type of arch gives off the common volar digital arteries, which extend distalwards, receive the volar metacarpal arteries from the deep arch and, at the level of the metacarpophalangeal joints, divide into the proper volar digital arteries for the adjacent surfaces of the first to fifth fingers. This is the main characteristic of Type I. It supplies the volar surfaces of all fingers. The proximal part of the superficial branch of the ulnar artery gives off the proper digital artery of the fifth finger on the ulnar side.

The superficial arch also gives off a variable

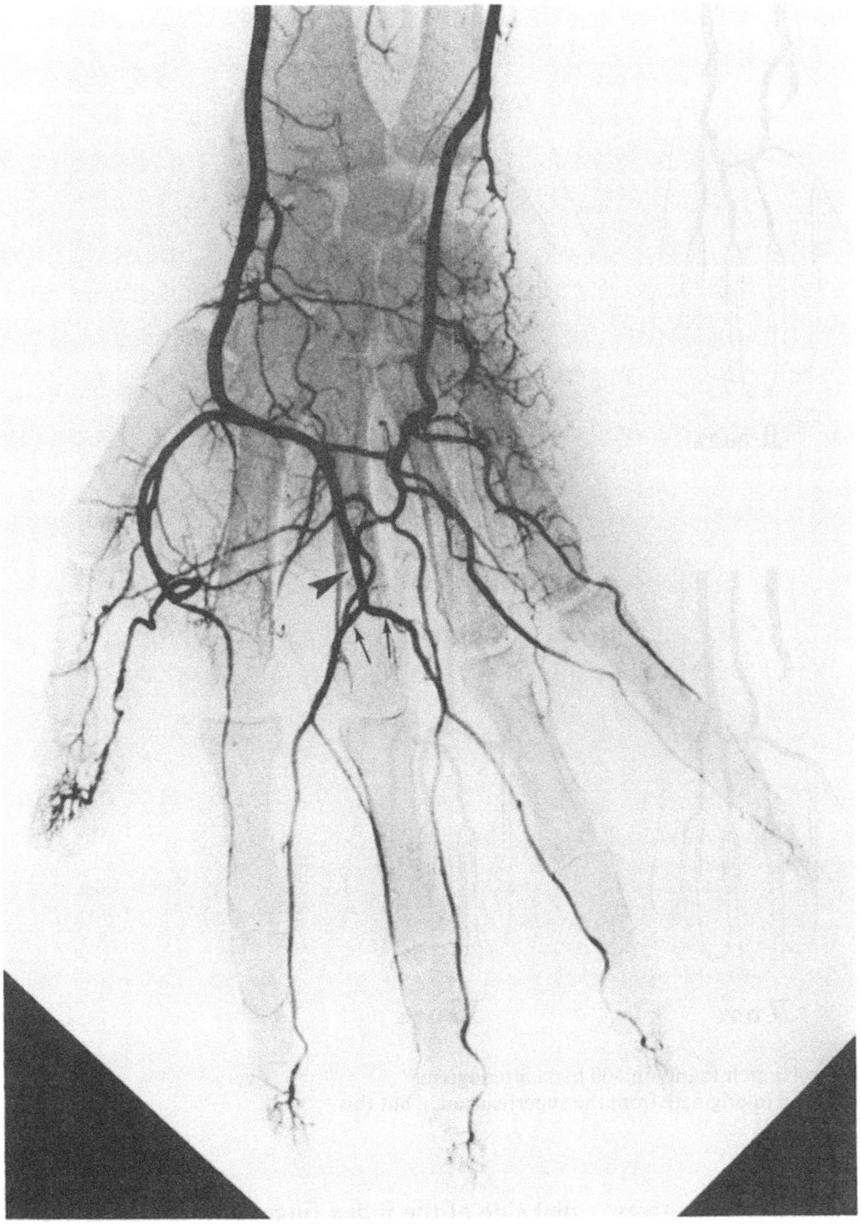

Fig. 74
The metacarpal artery from the second interosseous space (arrow head) divides into two branches which join the second and third common volar digital arteries of the superficial arch (small arrows). The second metacarpal artery is large while the corresponding common volar digital arteries from the second and third interspace are small in calibre.

number of small muscular and cutaneous branches, which will not be discussed here. Type I of the complete superficial arch was found in 35.4 percent of all cases (Table XVII).

Type II:
There is total radio-ulnar communication, from which three common volar digital arteries (II to IV) arise. It also gives off an artery which in turn is the origin of the arteria radialis indicis and a branch to the thumb to supplement the arteria princeps pollicis (see Fig. 77).

This type arch was present in 30.2 percent of the cases (Table XVII).

Type III:
This radio-ulnar arch contains two common volar digital arteries which extend to the volar surface of

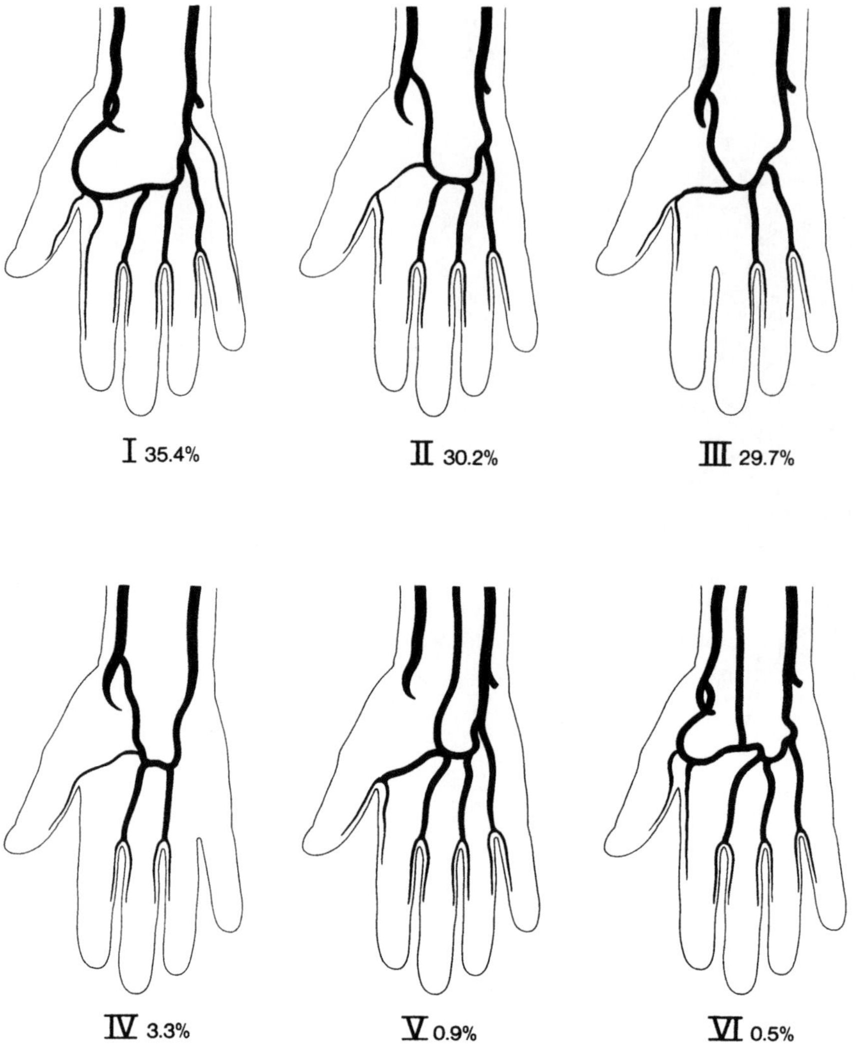

Fig. 75
Different types of complete superficial volar arch found on 500 hand arteriograms.
In type I, the arteria radialis indicis is drawn to originate from the superficial arch, but this occurs only in rare instances.

the third and the fourth interspaces. It also gives off a large artery which runs toward the first interspace where it divides into two branches for the radial side of the index finger and the ulnar side of the thumb (see Fig. 78).

This artery in fact represents the final termination of the superficial ramus of the ulnar artery in the palm. It was extensively analysed for the first time by Julius Tandler (1897) in a study of 130 specimens and therefore deserves to bear his name. Consequently in the following text this branch of the superficial arch will be called Tandler's artery. The common volar digital artery for the fifth finger sometimes arises from the ulnar side of the arch, but this is not a constant feature. On our hand arteriograms this type of arch occurred in 29.7 percent of the cases (see Table XVII).

TABLE XVII

Incidence of Different Types of Complete Superficial Arch.

Type	*Number*	*Percent*
I	75	35.4
II	64	30.2
III	63	29.7
IV	7	3.3
V	2	0.9
VI	1	0.5
Total	212	100

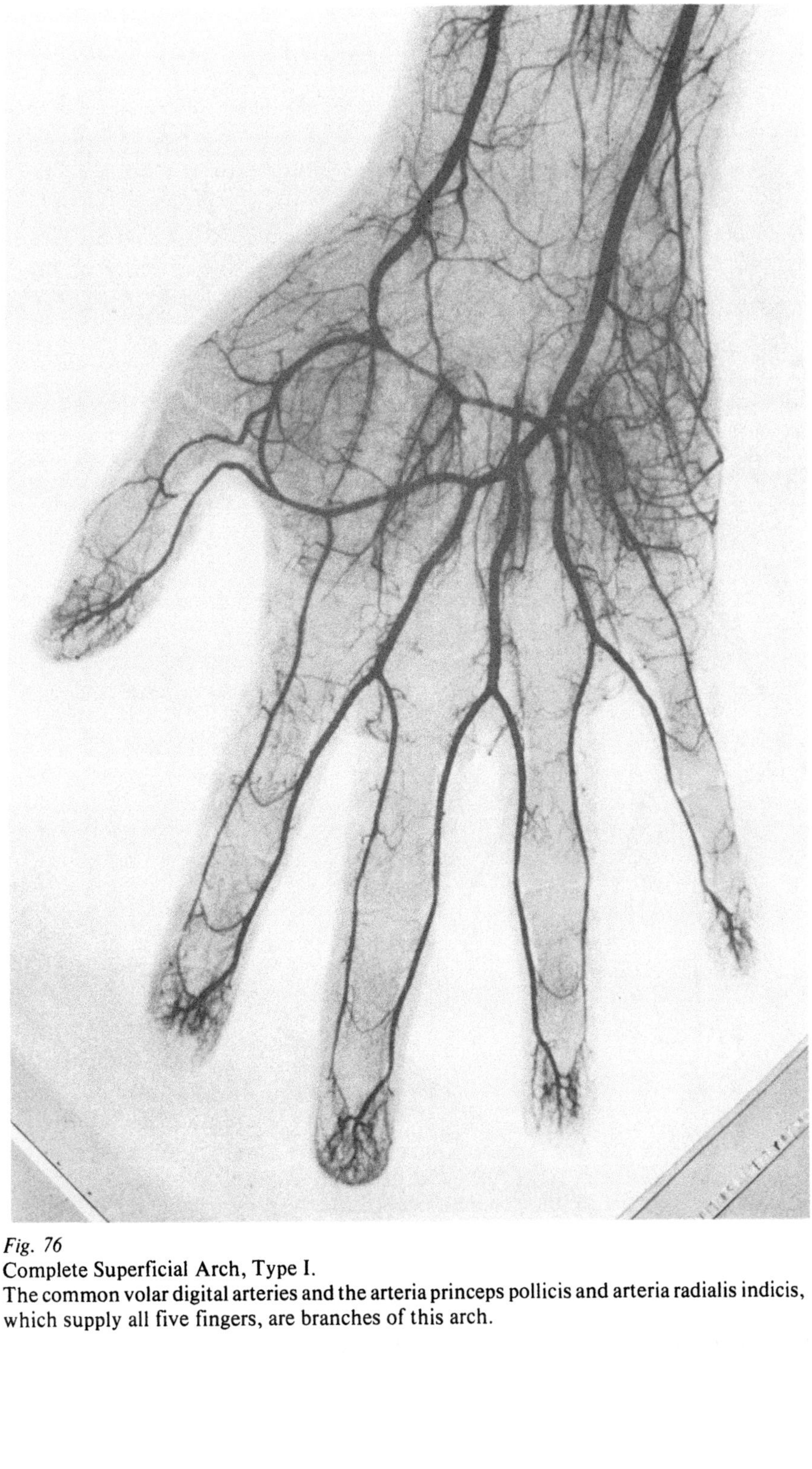

Fig. 76
Complete Superficial Arch, Type I.
The common volar digital arteries and the arteria princeps pollicis and arteria radialis indicis, which supply all five fingers, are branches of this arch.

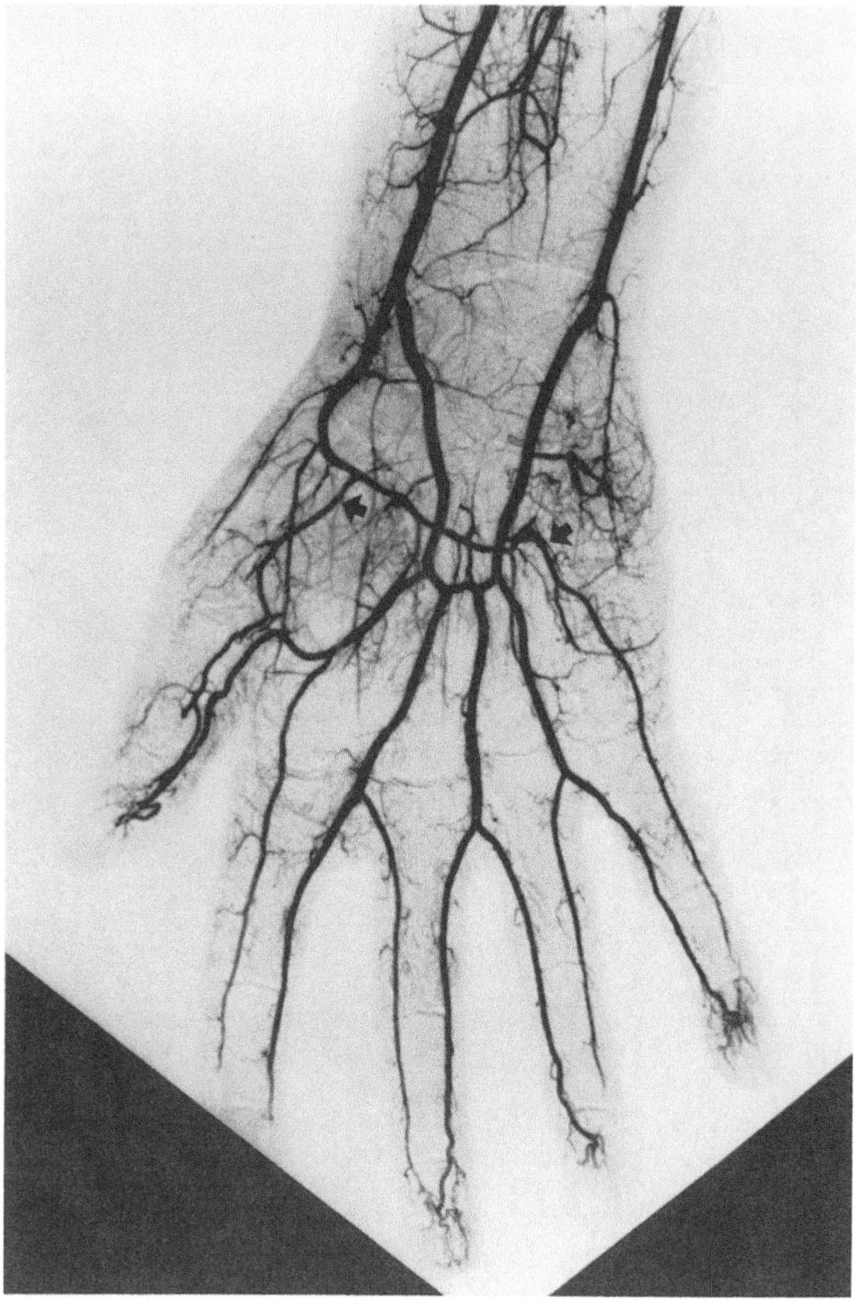

Fig. 77
Complete Superficial Arch, Type II.
The common volar digital arteries (II to IV), the radialis indicis and an artery to the thumb are the branches of this complete radioulnar arch.
The princeps pollicis artery and the fifth ulnar digital artery (arrows) originate from the deep volar arch.

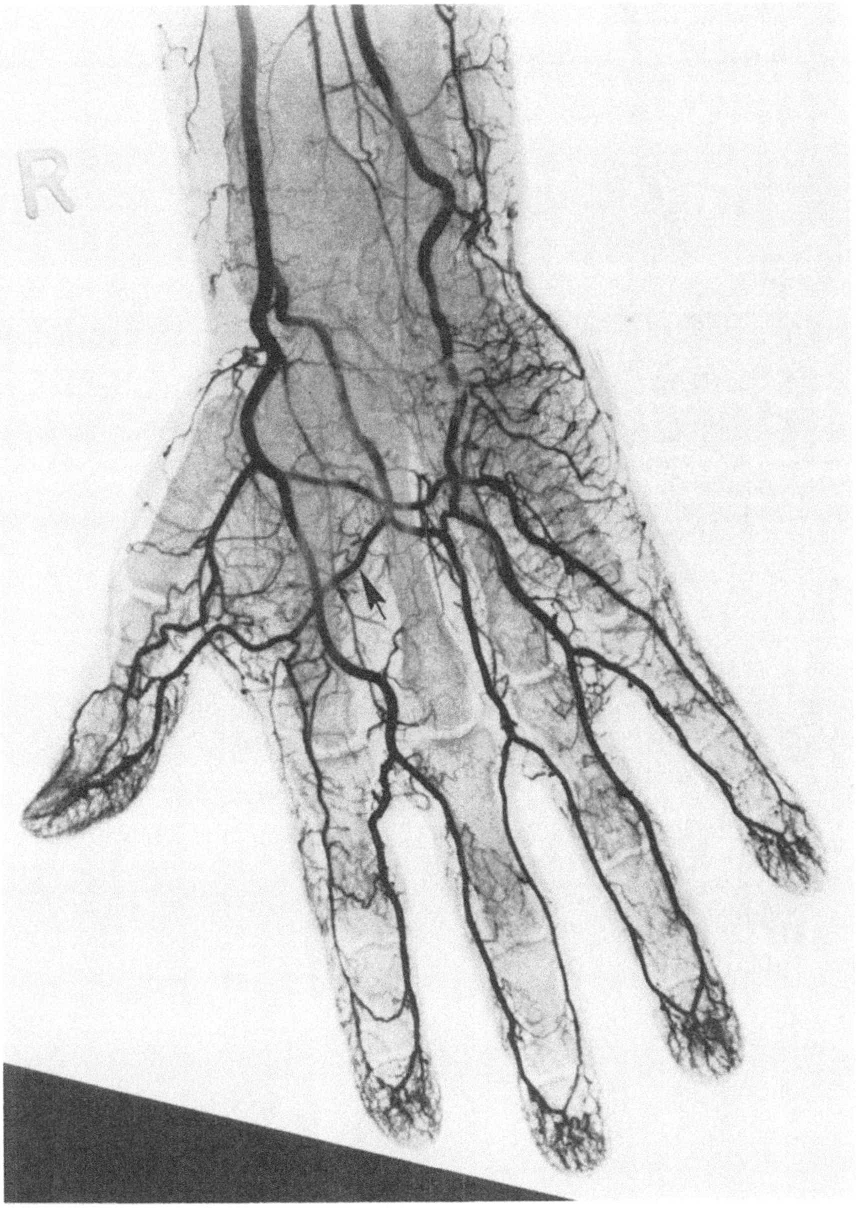

Fig. 78
Complete Superficial Arch, Type III.
This arch gives off two common volar digital arteries for the third and fourth interspace. It also gives off an artery (arrow) which later divides into a branch for the thumb and the arteria radialis indicis.

Type IV:
This arch of the radio-ulnar type gives off the common volar digital arteries for the second and third interspaces, and a small branch for the ulnar side of the thumb. This type of arch was seen in only 3.3 percent of the cases (Fig. 79).

Type V:
This type of arch is formed by the ulnar and median arteries. The latter replaces the radial artery seen in type II (see Fig. 80). Since the contributors to this arch are the median and ulnar arteries, it is also called the mediano-ulnar arch. Only two arteriograms (0.9%) showed this type of arch.

Type VI:
This is the so-called 'three vessels' arch, an arch consisting of three arteries: the radial, the ulnar

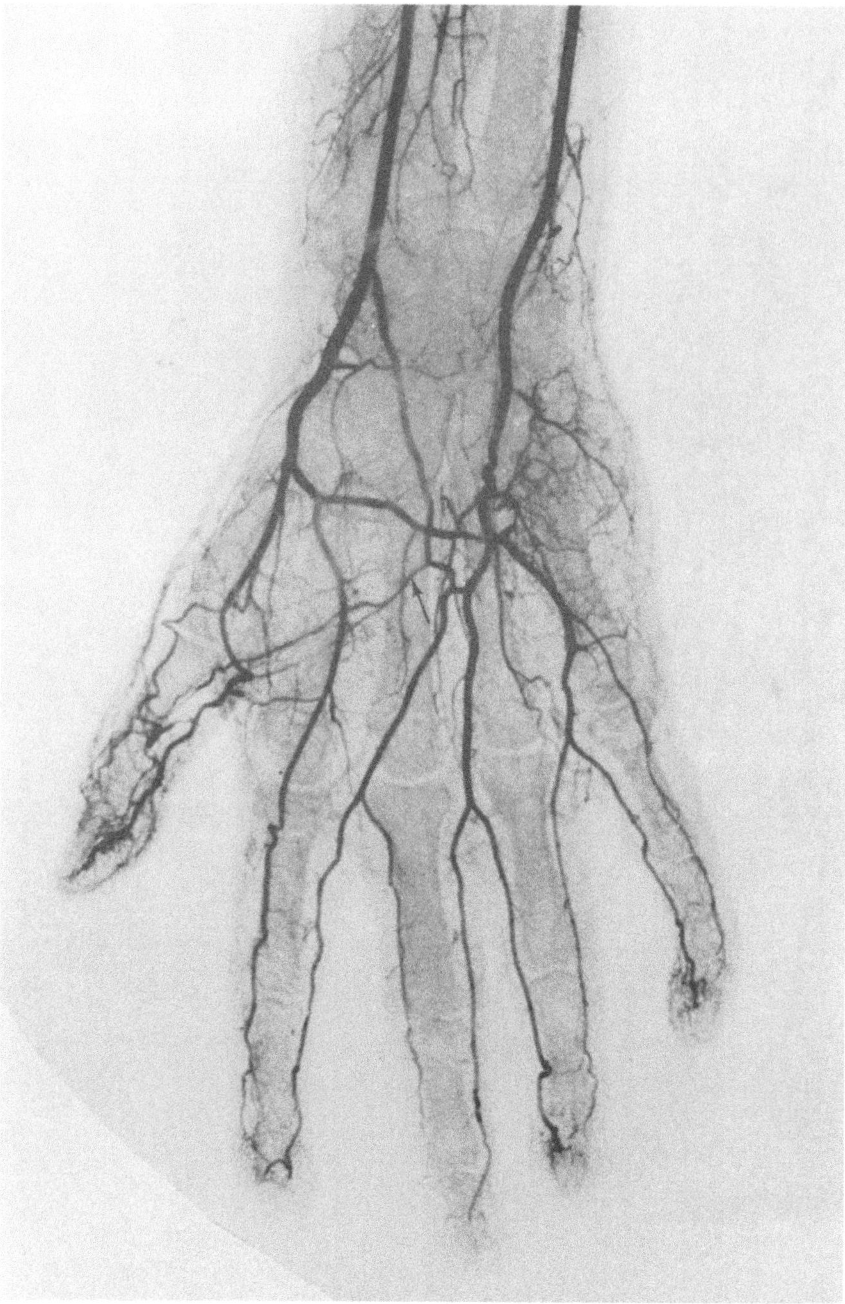

Fig. 79
Complete Superficial Arch, Type IV.
This arch gives off two common volar digital arteries for the second and third interspace. It also gives off a small branch to the thumb (arrow).

and the median arteries. This radiomediano-ulnar arch is usually formed by anastomoses of the radial and ulnar arteries. The median artery communicates at the centre of the arch (Fig. 81). This uncommon pattern was found on only one arteriogram (0.5%) (Table XVII).

6.8.2 Group II: Incomplete Arch

When the arteries contributing to the superficial arch do not anastomose with one another, the arch is incomplete. In most of the cases the superficial volar branch of the radial artery and the termina-

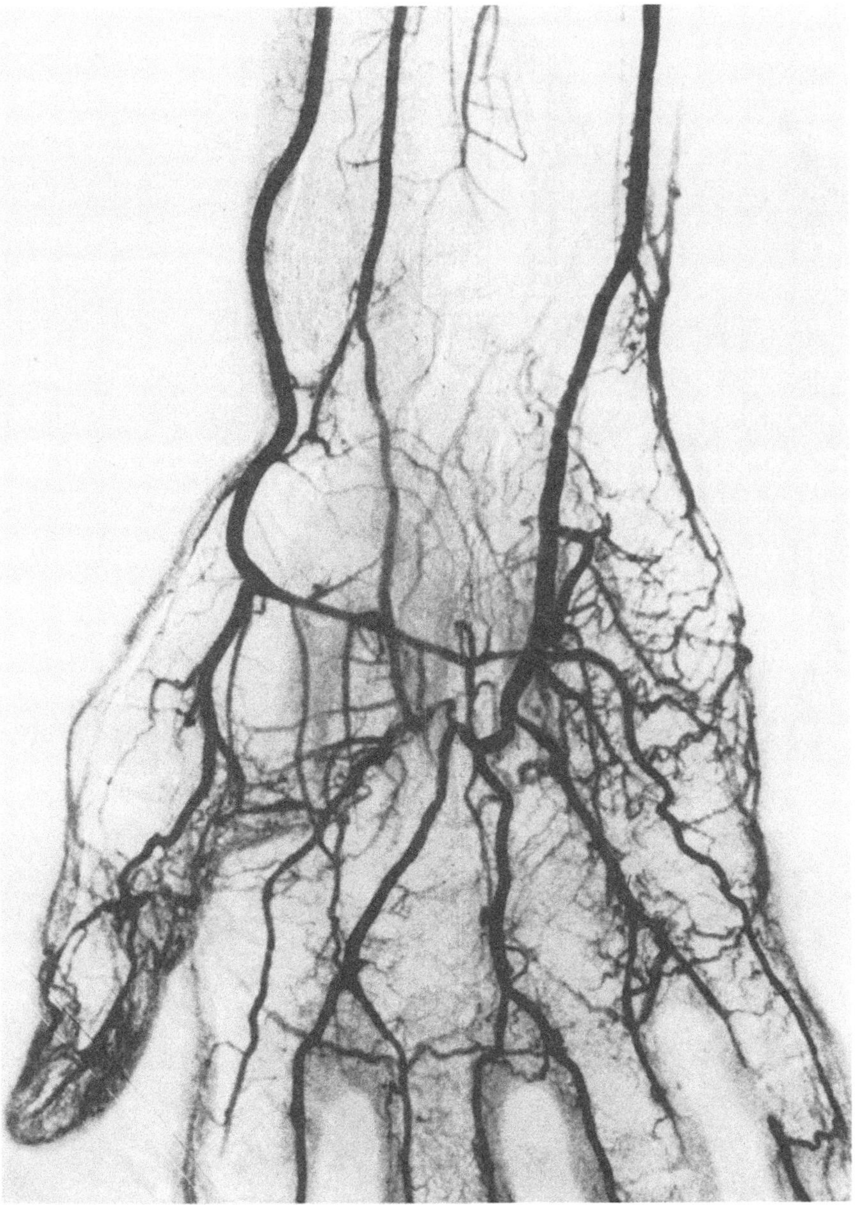

Fig. 80
Complete Superficial Arch, Type V.
This mediano-ulnar arch gives off the proper volar digital arteries for the last four fingers.
The principal artery of the thumb is the only vessel which arises from the deep arch.

tion of the ulnar artery supply the palm and fingers but, in doing so, fail to form an arch at the volar surface of the palm. In addition to these two vessels, in rare instances the median artery and even the volar interosseous artery may participate in the supply to the palm and fingers without anastomosing with the other vessels.

Since a large number of variations of the incomplete superficial volar arch was noted in our case material we decided to separate these patterns into four main categories according to the number of arteries which participate in the superficial volar supply to the palm and fingers.

a. Category I comprises those cases in which only one vessel forms the incomplete superficial volar arch (Fig. 82). This vessel is usually the ulnar artery. Incomplete superficial arches of category I

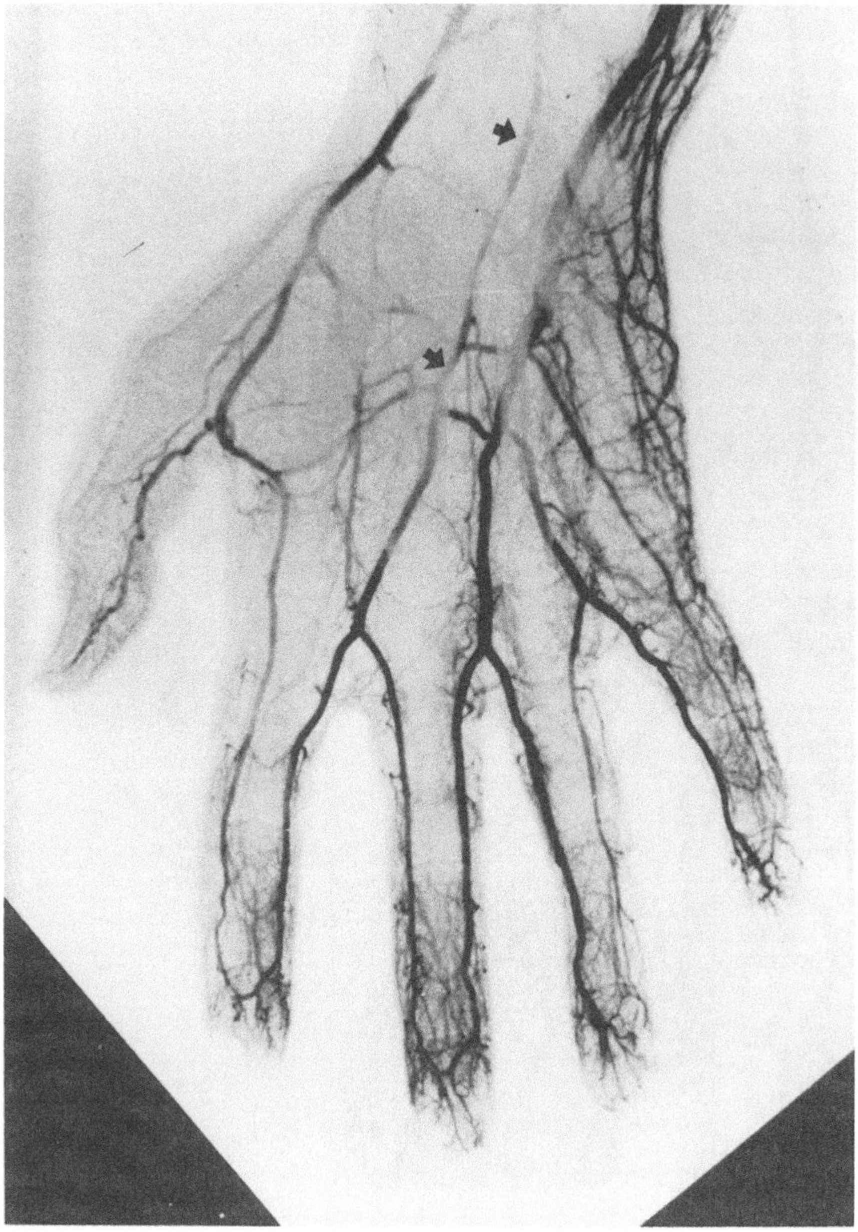

Fig. 81
Complete Superficial Arch, Type VI.
This radiomediano-ulnar arch gives off all digital arteries for the volar supply of all five fingers. The median artery (arrows) communicates at the centre of the arch.

appeared in 69.6% of our material (Table XVIII). The ulnar artery may give off one or more common volar digital arteries. According to the number of these branches several types of this category of arch can be distinguished.

Type A (Fig. 83) is an incomplete arch formed by the ulnar artery which gives off only one common volar digital artery; the latter divides into two appropriate digital arteries for the adjacent surfaces of two fingers. We found 17 cases (5.9%) of this type in our material (Table XVIII).

Type B (Fig. 84) is an incomplete arch in which the ulnar artery terminates by dividing into two common volar digital arteries which subsequently pass into the interdigital webs of the corresponding third and fourth interosseous spaces. At the bases

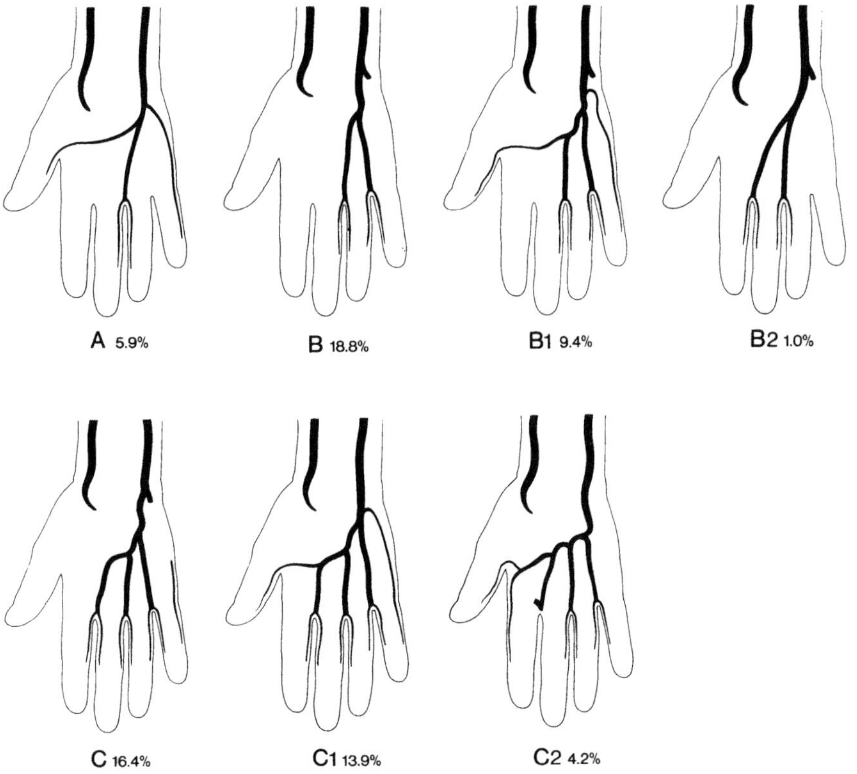

Fig. 82
Different types of incomplete superfical arch. Category I.

of the fingers they bifurcate into proper volar digital arteries for adjacent sides of the respective digits (III to V). Type B appeared in 18.8 percent of our cases (Table XVIII).

Type B1 is a modification of the preceding type. The ulnar artery gives off not only the last two common volar digital arteries but also two more branches for the thumb and the ulnar side of the fifth finger. This type appeared on 9.4 percent of our angiograms (Table XVIII).

Type B2 is the same pattern as type B, the only difference being that the common volar digital arteries originating from the ulnar artery pass into the interdigital webs of the second and the third interosseous spaces, and end by dividing into the appropriate digital arteries for the second and fourth digits (Fig. 85). This type of superficial arterial pattern was very rare. In our case material it was found only 3 times (1%) (Table XVIII).

Type C (Fig. 86) is a superficial arterial pattern in which the termination of the ulnar artery gives rise to three common volar digital arteries for the respective second, third and fourth interosseous spaces. The proper volar digital arteries, from the ulnar side of the second to the radial side of the fifth fingers, are branches of these arteries. This arterial pattern appeared in 16.4 percent of our case material (Table XVIII).

Type C1 is a modification of type C. Here, the ulnar artery gives off not only the three common volar

TABLE XVIII

Incidence of Different Types of Incomplete Superficial Arch on 288 Hand Arteriograms.

From Category I

Type	*Number*	*Percent*
A	17	5.9
B	54	18.8
B1	27	9.4
B2	3	1.0
C	47	16.4
C1	40	13.9
C2	12	4.2
Total	200	69.6

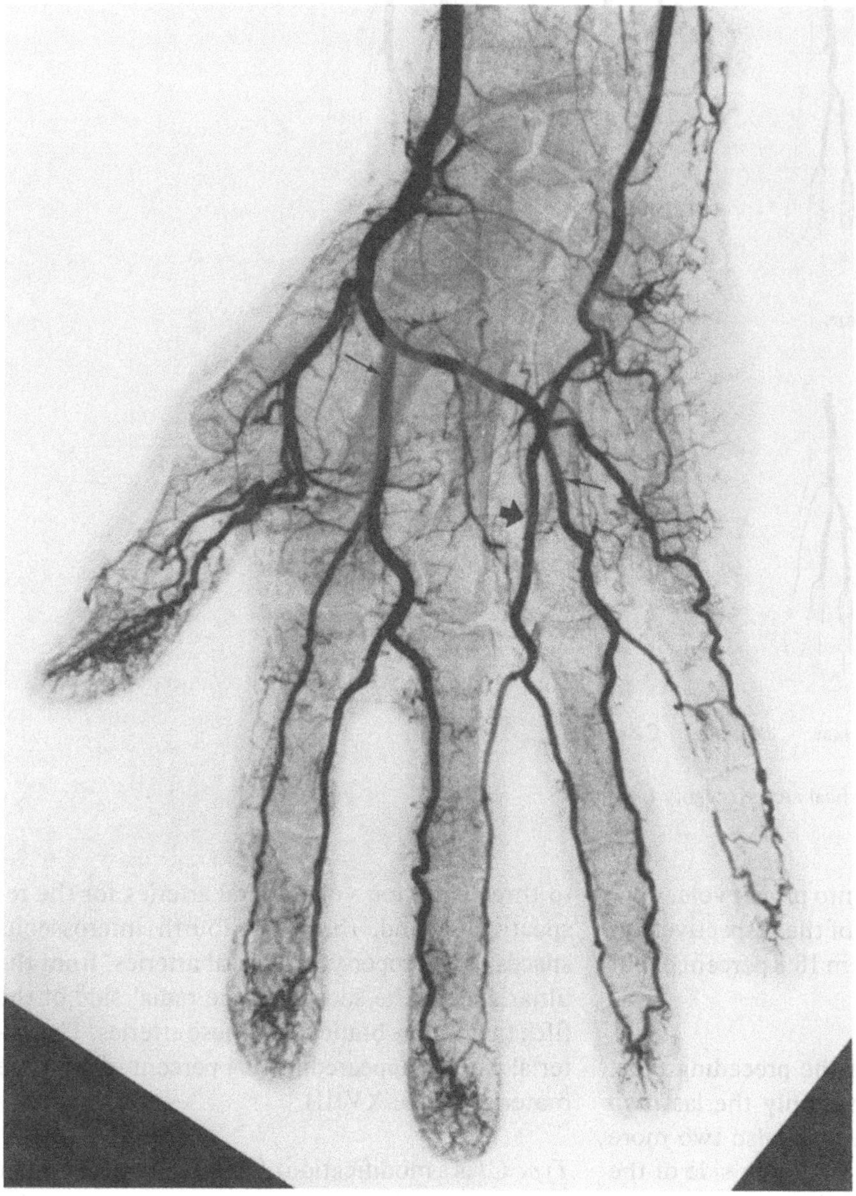

Fig. 83
Incomplete Superficial Arch, Category I, Type A.
The ulnar artery gives off only one common volar digital for the third interspace (arrow) and the proper volar digital arteries for the ulnar side of the third and radial side of the fourth fingers. The first and fourth metacarpal arteries (small arrows) are hypertrophic, because the corresponding common volar digital arteries are absent.

digital arteries, but also two other branches for the volar side of the thumb and ulnar side of the fifth finger (Fig. 82). This variation was found in 13.9 percent of our cases (Table XVIII).

Type C2 is the last type of category I; the branching pattern of the ulnar artery is more complex: two common volar digital arteries for the third and fourth interspaces and a small supplementary branch for the second interspace originate from the ulnar artery. The latter terminates on the lateral side of the hand in an artery which supplies the radial side of the index finger and ulnar side of the thumb (the so-called Tandler's artery). This superficial palmar arterial pattern was found on 4.2 percent of our arteriograms (Table XVIII, Figs. 87 and 88).

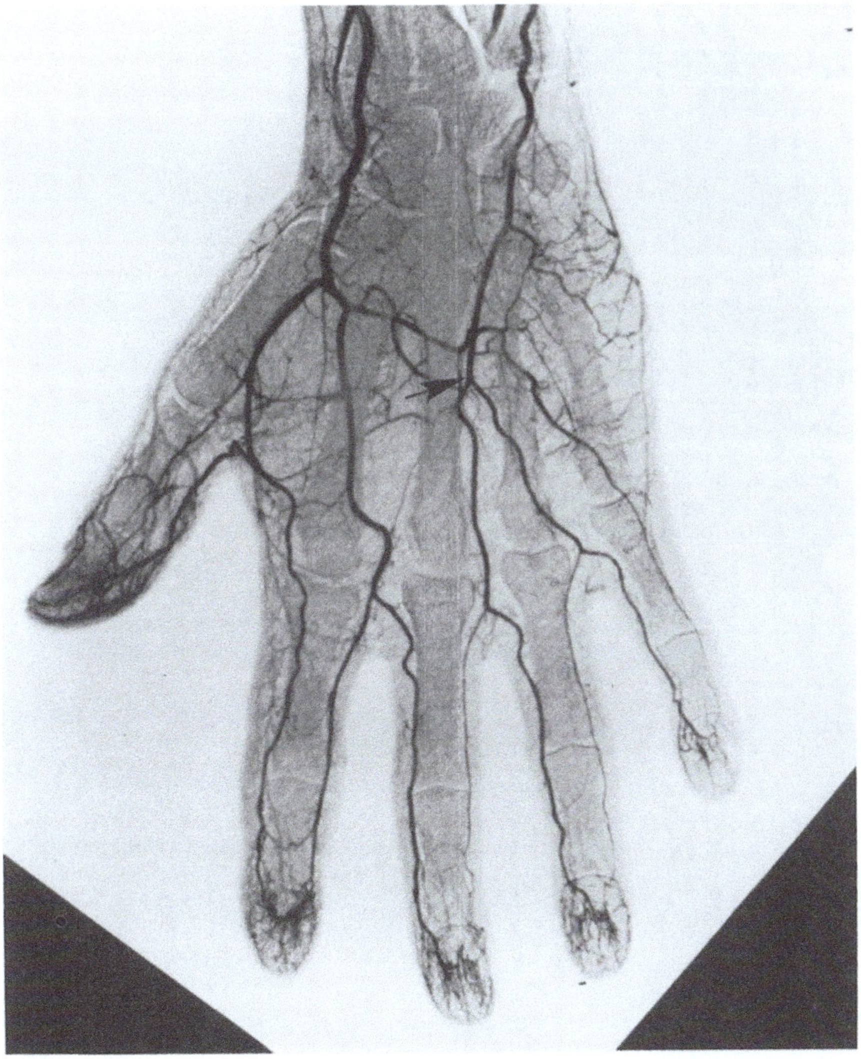

Fig. 84
Incomplete Superficial Arch, Category I, Type B.
The ulnar artery terminates by dividing into two common volar digital arteries (arrow), which give rise to the proper volar digital arteries, from the ulnar side of the third to the radial side of the fifth finger.

b. Category II. This category comprises all superficial volar arterial patterns involving the branches of both main arteries of the forearm, the radial and ulnar arteries. There are eight different arterial patterns in this so-called radio-ulnar category; they are illustrated in Figure 89. Altogether the different types of this category appeared in 27.6 percent of our cases (Table XIX).

Type D (Fig. 90). In this type the first and second common volar digital arteries are branches of the superficial volar ramus of the radial artery. The third and fourth common volar digital arteries arise from the termination of the ulnar artery. The final branches of these arteries (the proper volar digital arteries) supply adjacent sides of all five digits, except the ulnar side of the fifth finger. This arterial pattern turned out to be very uncommon; it was found in only 2 percent of our cases (Table XIX).

Type D1 is a modification of the preceding type. The only difference is that type D1 possesses one branch more than type D. It is an artery which arises from the most proximal part of the ulnar superficial ramus, descends toward the fifth finger

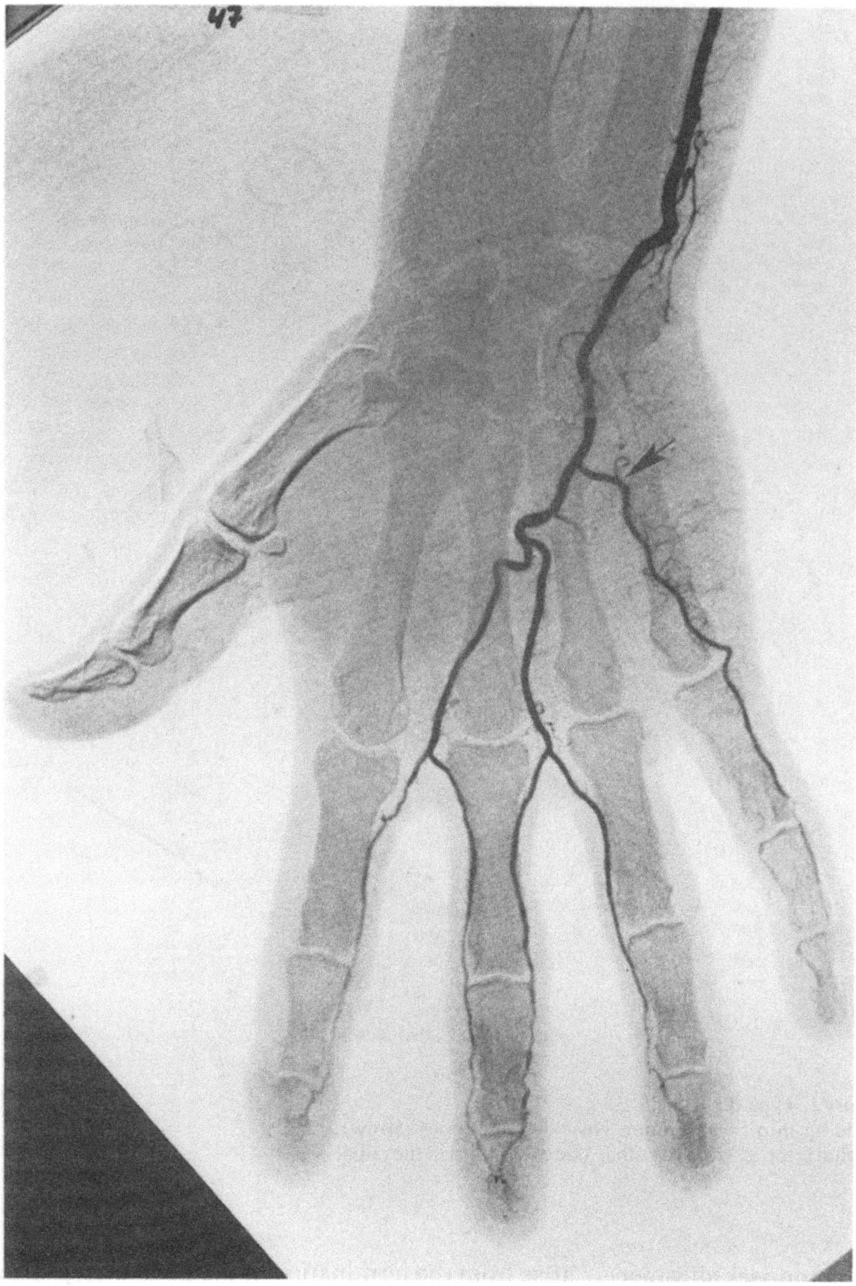

Fig. 85
Incomplete Superficial Volar Arch, Category 1, Type B2 (territorial arteriography).
The ulnar artery gives off two common volar digital arteries for the second and third interspaces with the corresponding proper volar digital arteries, as well as the digital artery on the ulnar side of the fifth finger (arrow).

and supplies the ulnar side of it. This uncommon pattern was found in only 2.8 percent of the cases (Table XIX).

Type E (Fig. 91) represents a radio-ulnar pattern in which the superficial volar ramus of the radial artery ends as the second common digital artery. Near the cleft of the second and third digits it is joined by a volar superficial branch of the ulnar artery and then divides into two appropriate digital arteries for adjacent sides of the corresponding fingers. The common volar digital arteries of the

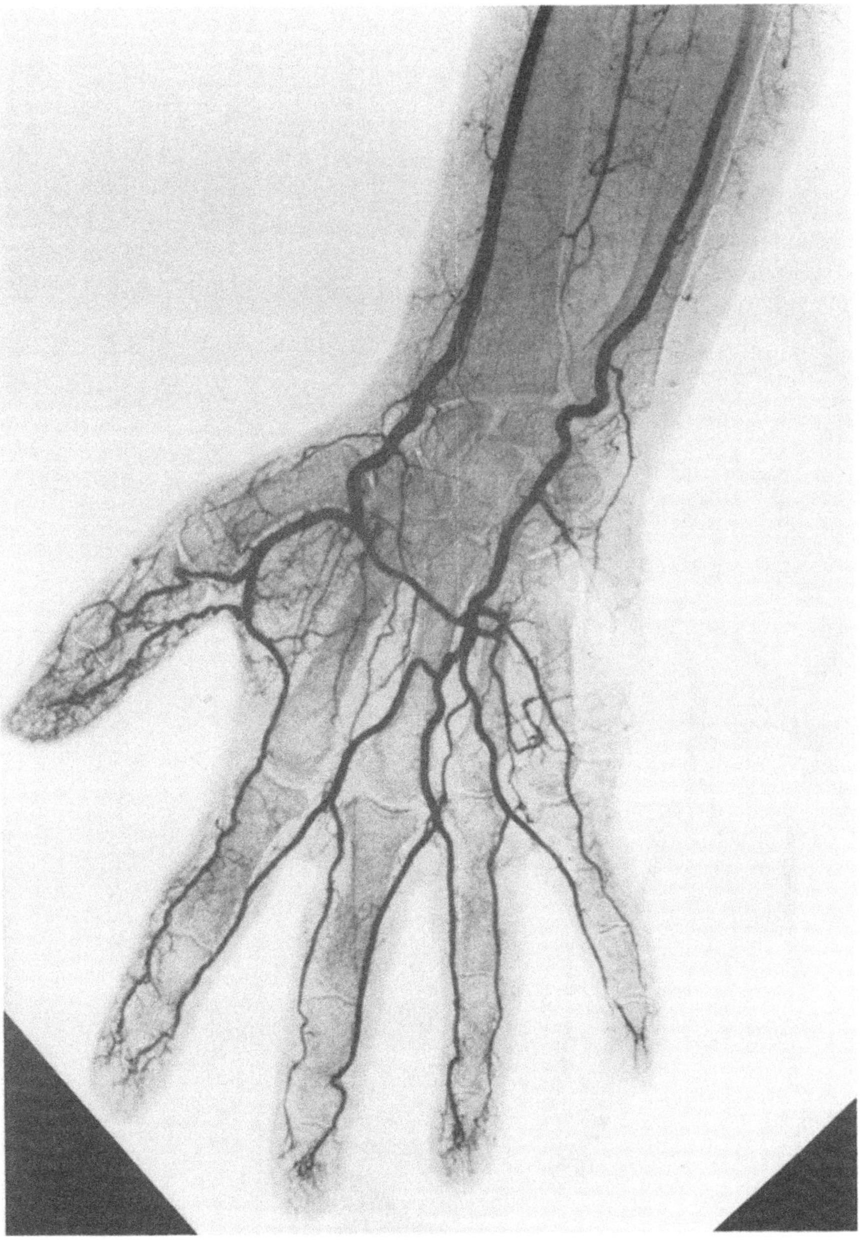

Fig. 86
Incomplete Superficial Arch, Category I, Type C.
The ulnar artery divides into three common volar digital arteries which give rise to the proper volar digital arteries to the last four fingers. The arteria radialis indicis and the ulnar digital artery of the fifth finger are branches of the deep volar arch.
Note the two principal arteries of the thumb arising separately from the termination of the radial artery.

third and fourth interspaces are also branches of the ulnar artery. Out of a total of 288 incomplete superficial arches, 9 percent showed this pattern (Table XIX).

Type F (Fig. 92). The superficial ramus of the radial artery in the first interspace divides into two branches for the volar surface of the thumb and radial side of the index finger. The ulnar artery gives off three common volar digital arteries (II to IV interspace) and the proper digital arteries for the corresponding fingers. This type occurred in 6.3 percent of the present series (Table XIX).

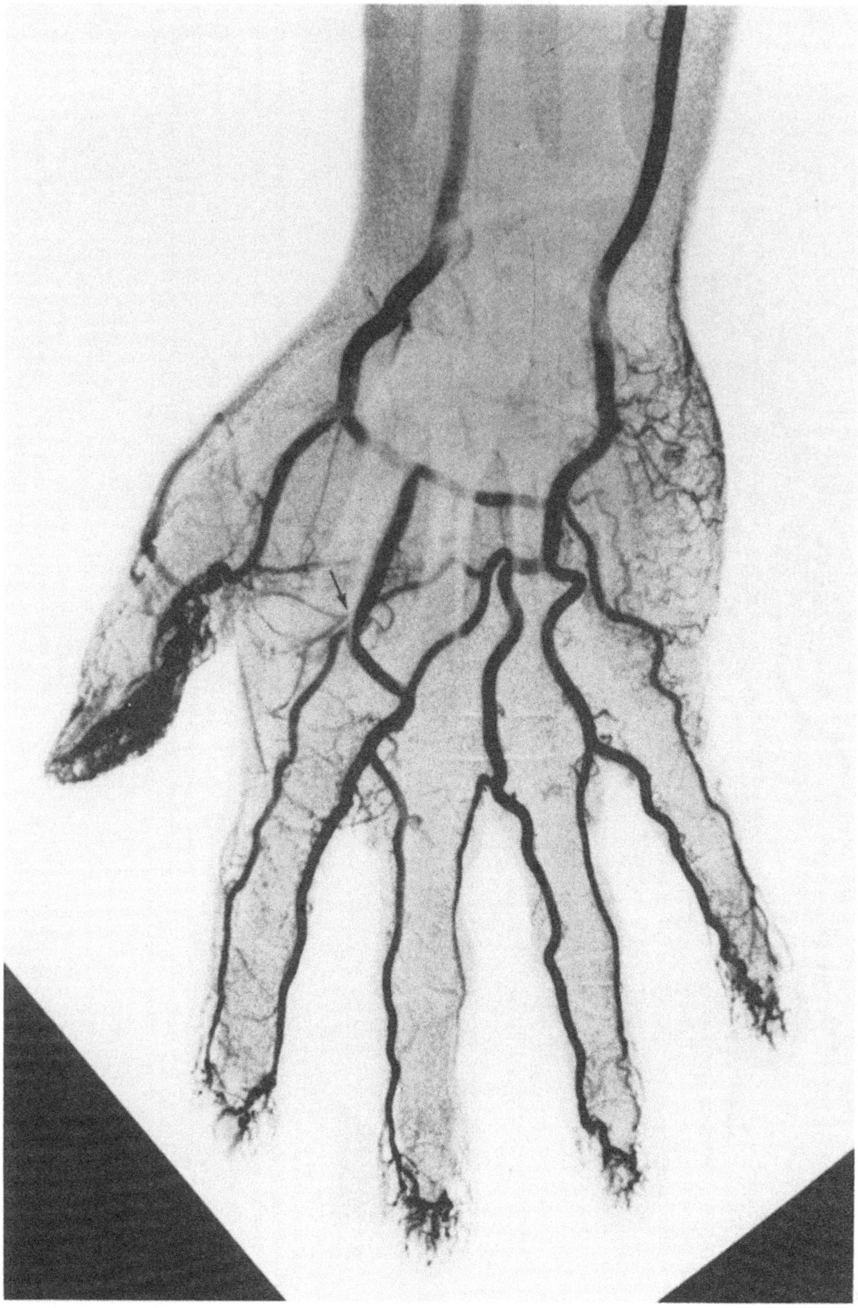

Fig. 87
Incomplete Superficial Arch, Category I, Type C2.
The ulnar artery gives off two common volar digital arteries for the third and fourth interspace and the corresponding proper volar digital arteries, from the ulnar side of the third to the radial side of the fifth fingers. It is also the origin of a small supplementary branch for the second metacarpal artery and terminates on the radial side of the palm in a very tiny artery (arrow), which divides into two small branches to the thumb and radial side of the index finger.

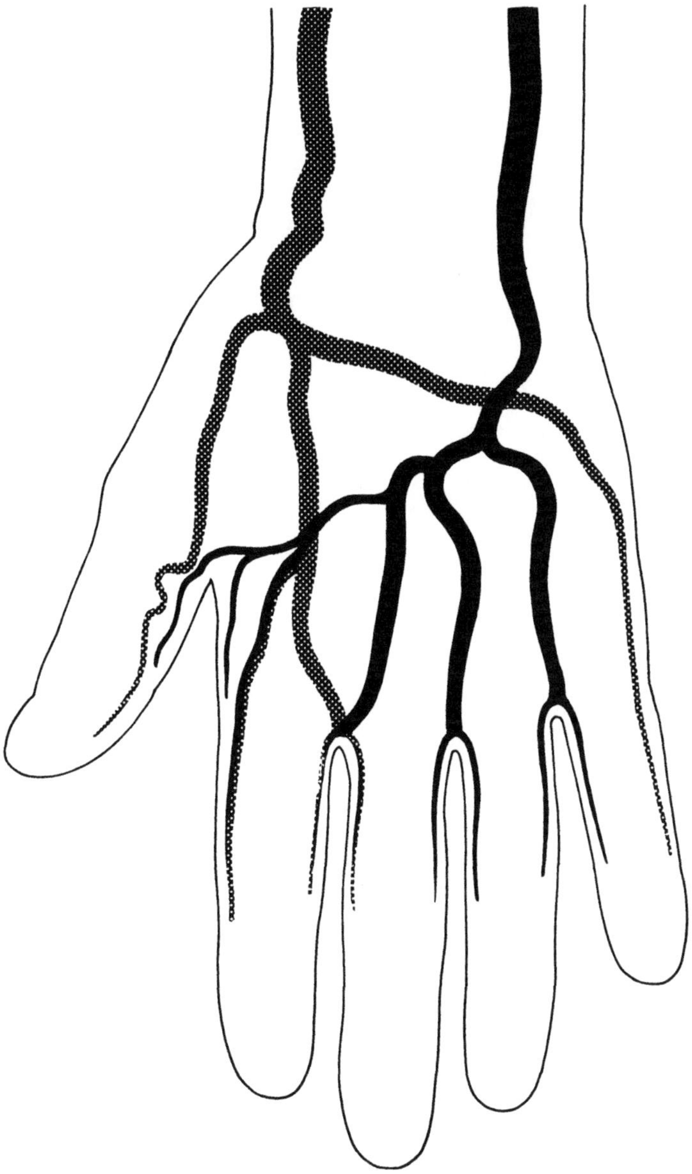

Fig. 88
Schematic diagram of the case illustrated in Fig. 87.
The superficial and the deep volar arches with their branches are drawn separately.

Type G is a radio-ulnar type in which the ulnar artery predominates. It gives off the common volar digital arteries for the second and third interspaces, the corresponding proper digital arteries, and an artery which supplies the ulnar side of the fifth finger. This vessel usually arises from the proximal part of the superficial ulnar ramus. The superficial ramus of the radial artery supplies the radial side of the index finger (Fig. 93). Only 2.0 percent of the cases fell into this category (Table XIX).

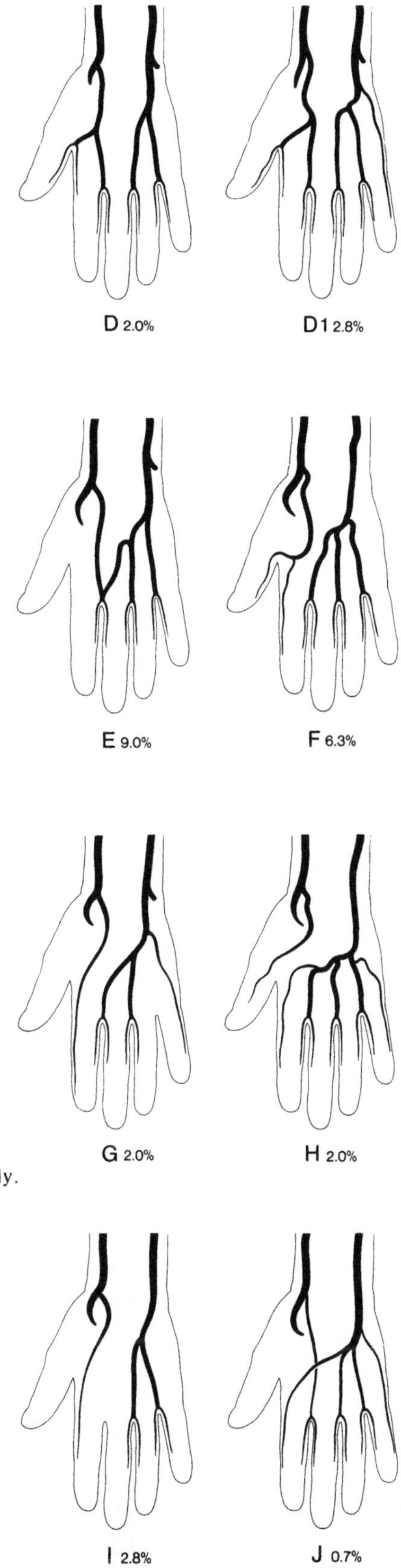

Fig. 89
Different types of incomplete superficial arch. Category II.

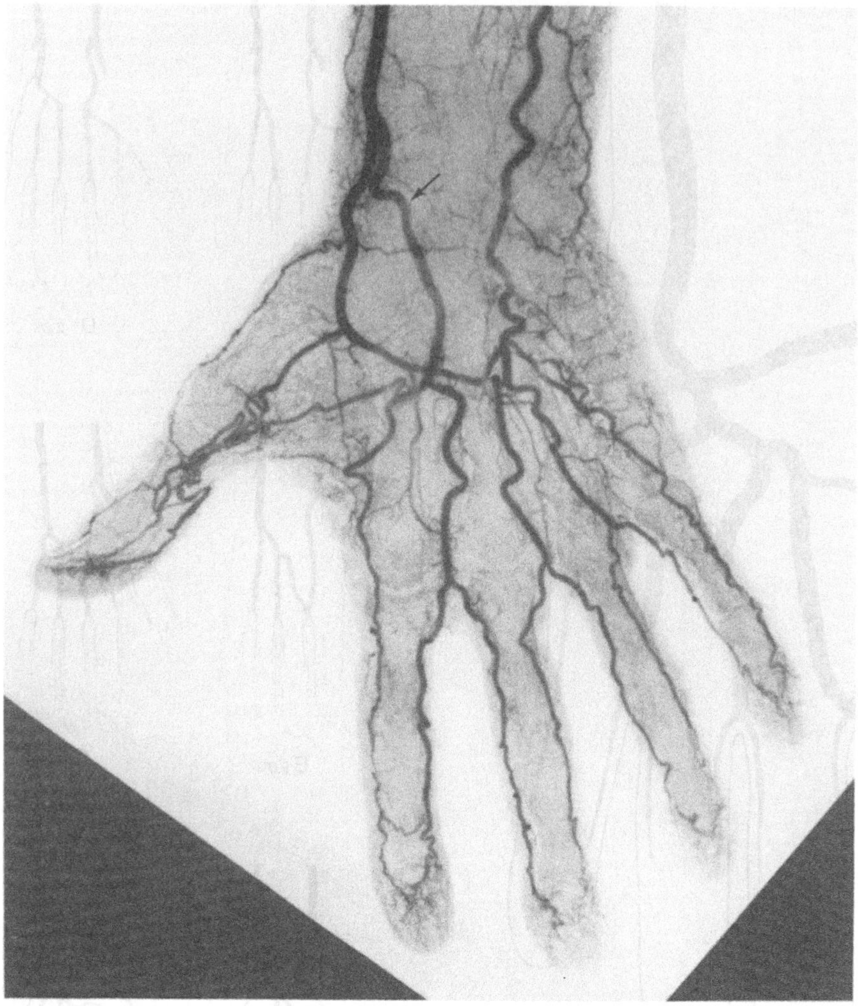

Fig. 90
Incomplete Superficial Arch, Category II, Type D.
The common volar digital arteries of the first and second interspace are branches of the superficial ramus of the radial artery (arrow). The third and fourth common volar digital arteries originate form the ulnar artery. Except arteria princeps pollicis and the digital artery on the ulnar side of the fifth finger, all other digital arteries are branches of this incomplete superficial arch.

TABLE XIX

Incidence of Different Types of Incomplete Superficial Arch on 288 Hand Arteriograms.

From Category II

Type	*Number*	*Percent*
D	6	2.0
D1	8	2.8
E	26	9.0
F	18	6.3
G	6	2.0
H	6	2.0
I	8	2.8
J	2	0.7
Total	80	27.6

Type H. In this type the ulnar artery gives off three common volar digital arteries (II to IV), a very tiny vessel for the radial side of the index finger and the artery for the ulnar side of the fifth finger (which usually arises from the proximal part of the fourth common volar digital artery) (Fig. 89). The superficial ramus of the radial artery supplies the volar surface of the thumb.

This type is also uncommon, occurring in only 2.0 percent of our material (Table XIX).

Type I (Fig. 89). This type is characterized by divi-

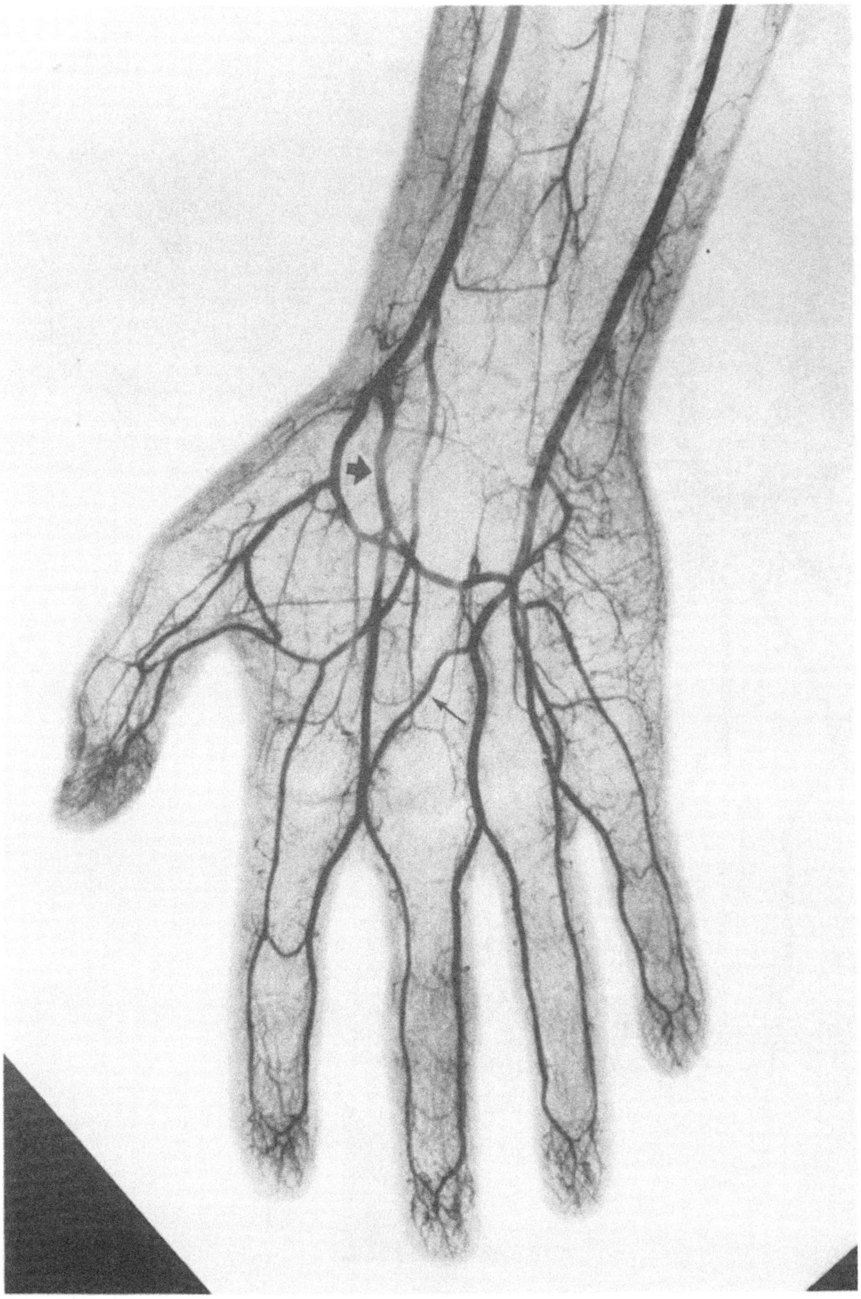

Fig. 91
Incomplete Superficial Arch, Category II, Type E.
The superficial ramus of the radial artery (large arrow) terminates as the second common volar digital artery. The ulnar artery gives off the last two common volar digital arteries and a branch (small arrow) which unites with the second common volar digital artery.
Note a second superficial branch of the radial artery, which arises at the level of the styloid process of radius and gives off the arteria radialis indicis and a small branch to the thumb.

sion of the ulnar artery into two common digital arteries for the third and fourth interspaces. The superficial branch of the radial artery supplies the radial side of the index finger. This type appeared in 2.8 percent of our cases (Table XIX).

Type J (Fig. 89). In this very uncommon type, the ulnar artery gives off two common volar digital arteries (III and IV) and two other branches to supply the radial side of the index finger and the ulnar side of the fifth finger. The superficial ramus of the ra-

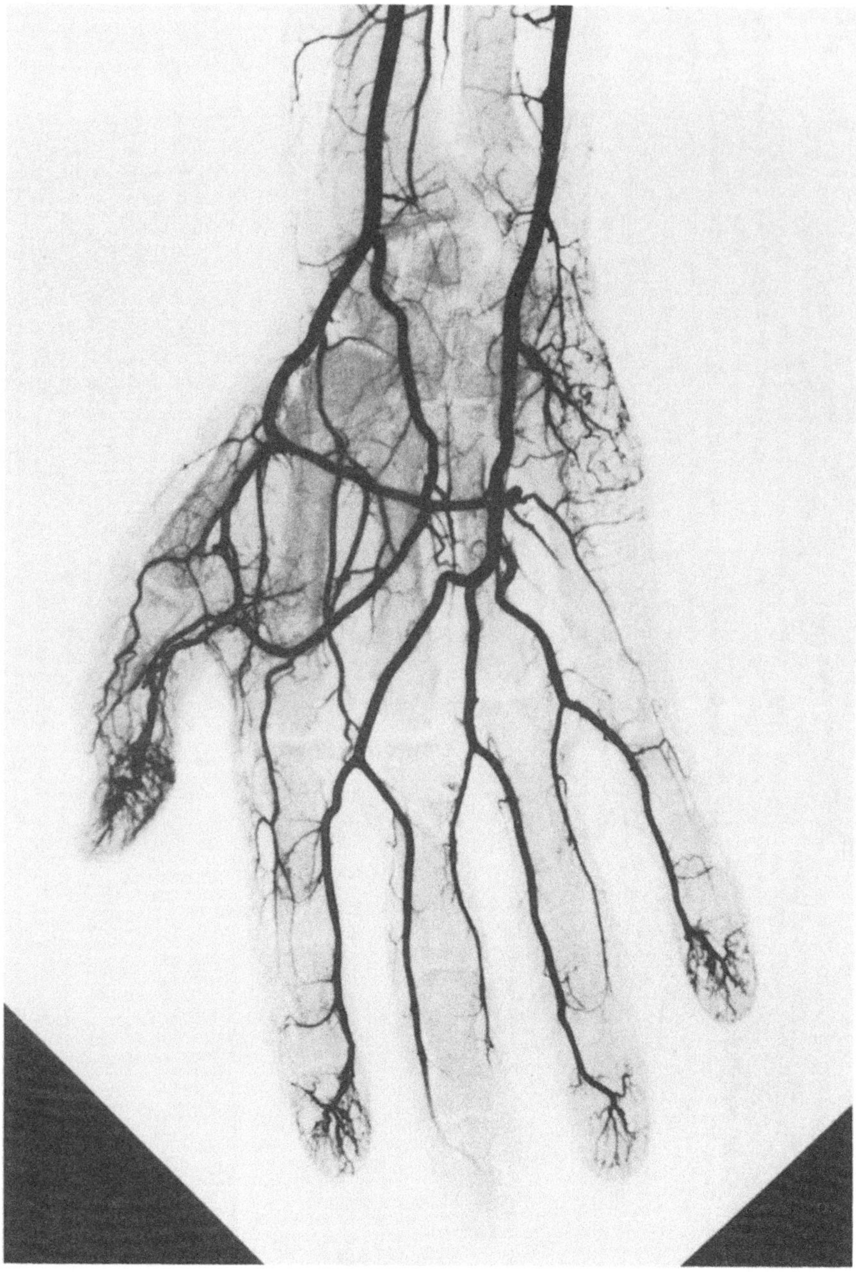

Fig. 92
Incomplete Superficial Arch, Category II, Type F.
The ulnar artery gives off the last three common volar digital arteries and the proper volar digital arteries for the corresponding fingers.
The superficial ramus of the radial artery is the origin of the arteria radialis indicis and an artery for the volar surface of the thumb.

dial artery terminates as the second common digital artery delivering the proper digital arteries for the ulnar side of the index finger and the radial side of the third finger. Type J is very uncommon; it was found in only 0.7 percent of the hands studied (Table XIX).

c. *Category III.* This category includes all cases in which three vessels take part in the palmar arterial supply: the radial, the ulnar and the median arteries. On all arteriograms of this type the median artery reaches the hand to furnish digital arteries without anastomosing with the radial and ulnar ar-

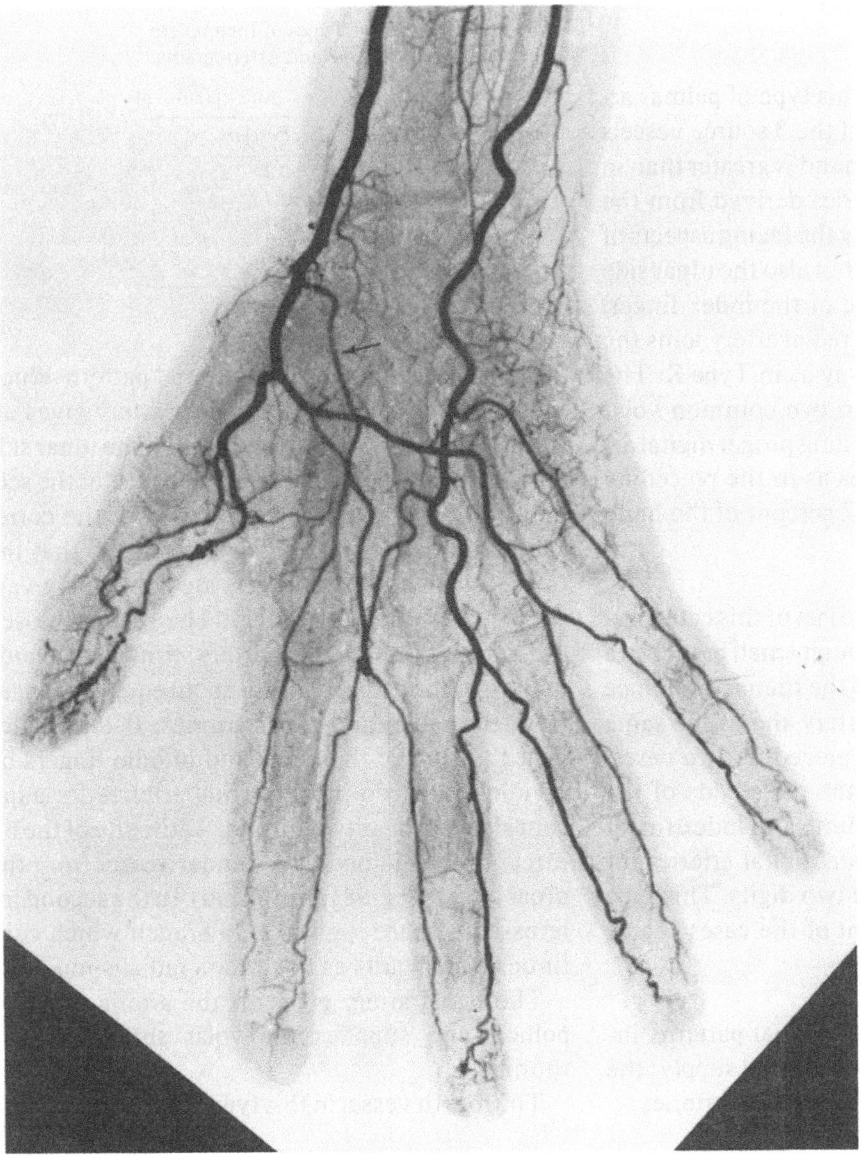

Fig. 93
Incomplete Superficial Arch, Category II, Type G.
The ulnar artery gives off the common volar digital arteries for the second and third interspace and the corresponding proper volar digital arteries as well as the digital artery on the ulnar side of the fifth finger. The superficial ramus of the radial artery (arrow) descends in the palm and continues as the arteria radialis indicis.

teries. On the basis of the arterial pattern three different types can be distinguished in this category: Type K, Type L and Type M (Fig. 94). Incomplete superficial arches of this category appeared in 2.1 percent of the present series (Table XX).

Type K is a radiomediano-ulnar type in which the ulnar artery is the origin of the common volar digital arteries for the third and fourth interspaces and the proper volar digital arteries for adjacent sides of the third, fourth and fifth fingers. The median artery together with the superficial ramus of the radial artery gives off the proper volar digital arteries for the ulnar side of the index finger and radial side of the middle finger. The two arteries anastomose near the cleft of these fingers (II and III) (Fig. 94). This type of arterial pattern and the remaining two of the same category appeared to be infrequent.

Each of them was found in only 0.7 percent of our cases (Table XX).

Type L (Figs 94 and 95). In this type of palmar arterial supply, the deviation of the 3 source vessels toward the radial side of the hand is greater than in the preceding type; the arteries derived from the median artery supply not only the facing aspects of the index and middle fingers but also the ulnar side of the thumb and radial side of the index finger. The superficial ramus of the radial artery joins the median artery in the same way as in Type K. The ulnar artery, by dividing into two common volar digital arteries and corresponding proper digital arteries, supplies the same area as in the preceding type. Type L was seen on 0.7 percent of the hand arteriograms (Table XX).

Type M (Figs. 94 and 96) is the last of this category; the radial artery supplies through small branches a very small superficial area of the thenar eminence and the thumb. The ulnar artery shows the same branching pattern as in the preceding two cases. The median artery reaches the radial side of the hand; near the cleft of the thumb and index finger it divides into two appropriate digital arteries for the adjacent aspects of these two digits. This type was also found in 0.7 percent of the cases (Table XX).

d. Category IV comprises all arterial patterns involving four arteries for palmar arterial supply: the radial, ulnar, median and interosseous arteries.

TABLE XX

Incidence of Different Types of Incomplete Superficial Arch on 288 Hand Arteriograms. From Category III

Type	*Number*	*Percent*
K	2	0.7
L	2	0.7
M	2	0.7
Total	6	2.1

Type N (Fig. 98) is the only arterial pattern which falls into this category. The ulnar artery gives off the digital artery of the fifth finger on the ulnar side and three common volar digital arteries for the second, third and fourth interspaces with the corresponding proper volar digital arteries, so that the third, fourth and fifth fingers are completely vascularized by the ulnar artery. The second vessel, the anterior interosseous artery, runs distalwards in front of the carpal bones at about equal distances from the radial and ulnar arteries. It terminates near the cleft of the index and middle fingers by dividing into two proper digital arteries for adjacent sides of these two fingers. At the site of the bifurcation it is joined by a slender vessel from the ulnar artery (Fig. 98; arrow head). In the second interosseous space it gives off a branch which continues distalwards as the arteria radialis indicis.

The radial artery gives off the arteria princeps pollicis and supplies the volar surface of the thumb.

The fourth vessel in this type of incomplete arch

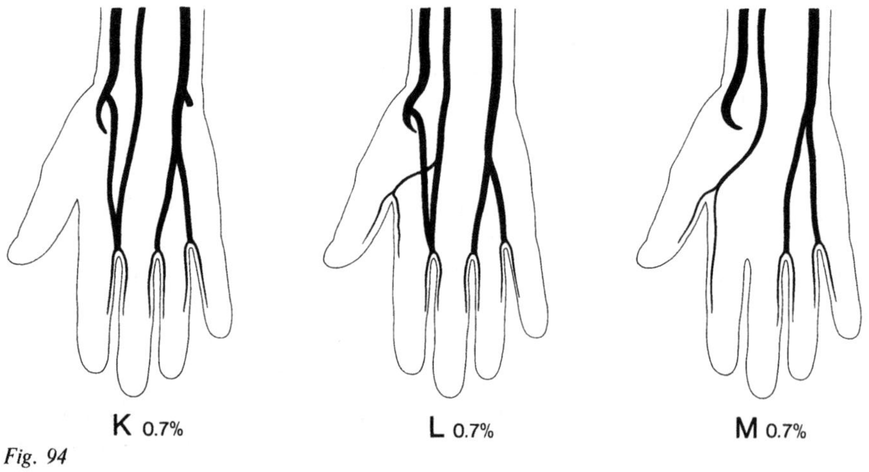

Fig. 94
Different types of incomplete superficial arch. Category III.

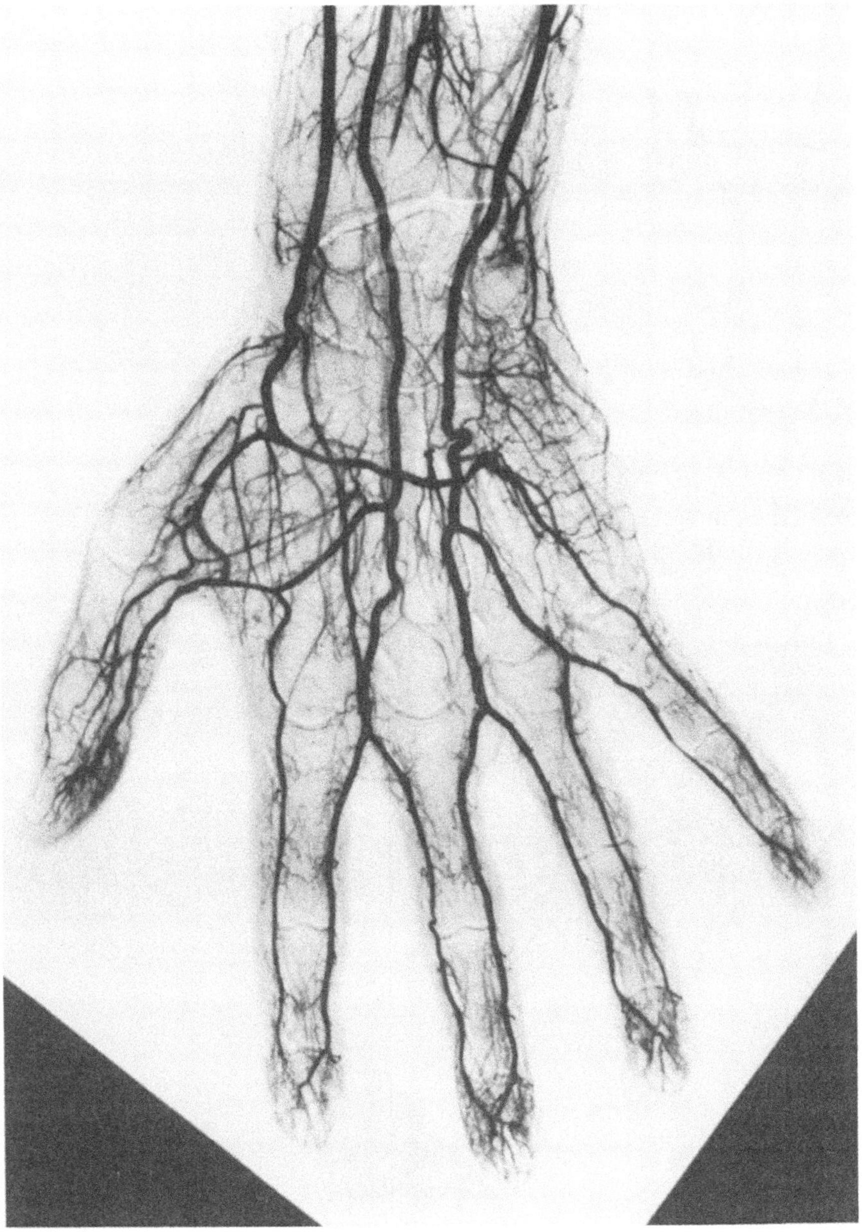

Fig. 95
Incomplete Superficial Arch, Category III, Type L.
In this variation of the superficial volar supply to the hand the ulnar artery gives off the third and fourth common volar digital arteries and the proper volar digital arteries for adjacent sides of the third, fourth and fifth fingers. The median artery supplies the index finger and part of the thumb. The superficial ramus of the radial artery joins the median artery near the cleft of the second and third fingers. The arteria princeps pollicis arises from the radial artery.

is the median artery. In the present case, it is a short slender vessel which terminates by dividing into two small branches: one for the proximal part of the volar surface of the thumb and another for the thenar eminence. This type, in which the volar interosseous artery takes part in the blood supply to the hand or contributes to the formation of the superficial arch, represents according to Manners-Smith (1910) a very primitive condition. In the present series two examples of this pattern were found (0.7%), in both hands of the same individual (Table XXI).

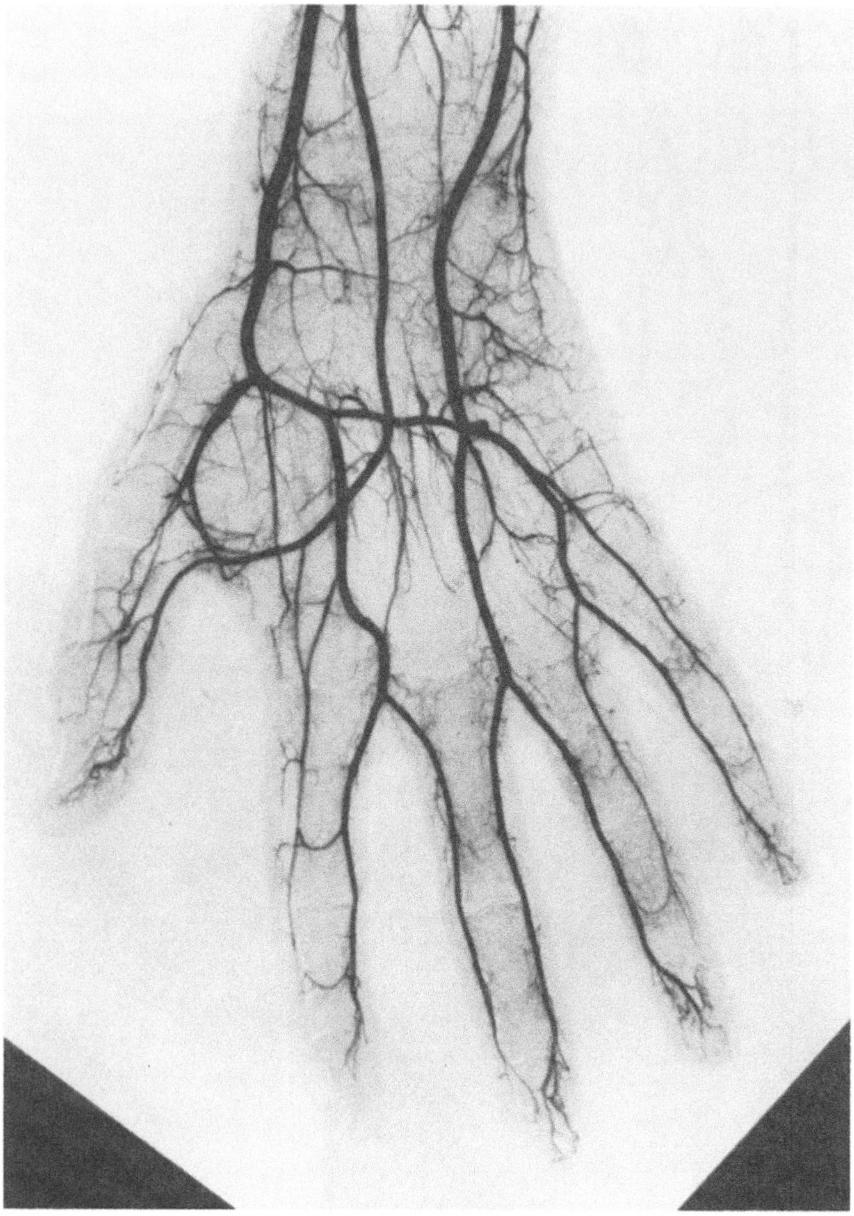

Fig. 96
Incomplete Superficial Arch, Category III, Type M.
The ulnar artery gives off the third and fourth common volar digital arteries, which in turn divide into the appropriate digital arteries for the adjacent surfaces of the third, fourth and fifth fingers. It also is the origin of the digital artery for the fifth finger on the ulnar side. The median artery gives off the arteria princeps pollicis and a small branch to the radial side of the index finger. The radial artery supplies the thenar eminence and gives off branches to the volar side of the thumb.

6.9 Other Observations and Discussion

6.9.1 The Calibre of The Deep and The Superficial Volar Arches

Out of 500 hand arteriograms, 245 (49%) were used for a comparison of the calibre of the deep and superficial volar arches. The measurements were taken at the midline of the palm at the point where the convexity of the arches is usually most pronounced.

It has been found that the deep volar arch had

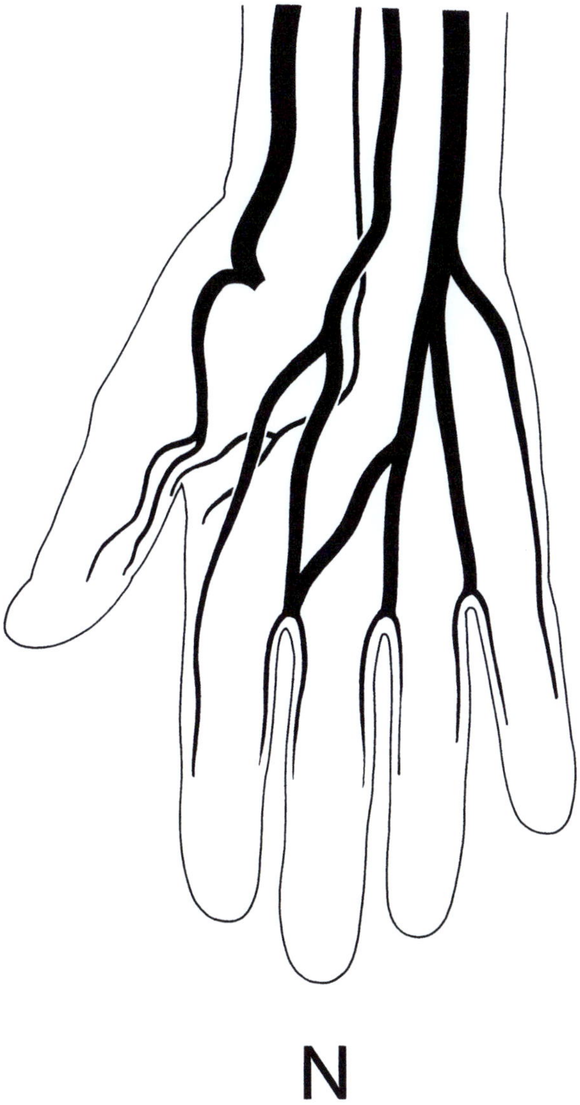

Fig. 97
Schematic diagram of incomplete superficial arch. Category IV. Type N.

the larger calibre in 130 cases (53.0%). The superficial volar arch had the larger calibre in 45 cases (18.4%). In 70 cases, or 28.6 percent of the cases, the arches were of the same calibre. It was noted in almost all cases of unequal diameters, that an inverse ratio between the calibre of the deep volar arch and that of the corresponding superficial arch existed.

TABLE XXI

Incidence of Different Types of Incomplete Superficial Arch on 288 Hand Arteriograms.

From Category IV

Type	*Number*	*Percent*
N	2	0.7
Total	2	0.7

6.9.2 Branches of the Superficial Volar Arch

In all cases of a complete superficial volar arch, the arch is the origin of a variable number of small branches to the surrounding muscles and skin as well as the common volar digital arteries.

6.9.3 The Common Volar Digital Arteries
(Aa. digitales volares communes) (Fig. 61)

In the majority of cases these arteries are three in number. They arise from the convexity of the superficial arch, extend distalwards through the interdigital webs of the second, third and fourth interosseous spaces and unite with the corresponding volar metacarpal arteries to form short trunks which divide at the level of the metacarpophalangeal joints, each into two proper volar arteries for adjacent sides of the respective digits.

a. Variations

It is customarily stated that there are three common volar digital arteries. In our experience, a great variation in the number of these arteries exists. We found three arteries on 58 percent of the hand arteriograms, two on 40.4 percent and only one artery on 1.6 percent (Table XXII).

It has also been noted that an inverse ratio exists between the calibre of a common volar digital artery and that of the corresponding volar metacarpal artery, *e.g.* if a common volar digital artery is small in calibre, then the corresponding metacarpal artery is usually larger. When a common volar

TABLE XXII

Number of Common Volar Digital Arteries Found on 500 Hand Arteriograms.

Number of arteries	*Number of arteriograms*	*Percent*
One	8	1.6
Two	202	40.4
Three	290	58.0
Total	500	100

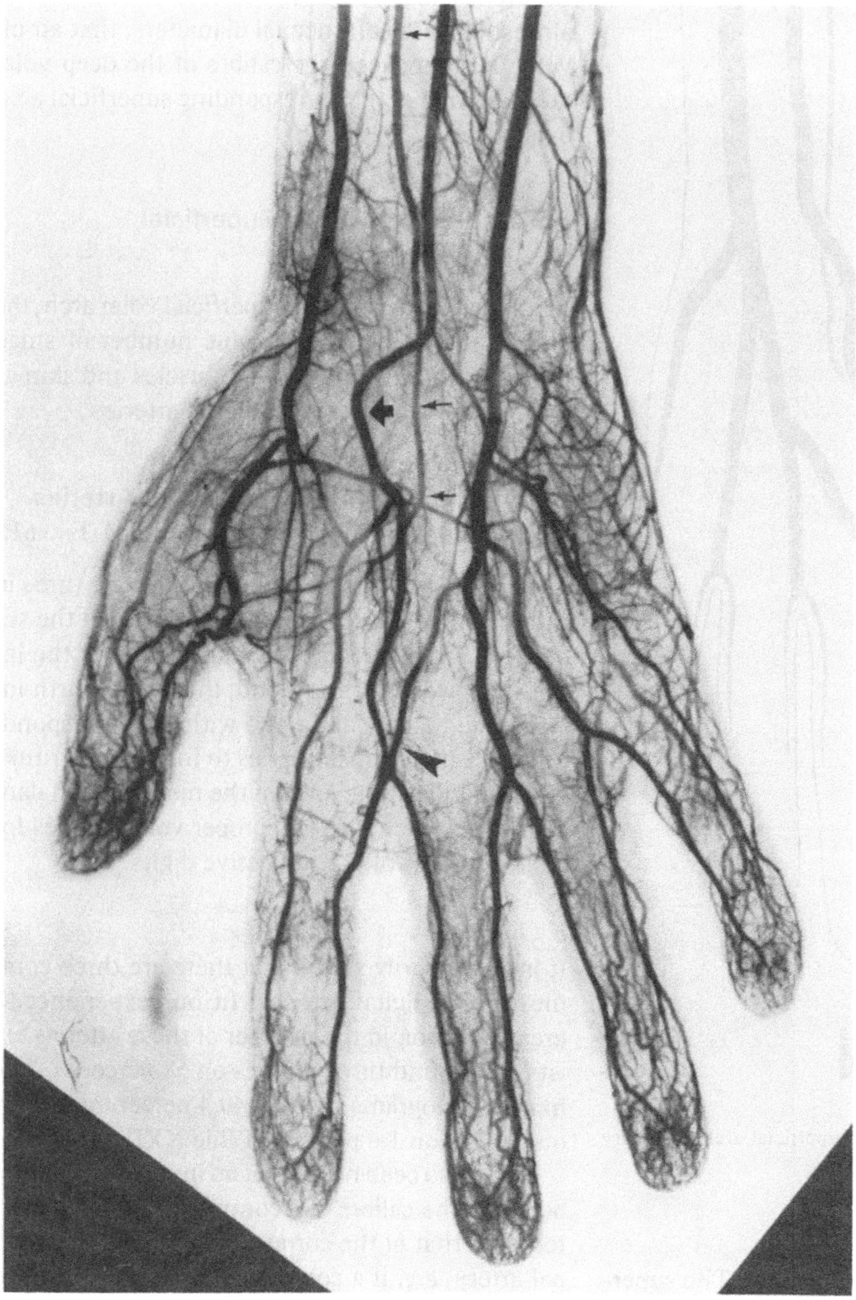

Fig. 98
Superficial Incomplete Arch of Category IV, Type N.
In this 'four vessel' type the ulnar artery completely supplies the last three fingers. The volar interosseous artery (large arrow) supplies the index finger. The radial artery gives off the arteria princeps pollicis and small branches to the thenar eminence. The median artery (small arrows) gives off a small branch to the thumb and another to the thenar eminence. Arrow head indicates a small branch of the ulnar artery extending to the termination of the volar interosseous artery.

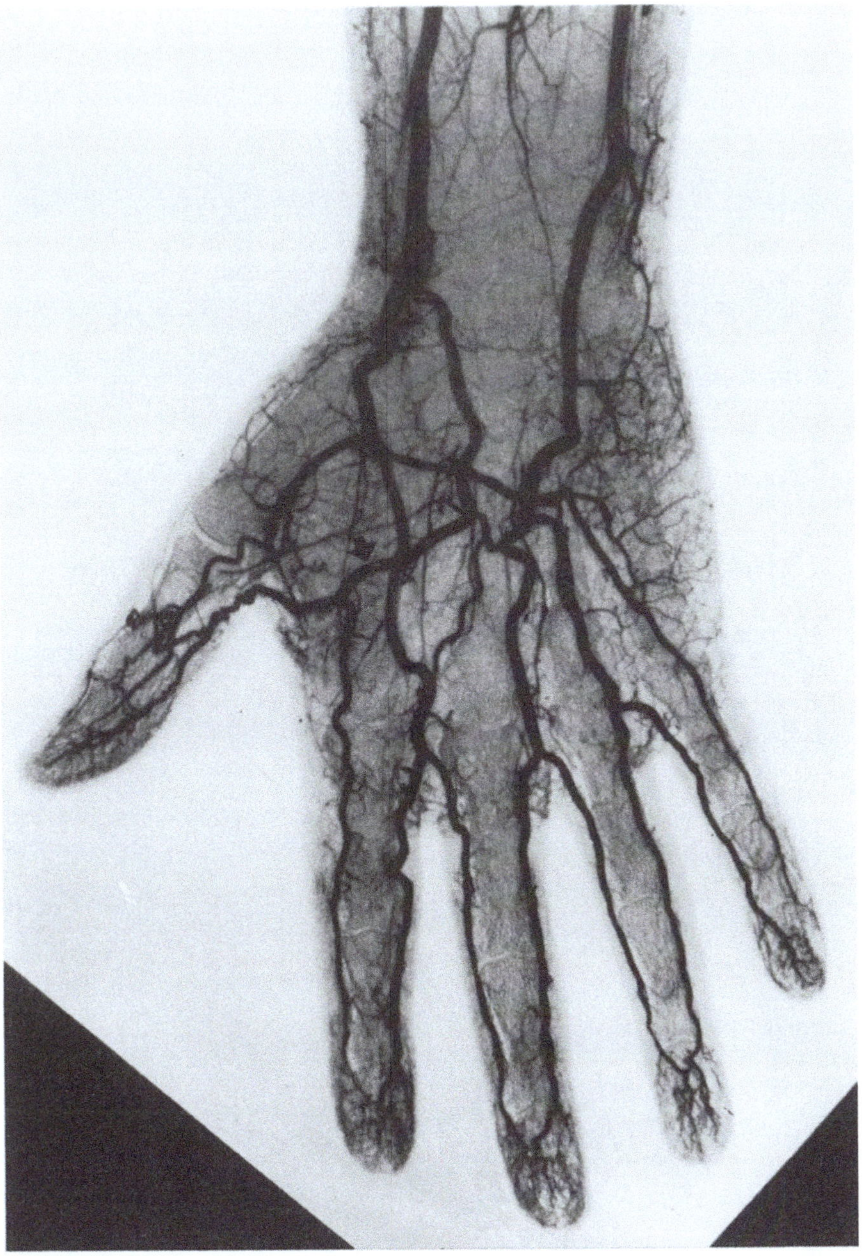

Fig. 99
Tandler's artery in a complete superficial volar arch is the last branch of the superficial arch (arrow) on the radial side, which gives off the arteria radialis indicis and a second artery for the volar side of the thumb.

digital artery is completely absent, then its area of supply is nourished by the corresponding volar metacarpal artery, which in such cases is always hypertrophic (Fig. 83).

We have observed that the digital artery which supplies the ulnar side of the fifth finger arises in 41.0 percent of the cases from the medial side of the superficial arch just below the place where the ulnar artery turns to the radial side to form the superficial volar arch. The same artery was seen to arise more often from the deep volar arch, namely in 59.0 percent of the cases.

6.9.4 Tandler's Artery (Figs. 99 and 100)

The last branch of the superficial arch on the radial

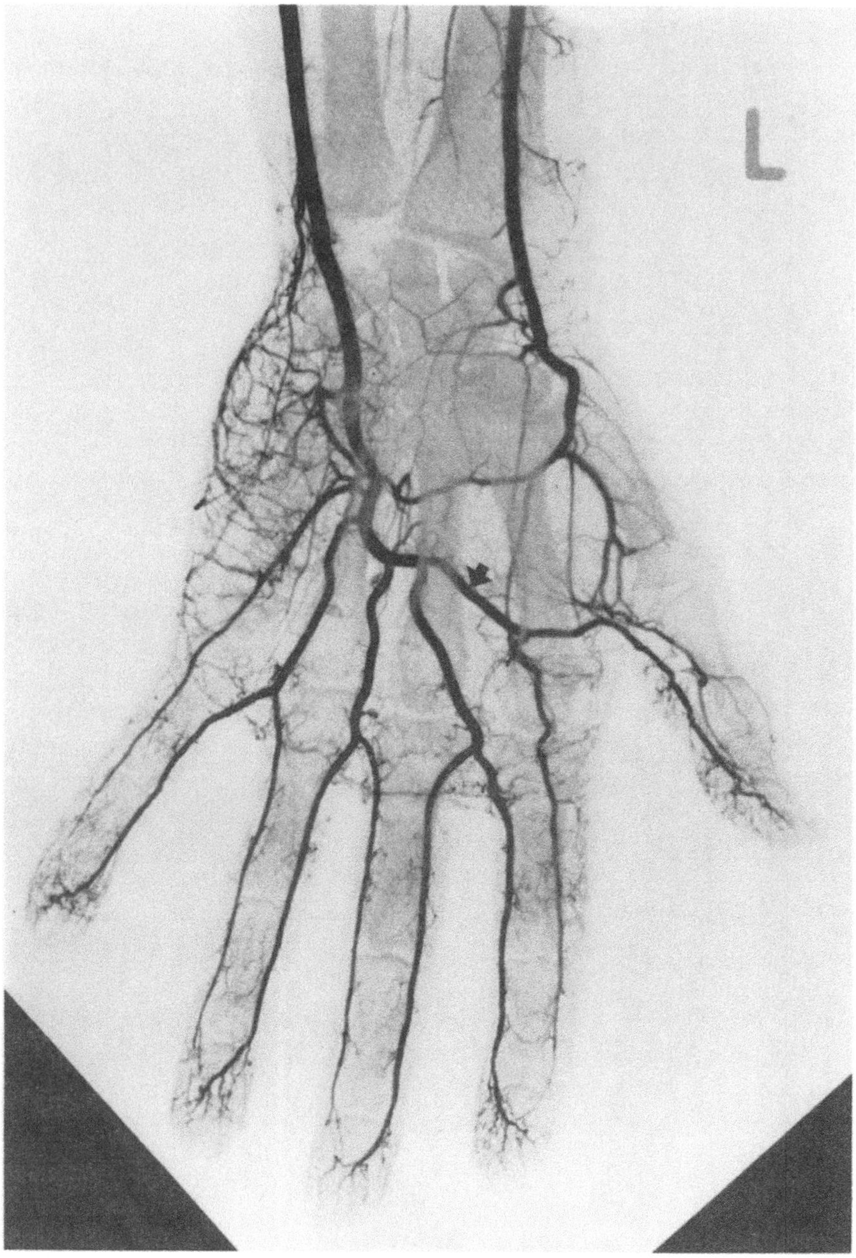

Fig. 100
Tandler's artery in an incomplete superficial volar arch is the termination of the ulnar artery (arrow), which by dividing into two arteries supplies the radial side of the index finger and the ulnar side of the thumb.

side, or the final termination of the ulnar artery in the palm in cases of incomplete superficial arches, is often an artery which by dividing into two branches supplies both the radial side of the index finger and the ulnar side of the thumb.

This artery is usually smaller compared with other common volar digital arteries of the superficial arch. In rare cases it may have the same calibre or even be larger.

In 1897 Julius Tandler called this vessel the first common volar digital artery (arteria digitalis volaris communis prima). This name is generally not accepted, because of the divergent opinions regarding the connections of the superficial volar arch in the first interspace. In our angiographic material Tandler's artery was seen on 14.5 percent of the arteriograms.

6.9.5 Persistent Median Artery

The median artery usually arises from the proximal part of the anterior interosseous artery and is a long slender vessel which descends approximately in the middle of the forearm between the radial and ulnar arteries. In its distal part it may become very small and may end by anastomosing with the termination of the anterior interosseous artery. When this artery is large, it descends as far as the palm and joins in the formation of the superficial volar arterial arch. In the event of a complete superficial volar arch it may replace the radial artery, as seen in type V (Fig. 80), or it may contribute to the formation of the so-called 'three vessels' complete superficial arch, as seen in type VI (Fig. 81). In these arches the median artery appeared on 1.4% of our arteriograms (Table XVII).

In the event of incomplete superficial arches, as described and illustrated in 6.8.2, the median artery was observed in several types of categories III and IV. In all incomplete superficial arches together, the median artery persisted in 2.8 percent of the cases (Tables XX and XXI).

The participation of the median artery in the formation of the superficial volar arch is called by some authors an atavistic characteristic because the median artery is normally found in the volar arch of certain lower animals, and at a late stage in the development of the arteries of the human hand. In the present series of 500 arteriograms, the frequency with which the median artery was involved in the volar supply to the hand was found to be 2.2 percent.

6.9.6 The Proper Volar Digital Arteries
(Aa. digitales volares propriae)

These arteries are terminal branches derived from the common volar digital arteries of the superficial arch. They supply the volar surface of the radial side of the little finger, both sides of the second and third fingers and the ulnar side of the index finger. The radial side of the index finger is supplied by the arteria radialis indicis or (in 14.5 percent) by the medial branch of Tandler's artery. The thumb is supplied by the arteria princeps pollicis.

The proper volar digital arteries pass distalwards towards the ends of the fingers. On their way to the fingertips they anastomose by small transversal branches forming a bridge across the front of the bones on the proximal side of each interphalangeal joint. These anastomoses provide very important collateral connections, in case of occlusion of the contralateral proper digital artery. Each appropriate artery of the finger terminates in a plexus by anastomosis with the proper digital artery from the contralateral side.

6.10 Conclusions

6.10.1 Brachial and Antebrachial Arteries

The variations in the origin and course of the arteries of the upper extremities have long received the attention of anatomists.

The first study was carried out by Laurentius (1600). In 1831 Tiedeman systematically described the variations in the arterial pattern of the upper extremities. Henle (1868) provided an analysis of the large European series studied prior to his time and Poynter in 1920 summarized all series which had appeared up to 1920, adding his own series of 250 specimens.

A complete angiographic study of the variations in the arteries of the upper extremity has not yet been published. Most of the articles which have appeared in the literature were concerned chiefly with single examples of anomalies.

In the present series of 250 arteriograms of the shoulder and arm, variations in the origin and the course of the major branches of the brachial and antebrachial arteries occurred in 32.8% of the cases.

The vertebral artery had an abnormal origin on the left side in 5.5% (see Table IV) and a bifid origin on the same side in 0.6% of the cases. The right vertebral artery had an abnormal origin in two cases (0.6%) where it arose from the right common carotid artery. In both cases an aberrant right subclavian artery was present.

An incomplete thyrocervical trunk, with one of its branches originating directly from the subclavian artery, was found in 16.4% of the cases. The trunk was absent in 31.2 percent; the remaining 52.4% represent a single trunk with all its branches. The costocervical trunk was absent in 11.6% of our series. The highest thoracic artery showed variations on 24% of the arteriograms (absent 16.4%; double 3.6%; triple 0.4% and originating together with thoracoacromial artery in 3.6%).

The thoracoacromial, lateral thoracic and subscapular arteries showed similar variations in their origin. The origin of the lateral thoracic artery was different in 35.6% and that of the subscapular artery in 20.4% of the cases.

The anterior and posterior humeral circumflex arteries arose from a common trunk in 70% of the cases, the remaining 30% showed a variable origin. In most cases they arose separately from the axillary artery, or in common with the deep brachial artery.

In relatively rare cases both humeral circumflex arteries were represented by three of four small branches.

A separate superficial brachial artery was present in 2.4% of the patients. It can be recognized by its proximal origin from the brachial artery and its superficial course along the medial aspect of the arm. McCormack *et al.* (1953) in their series of 750 specimens found this artery 8 times (1.07%). In one of their cases the superficial brachial artery arose from the axillary artery; Gruber (1852) reported 5 cases of a superficial brachial artery in 1200 arms; Quain (1844) found one in 506 and Muller (1903) one in 100 specimens.

The variation in the origin of the radial artery proximal to the elbow joint formed by far the largest group of gross variations. This pattern was observed on 61 arteriograms (24.4%). Within this group the radial artery arose from the axillary artery 13 times (5.2%) (6 on the right side and 7 on the left) and it arose from some part of the brachial artery 48 times (19.2%). The higher origin of the radial artery is indicated in Table XII as a high bifurcation of the brachial artery. It occurred more frequently on the right side (12.4%) than on the left (6.8%) (see Table XII).

McCormack *et al.* (1953) observed this pattern in 14.27 percent of their series.

If the antebrachial arteries are studied, differences in the calibre of the radial and ulnar arteries can be noted. Once we observed a total aplasia of the ulnar artery and once total aplasia of the radial artery. The area of the ulnar artery in the former case was supplied by the branches of the interosseous artery.

The presence of a median artery and other variations closer to the wrist will be discussed together with the variations of the hand arteries.

6.10.2 Arteries of the Hand

The present study shows that the arteries of the hand, despite their many diversified patterns, can be classified into well-defined categories.

On the 500 hand arteriograms analysed in this study, the deep volar arch appeared in its complete form in 95.2 percent of the cases; it was therefore incomplete on only 4.8 percent of the arteriograms. In the recent series of Coleman and Anson (1961) a complete deep volar arch was found in 97.0% of the cases.

In the present series four main types of complete deep volar arch and seven other subtypes were observed. The incomplete deep arch appeared to be less variable; only four patterns were identified.

There are six types of complete superficial arch, divided according to the contributing arteries and the number of common volar digital arteries arising from it. The incomplete superficial arch showed a large number of different patterns, which were classified into four main categories and nineteen types. The complete superficial volar arch appeared in 42.4 percent of the cases, and the incomplete arch in 57.6 percent. Coleman and Anson (1961) found that 78.5 percent of their subjects had a complete superficial arch and 21.5 percent had an incomplete superficial volar arch. These relatively large differences in the percentage with a complete superficial arch noted between an anatomical and a roentgenological study can be explained partially by the observation of some anatomists: that the superficial ramus of the radial artery, in some instances, joins the superficial arch as a fibrotic thread or as a very tiny vessel which probably cannot be opacified at angiography.

The same anatomical findings have been reported for the median artery.

The calibre of the complete deep volar arch was usually the opposite of that of the corresponding superficial arch.

The volar metacarpal arteries, with the exception of those in the first and second interspace, are exceedingly variable as far as number, size and course of distribution are concerned. Most hands (54.6%) have three metacarpal arteries. On the average there are two to four metacarpal arteries in each hand.

A volar metacarpal artery may divide into two branches to join two common volar digital arteries, or it may fail to join its corresponding common volar digital artery. On the other hand, two volar metacarpal arteries may join the same common volar digital artery.

When a volar metacarpal artery is enlarged, the corresponding common volar digital artery from the superficial arch is usually small in calibre. If a branch of the superficial arch is completely absent, the area of supply of that artery may be nourished by a volar metacarpal artery.

The arteria princeps pollicis is a single vessel in 47.6 percent of the cases, but it can be double (52.0%) and even triple (0.4%). It usually arises separately from the radial artery but may originate from a common trunk in some instances. A common origin with the arteria radialis indicis was found in 48 percent of the cases.

The arteria radialis indicis shows a marked variation in its origin; in 30.8 percent of the cases it originated from the metacarpal artery of the first interspace. Occasionally it may originate from the ulnar side of the deep volar arch. The artery may be completely absent; in such instances the area of supply is usually nourished by the medial branch of Tandler's artery.

The common volar digital arteries vary as far as their number is concerned. In most cases there are three arteries (58.0%); two common volar digital arteries were found in 40.4 percent and one artery in 1.6 percent of the cases.

A persistent median artery in the palm of the hand is not a frequent feature. This artery together with the radial and ulnar arteries may participate in the supply of the hand, either with or without forming an anastomosis.

The reported frequency with which the median artery takes part in the formation of the superficial arch varies in the literature; Tandler (1897) in his 160 specimens found 27 cases or 16.1 percent; Jaschtschinski (1897), 7.5 percent; Adachi (1928), 8.0 percent; Gray (1944) 1.1 percent in 452 specimens; Coleman and Anson (1961) in their series of 650 specimens found 64 cases or 9.9 percent. In the present series of 500 arteriograms it was found in 11 cases or 2.2 percent.

The radial, the ulnar, the median and the interosseous arteries may all contribute to the blood supply of the hand. The anterior interosseous artery only contributed twice (1.4%) to the supply of the hand without forming an anastomosis; the artery was present in both hands of the same individual.

This condition is a very rare anomaly. According to Manners-Smith (1910) it represents a much earlier stage of evolution, since it is not even a mammalian characteristic but an amphibious one. Other investigators have also stated that this represents a very primitive condition.

In the present series two examples of this pattern occurred.

The proper volar digital arteries did not show any variations on our 500 hand arteriograms.

REFERENCES

ABBOTT, M. E.: Coarctation of the aorta of the adult type. *A. Heart J., 3: 574-618. 1928.*

ADACHI, B.: Das Arteriensystem der Japaner. *Kyoto, Maruzen Co., Band 1: 29-103, 1928.*

ARKIN, A.: Totale Persistenz des rechten Aortabogens im Röntgenbild. *Wien. Arch. in. Med., 12: 385-416, 1926.*

BOSNIAK, M. A.: An Analysis of some Anatomic-Roentgenologic Aspects of the Brachiocephalic Vessels. *Amer. J. Roentg., 91: 1222-1231, 1964.*

COLEMAN, S. S. and B. J. ANSON: Arterial Patterns in the Hand Based Upon A Study of 650 Specimens. *Surgery Gynec. & Obst., 113: 409-442, 1961.*

FISHMAN, N. H., M. H. BERMAN, W. BENSON, R. B. EDMUNDS Jr., L. H. ROBINSON and A. M. RUDOLPH: Surgical management of severe aortic coarctation and interruptured aortic arch in neonates. *J. Thor. cardiovasc. Surg. 71: 35-47, 1976.*

GRAY, H.: Anatomy of The Human Body. Edited by *W. H. Lewis, Lea & Febiger, 24th ed. Philadelphia, 1944.*

GRUBER, W. L.: Cited by Henle (1868) and McCormack *et al.* (1953).

HAUGHTON, V. M., K. E. FELLOWS and A. E. ROSENBAU: The cervical aortic arches. *Radiology, 114: 675-681, 1975.*

HENLE, J.: Handbuch der systematischen Anatomie des Menschen. *Vol. 3., Braunschweig: Vieweg, 1868.*

JASCHTSCHINSKI, S. N.: Morphologie und Topographie des Arcus Volaris Sublimis und Profundus. *Anat. Hefte, 7: 163-188, 1897.*

KELLER, F. S., J. RÖSCH, C. DOTTER and J. M. PORTER: Proximal Origin of Radial Artery: Potential Pitfall in Hand Angiography. *Am. J. Roentg., 134: 169-170, 1980.*

KLINKHAMER, A. C.: Het vaststellen van aberante arterieën in het mediastinum superius d.m.v. het oesophagogram. *Thesis, Leiden 1-187, 1962.*

KLINKHAMER, A. C.: Oesophagography in anomalies of the aortic arch system. *Baltimore, The Williams & Wilkins Co. 1969.*

KOMMERALL, B.: Verlagerung des Oesophagus durch eine Abnormal verlaufende A. subclavia dextra (A. lusoria). *Fortschr. Röntgenstr. 54: 590-595, 1936.*

LANZ von, T. und WACHSMUTH: Praktische Anatomie. *Band: 1, Teil 3 Arm. 195-217, 1959.*

LAURENTIUS (1600): Cited by F. Tiedeman (1831) and L. J. McCormack *et al.* (1953).

LIE, T. A.: Congenital Anomalies of the Carotid Arteries. *Amsterdam. Excerpta Med. Found. 1-30, 1968.*

MCCORMACK, L. J., E. W. CAULDWELL and B. J. ANSON: Brachial and Antebrachial Arterial Patterns. *Surg. Gynaecol. Obst., 96: 43-54, 1953.*

MANNERS-SMITH, T.: The Limb Arteries of Primates. *J. Anat. Physiol., 45: 23-64, 1910.*

MOLZ, G.: Abnormaler Abgang der Aa. Subclaviae, Häufigeres Vorkommen beim weiblichen Geschlächt. *Bas. Res. Cardiol. 71: 420-427, 1976.*

MOLZ, G. and B. BURRI: Aberrant subclavian artery (Arteria Lusoria): Six differences in the Prevalence of Various Forms of the Malformation. *Virchows Arch. Path. Anat. and Histol. 380: 303-315, 1978.*

MOORE, T. S.: Aortic Arch Vessels Anomalies Associated with Persistent Trigeminal Artery. *Am J. Roentg., 133: 309-311, 1979.*

MULLER, E.: Die Arm Arterieën des Menschen. *Anat. Hefte, 22: 379-574, 1903.*

NATH, P. H., CASTANEDA-ZUNIGA and C. L. ZOLLIKOFER: Anusual Aberrant Left Subclavian Artery. *Radiology, 134: 17-18, 1980.*

PATURET, G.: Traité D'Anatomie Humaine. *Paris, Masson & C, éd., Tome 2: 375-428, 1951.*

POYNTER, C. W. M.: Congenital anomalies of the arteries and veins of the human body. *University studies. Univ. of Nebraska, 22: 1-106, 1920.*

PRAAGH, van R., W. F. BERNARD, A. ROSENTHAL, L. F. PARISI and D. C. FYLER: Interrupted aortic arch: Surgical Treatment. *Am. J. Cardiol. 27: 200-211, 1970.*

QUAIN, R.: The Anatomy of the Arteries of the Human Body. *Taylor & Walton, London, 1844.*

QUIRING, D. P.: Collateral Circulation (Anatomical Aspects). *pp. 108-119, Lea and Febiger Co., Philadelphia, 1949.*

RADKE, H. M.: Arterial Circulation of the Upper Extremity. In Collateral Circulation in Clinical surgery, by *D. E. Strandness jr. pp.: 294-307, W. B. Saunders, Philadelphia, 1969.*

RAIDER, L.: Aberrant Right Subclavian Artery. *S. Med. Jour., 60: 145-151, 1967.*

RICHTER, K., G. WILLAMOWSKI and K. MOTSCH: Über die Bedeutung der A. lusoria bei Koarktation der Aorta. *Fortschr. Röntgenstr. 104: 766-772, 1966.*

SHUFORD, W. H., R. G. SYBERS and P. C. SCHLANT: The cervical aortic arch. *Am. J. Roentg. Radiom. ther. Nucl. Med. 116: 519-527, 1972.*

SHUFORD, W. H., R. G. SYBERS and F. K. EDWARDS: The Three Types of Right Aortic Arch. *Am. J. Roentg. 109: 67-74, 1970.*

TANDLER, J.: Zur Anatomie der Arterien der Hand. *Anat. Hefte, 7: 264-288, 1897.*

THOMAS, T. V.: Looped Innominate Artery. *J. Thor. Card., 54: 719-722, 1967.*

TIEDEMAN, F.: Manual of Angiology. (Trans. by R. Knox). *MacLachlan and Stewart, Edinburgh, 1831.*

WARWICK, R. and P. L. WILLIAMS: Gray's Anatomy. *35th edition, Longman 6: 645-656, 1973.*

Chapter 7

VASCULAR INJURIES OF THE UPPER EXTREMITY

General Remarks

Many injuries involve the arteries of the upper extremity. It is most important to recognize such injuries and institute proper treatment, since delayed or no treatment frequently results in loss of limb or permanent disability (Gill *et al.*, 1976).

Arterial injuries frequently accompany major fractures or dislocations of the upper extremities. In more than 50 percent of the cases they are caused by blunt trauma resulting from traffic accidents.

The anatomical vascular alterations include arterial spasm, external compression, partial laceration with subsequent formation of a false aneurysm, arterial thrombosis due to contusion, intimal disruption with vascular occlusion, injury to neighbouring artery and vein with formation of an arteriovenous fistula and total transection of the artery (Shuck *et al.*, 1972; Slaney and Ashton, 1971; Louis *et al.*, 1974).

7.1 Different Types of Injury: Signs and Symptoms

Penetrating as well as blunt trauma of an extremity can cause several different forms of arterial damage.

A contused artery immediately constricts resulting in a severe arterial spasm and total occlusion of the arterial lumen. Signs of excessive bleeding such as shock or formation of a massive haematoma are unusual in this type of injury. The clinical and physical signs are ischaemic pain and pallor, absence of distal pulses and neurological symptoms such as paraesthesia and paralysis.

A blunt injury of the tissues may result in oedema and haemorrhage to such an extent that compression or displacement of an artery occurs.

Partial laceration of an artery is characterized by excessive bleeding, because the intact portion of the arterial wall effectively holds the defect open permitting continued or recurrent haemorrhage. The soft tissue contains the blood around the partially transected vessel. Progressive bleeding leads to enlargement of the haematoma and the simultaneous formation of a pseudo-encapsulation in the soft tissue. Finally the organized haematoma which surrounds the arterial injury develops a large central cavity in communication with the arterial lumen, forming a so-called 'false aneurysm' (Saletta *et al.*, 1970; Louis *et al.*, 1974).

An arteriovenous fistula can develop if the false aneurysm ruptures into a vein or the adjacent artery and vein are perforated simultaneously.

If a pseudoaneurysm or arteriovenous fistula is suspected, careful auscultation of the area of injury is mandatory. A systolic bruit is frequently symptomatic of a partial arterial injury with an accompanying false aneurysm.

If an arteriovenous fistula is present a continuous bruit is heard, particularly if the former is quite large (Saletta and Freeark, 1970).

A posttraumatic false aneurysm may occur directly after the trauma or within hours, days or weeks after the trauma. In some instances distal oedema of the limb can be observed, as a result of venous obstruction by the mass (Crawford *et al.*, 1959). Another form of arterial injury is *intimal dis-*

ruption. This usually follows blunt trauma such as dislocation of a major joint. In this situation a crack in the intima develops but the tunica media and the adventitia remain intact. The arterial stream may then dissect the intima from the tunica media which can result in occlusion and thrombosis of the vessel.

On physical examination immediately after the trauma the distal pulses may be normal but this can gradually change to severe impairment of the circulation.

The last form of arterial injury is total *transection* of an artery. A history of excessive blood loss at the time of the accident will be the first clue that a major vascular injury has occurred, particularly if the bleeding was noted to be pulsatile (Spencer, 1962). On physical examination the most constant finding accompanying an arterial transection is the presence of an unusually large or expanding haematoma at the site of the vascular injury. On occasion, the haematoma may be pulsatile, making the diagnosis more obvious.

Aneurysms that develop as a result of trauma can be classified as true aneurysms and false aneurysms.

True aneurysms resulting from traumatic degeneration of the arterial wall are very rare (Green, 1973).

False aneurysms usually develop after penetrating trauma of the vessels, less frequently as a consequence of severe blunt trauma. Several authors have reported the high incidence of false aneurysms following penetrating and blunt wounds (Bowie and Kay, 1949; Seeley *et al.*, 1952; Spittal, 1958; Narsete, 1964; Engelman *et al.*, 1969; Rich *et al.*, 1970; Winegarder *et al.*, 1970; Kleinert *et al.*, 1973).

False aneurysms may occur at any location where the vessel is perforated but in the upper extremity they have been reported most often in the antecubital fossa and in the radial artery at the wrist.

7.2 Traumatic Diseases of the Arteries of the Proximal Part of the Upper Extremity

Literature

Traumatic arterial injuries of the upper extremity can be classified as open and closed arterial injuries.

The open arterial injuries are usually obvious, because of severe haemorrhage, distal ischaemia, paralysis, anaesthesia and absence of pulses. Closed arterial injuries usually follow crushing and are most commonly associated with fractures.

7.2.1 Injuries of the Innominate and Subclavian Arteries

Injuries of the innominate and subclavian arteries are relatively uncommon compared to trauma of the peripheral arteries. These vessels are protected by surrounding bony structures including the clavicle, costal cartilages and ribs. On the other hand, when these bony structures are fractured or dislocated they may contribute to the trauma of the vessels (Rich *et al.*, 1973).

At the thoracic aperture the innominate artery runs upwards and then lateralwards behind the right sternoclavicular joint. A retrosternal dislocation of the clavicle, which is an uncommon injury compared to acromioclavicular dislocation, may result in injury or compression of the innominate, the subclavian or the right common carotid artery (Patterson, 1965).

The subclavian artery passes between the middle third of the clavicle and the first rib into the axilla. In this costoclavicular space the artery is accompanied by the subclavian vein and the brachial plexus. Injuries in or close to the costoclavicular space may damage this neurovascular bundle. The vascular injuries at this site include complete transection of the subclavian vessels, external compression, thrombosis, aneurysmal dilatation and arteriovenous fistulae. These complications may appear after fractures of the middle and medial third of the clavicle, posterior sternoclavicular dislocation and proliferative callus formation (Wholey *et al.*, 1967).

Several well recognized injuries of the subclavian artery associated with medial clavicular fractures have been reported in the literature.

Complete transection of the subclavian artery associated with a clavicular fracture was reported by Gryska in 1962. Subclavian artery thrombosis as a complication of nonunion of a clavicular fracture was reported by Guilfoil *et al.* (1967). De Bakey *et al.* (1965) recorded a case of a clavicular fracture complicated by aneurysmal dilatation of the subclavian artery.

Lateral clavicular fractures are usually not associated with trauma of the subclavian vessels, the major complicating factors in these fractures are cosmetic deformation of the clavicle or pseudoarthrosis (Neer, 1970).

7.2.2 Injuries of the Axillary Artery

Numerous cases of rupture of the axillary artery in association with humerus fractures characterized by considerable dislocation of the fragments and anterior dislocation of the shoulder joint have been reported by several authors. In a review of the literature, Johnson and Lowry in 1962 stated that approximately 100 cases of arterial injury associated with fractures and anterior dislocation of the head of humerus have been reported since 1825. The axillary artery or its circumflex humeral branch are the vessels most commonly involved. In isolated uncomplicated shoulder dislocations, injuries of the axillary artery are relatively rare. Approximately 90 percent of the shoulder dislocations are anterior, with the common site being in front of and inferior to the coracoid process in the recessus subscapularis. A subsequent injury of the axillary artery is uncommon, since the muscles which arise from the coracoid process act as a protective cushion (Wholey and Bocher, 1967).

Injuries of the axillary artery resulting from a simple fracture of the neck of humerus without shoulder dislocation are relatively rare. De Bakey and Simeone (1946), in their series of 2,471 cases of acute arterial lesions, reported seven cases of injury of the axillary artery associated with fractures of the humerus. Their survey concerned multiple war wounds and it is not clear how many injuries of the axillary artery occurred in association with simple fractures of the neck of humerus. Morris did not mention one single case of an arterial lesion resulting from a fracture of the neck of humerus in his series of 220 acute arterial injuries in civilian practice (Morris *et al.*, 1960). In recent literature five other cases of injury of the axillary artery together with a fracture of the neck of humerus have been reported by Smyth (1960), LeBorgne *et al.* (1973) and Theodorides *et al.* (1976). This illustrates the low frequency of injuries of the axillary artery together with fractures of the neck of humerus.

7.2.3 Injuries of the Brachial Artery

The proximal part of the brachial artery descends on the medial side of the humerus while the distal section passes in front. The course of this artery along the medial aspect of the arm is quite superficial. It lies anterior to the medial muscular septum, between the biceps and brachial muscles. Because of its superficial course, injuries most commonly occur following penetrating or blunt trauma of the extremity. The most common types of fracture of the humerus, namely an impacted neck fracture or spiral fracture of the humeral shaft, do not normally cause vascular injury. However, a severe blunt trauma of the extremity may result in compression of the brachial artery against the shaft of the humerus with subsequent contusion of the vascular wall and complete occlusion of the vessel. This is the most frequently seen injury of the brachial artery (Makin *et al.*, 1966).

The distal brachial artery may be injured by a fracture or dislocation of the elbow joint. Supracondylar fractures of the humerus are the most common type, particularly in children. In these fractures the distal fragment is usually displaced posteriorly while the anterior aspect of the proximal part occasionally protrudes through the brachial muscle, severing the brachial artery. There are reports in the literature that the brachial artery in oblique supracondylar fractures may be displaced behind the distal end of the proximal fragment, with no evidence of disturbed circulation. When closed repositioning is attempted by traction, the vessel may be compressed between the fragments resulting in circulatory ischaemia of the distal extremity. This ischaemia is relieved when traction is released (Staples, 1965).

Dislocation of the elbow is a relatively common traumatic injury (Kilburn *et al.*, 1962). There are many cases reported in the literature of injury of the brachial artery associated with dislocation of the elbow. In most of these cases the dislocation of the elbow is a closed injury. Open dislocations of the elbow are almost always complicated, with total *transection* of the brachial artery (Marnham 1934; Jackson 1940; Spear and Janes, 1951; Henderson and Robertson, 1952; Friedmann, 1961; Kilburn *et al.*, 1962).

Linscheid and Wheeler (1965) reviewed the Mayo Clinic patient material involving 110 elbow dislocations and found laceration or thrombosis of the brachial artery in six cases or 5.5 percent.

Because the collateral arterial network of the upper extremity is particularly extensive around the elbow, an interruption of the brachial artery just above the bifurcation usually will not lead to severe ischaemia (Aufranc *et al.*, 1966). The classical review by De Bakey and Simeone (1946) of arterial war wounds reports that combat injuries involving interruption of the brachial artery ended in amputation in 54 out of 209 cases (26%). When the lesion of the brachial artery was so proximal that it included the deep brachial artery, the incidence of amputation was approximately doubled. The authors pointed out that war injuries are usually complicated by gross contamination and by unavoidable delay in definitive surgical care.

In recent years it has been shown experimentally that in the event of posterior dislocation of the elbow, not only the brachial artery can be disrupted but also the anterior collateral arteries of the elbow. In 1974 Louis *et al.* performed an anatomical post mortem study of the elbow collaterals in 14 fresh upper extremities in which a posterior dislocation of the elbow was produced by forceful hyperextension.

After dissection of the vascular anastomoses around the elbow, they found in thirteen specimens a disruption of the anastomosis between the inferior ulnar collateral and anterior ulnar recurrent branch, which runs ventral to the elbow joint. In one specimen in which a posteromedial dislocation was produced, the anastomotic vessels were not disrupted.

When an isolated occlusion of the brachial artery occurs at the elbow, the two anterior and two posterior collateral channels are probably sufficient to maintain the distal flow. Therefore injuries of the distal brachial artery carry in general a much more favourable prognosis than those of the subclavian or axillary artery.

However, if the arm is markedly ischaemic and surgical exploration reveals no evidence of collateral pulsatile arterial flow, arterial reconstruction is clearly indicated (Aufranc *et al.*, 1966).

7.2.4 Angiography

The value of arteriography in peripheral vascular injuries has been stressed in several reports (Lumpkin *et al.*, 1958; Sinkler and Spencer, 1960; Love and Braun, 1968; Wenz, 1968; Smith, 1963; Piyachon *et al.*, 1973; Enge, 1975).

In all instances when clinical differentiation between thrombosis, spasm and laceration is not possible, arteriography is indicated (Wholey and Bocher, 1967). Suspected injuries of the proximal

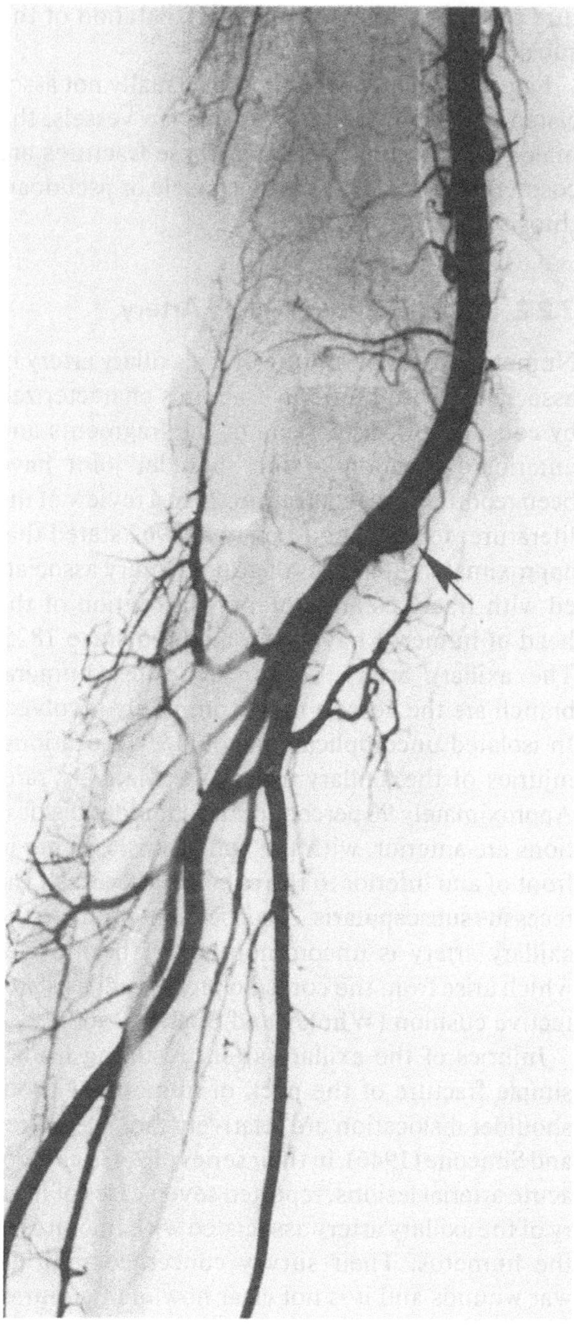

Fig. 101
Small aneurysm of the medial wall of the distal brachial artery in patient with history of blunt trauma of the elbow in the past (arrow).

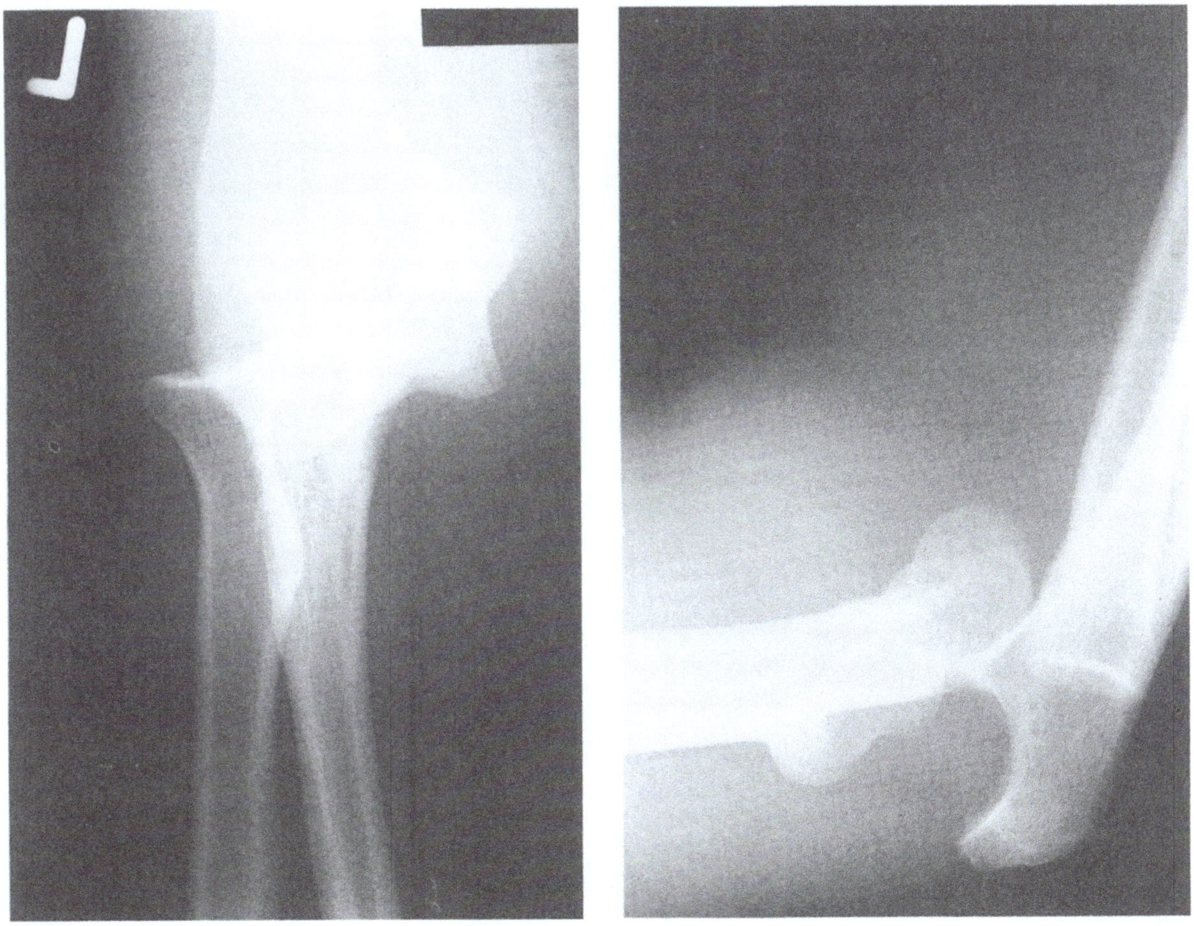

a b

Fig. 102
Initial roentgenograms of the left elbow in two projections show an obvious posterior dislocation.

vessels are best evaluated by the catheterization technique, which permits selective cannulation of an injured vessel under direct fluoroscopic control as well as pressure injection and multiple exposures. Injuries of the brachial and forearm arteries can be evaluated either by the catheterization technique or by direct needle puncture. In these cases the injection of contrast medium is usually administered manually.

Angiographic studies permit localization of the site of the arterial injury and demonstration of the collateral circulation, which undoubtedly is very helpful for planning proper treatment. Arteriograms may also demonstrate multiple unsuspected arterial lesions due to small penetrating wounds.

On angiograms the following signs of arterial trauma may be encountered.

In the case of *complete transection* of the artery an abrupt termination of the contrast medium column is usually seen on the arteriograms. The collaterals which fill the artery distal to the transection may also be demonstrated.

In traumatic *thrombosis* arteriography demonstrates a blockage of the flow of the contrast medium. At the proximal end of the thrombus a convex or polypoid filling defect in the contrast column can be seen.

Acute *bleeding* into the soft tissue is demonstrated by extravasation of the contrast medium.

A circumferential compression of an artery with or without displacement of the vessel is characteristic of oedema and haemorrhage within a closed compartment.

Arteriovenous fistula is demonstrated on the arteriograms by early dense opacification of the veins, which are often enlarged.

A *pseudoaneurysm* can be seen as an extralumi-

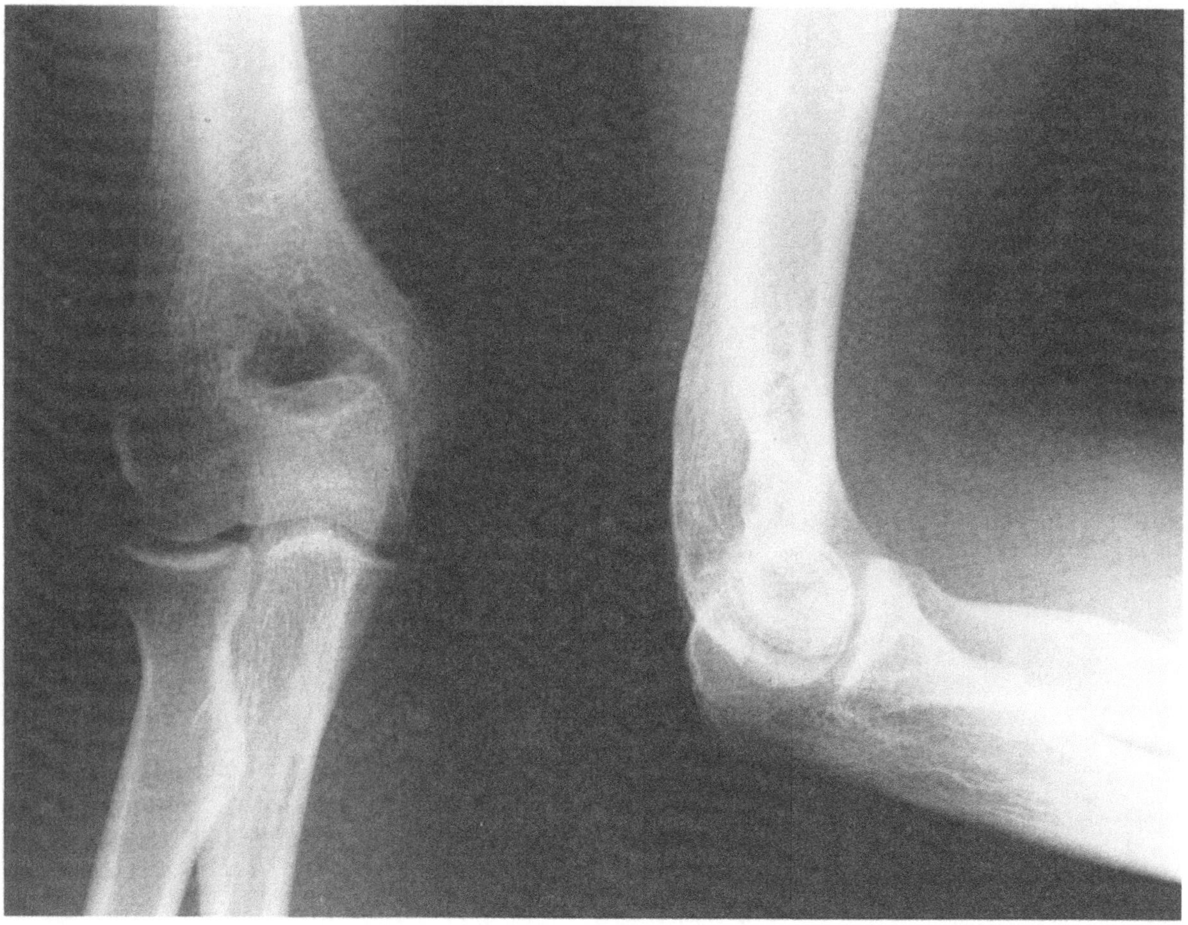

Fig. 103
The control roentgenograms following reduction of the dislocation show normal positioning of the elbow bones.

nal, usually round collection of contrast material with a prolonged opacification of the sac. Depending upon the size, displacement of the adjacent vessels may be seen.

7.2.5 Report of Our Cases

Out of many patients examined for traumatic lesions of the arteries of the upper extremity in the last ten years in our department two cases which we regard as illustrative will be reported below.

Case 1, small true aneurysm of the right brachial artery.
The patient was a 28-year-old woman with a small pulsating mass in the right antecubital fossa. The swelling was noticed ten months before admission. In that time, according to the patient, there had been no change in the size of the mass. Associated pain, tenderness, coldness and numbness of the fingers were not present.

The patient had a history of local blunt trauma due to a traffic accident. There was no history of any disease. The only positive physical finding was a pulsatile tumour in the right antecubital fossa, 1 cm in diameter.
The brachial arteriogram demonstrated a small aneurysm in the medial wall of the distal brachial artery just proximal to the elbow joint. The aneurysm showed smooth contours and no signs of the presence of a thrombosis (Fig. 101, arrow).

Case 2, arterial trauma due to elbow dislocation.
A 24-year-old man fell on his extended left upper extremity. Physical examination revealed a closed posterior left elbow dislocation with resulting deformity and soft tissue swelling. The radial and ulnar pulses were just palpable. The neurological

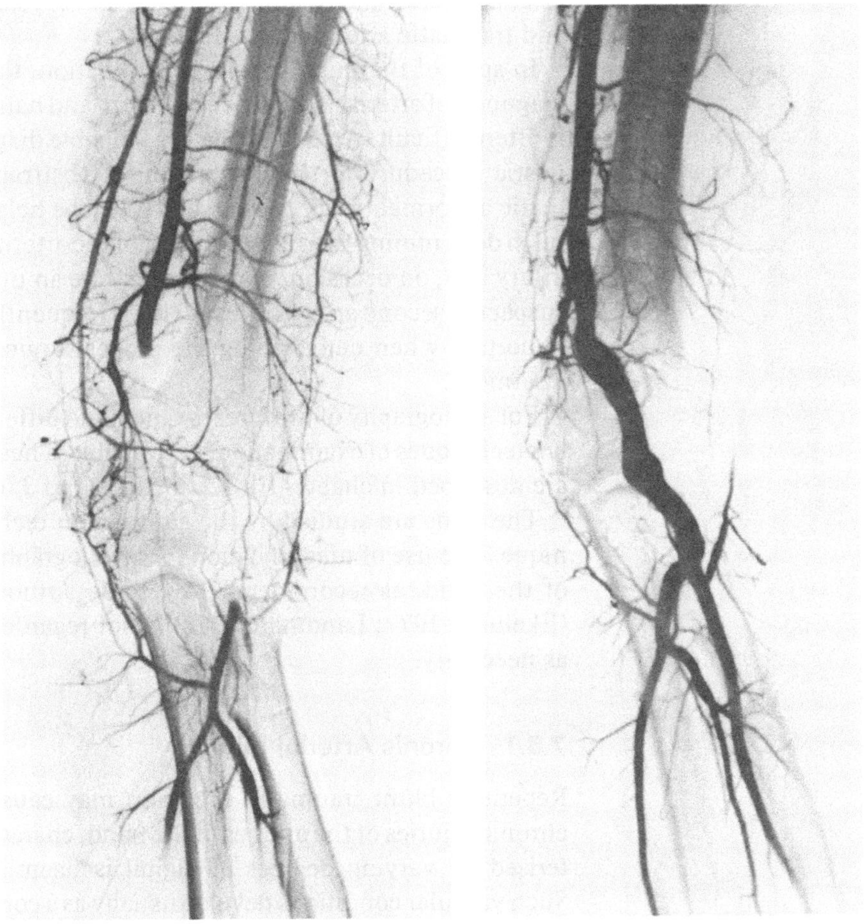

Fig. 104

a b

A. Left brachial arteriogram on arrival at the hospital demonstrates complete occlusion of the brachial artery. There is collateral filling of the vessel below the elbow joint. Most of the collaterals around the elbow show slight displacement and rounded course, probably due to soft tissue swelling.

B. A control brachial arteriogram two years after the operation demonstrates complete re-establishment of the vascular continuity by means of a normally functioning venous graft.

Note the paucity of collateral vessels around the elbow.

function was intact. The roentgenograms showed a posterior dislocation of the elbow joint, without fractures (Fig. 102); under general anaesthesia the dislocation was reduced. Subsequent roentgenograms showed normal positioning of the elbow bones (Fig. 103).

Three hours after the reduction of the dislocation, the radial and ulnar pulses were not palpable. The hand showed signs of ischaemia i.e. coldness, pallor and pain. An arteriography was performed by the transfemoral technique, the catheter being placed in the proximal brachial artery.

The arteriograms revealed total occlusion of the brachial artery with marked collaterals about the elbow and collateral filling of the brachial artery distal to the elbow joint (Fig. 104A).

At surgery the brachial artery was found to be totally lacerated about seven centimetres proximal to the bifurcation. The median nerve was intact. The damaged brachial artery was resected and a saphenous vein graft about 10 centimetres long was used to re-establish arterial continuity. An intraoperative arteriogram revealed good flow to the distal part of the forearm and the hand.

Two years after the injury the patient was seen again. He complained of a feeling of tightness at the extremes of motion and slight claudication. The brachial arteriogram was repeated and dem-

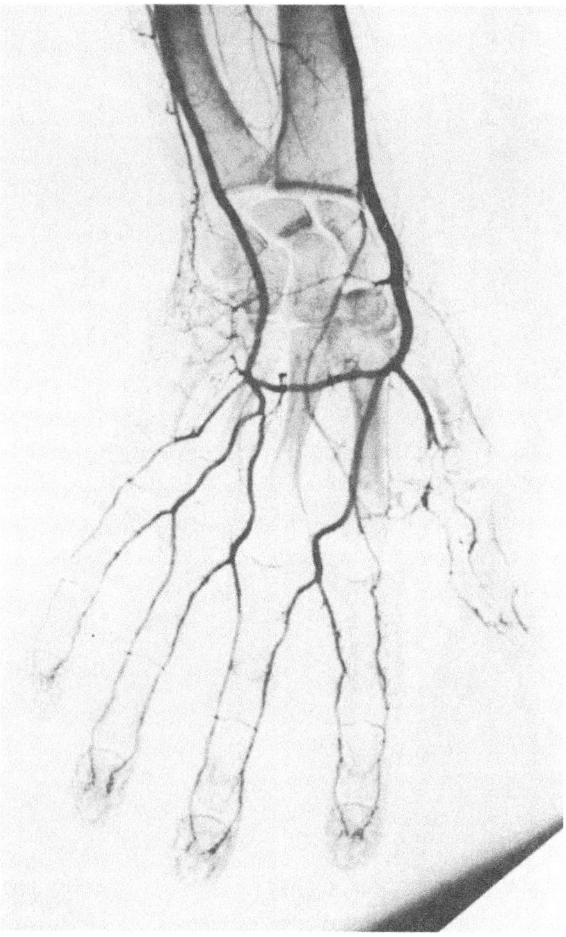

Fig. 105
Normal left hand arteriogram of the same patient as in Figure 104 A and B.

onstrated a normally functioning venous graft (Fig. 104B). The additional hand arteriograms showed no evidence of distal emboli (Fig. 105).

7.3 Traumatic Arterial Injuries of the Forearm and Hand

Literature

Traumatic arterial injuries of the forearm and hand may be classified as acute or chronic. Penetrating or crushing trauma to the extremity are the main causes of acute damage of the vessels in the forearm and hand.

The acute vascular injuries may consist of arterial laceration of transection with subsequent total arterial occlusion, traumatic arterial aneurysms and traumatic arteriovenous fistulae.

In spite of thorough physical examination, the diagnosis of arterial injury of the forearm and hand is often difficult. Arteriography is a valuable diagnostic procedure for the evaluation of posttraumatic abnormalities of the vessels. It can be helpful in determining the site and extent of the arterial injury and, on occasion, may demonstrate an unsuspected second arterial injury. This is frequently important when determining the proper surgical treatment.

For angiography of the forearm and hand different techniques of examination are available. These are described in chapter III, sections 3.5 and 3.6.

The films are studied by the subtraction technique. The use of magnification for arteriography of the hand, as recommended by some authors (Ekelund, 1977; Landman, 1978) is not regarded as necessary.

7.3.1 Chronic Arterial Injuries

Repetitive blunt trauma to the palm may cause chronic injuries of the arteries of the hand, characterized by varying degrees of digital ischaemia. Such vascular conditions develop usually as a consequence of injuries of the distal radial and ulnar arteries or the superficial palmar arch.

There are two syndromes of a morbid vascular condition of the hand caused by chronic trauma.
1. The Hypothenar Hammer Syndrome
2. The Thenar Hammer Syndrome (traumatic thenar ischaemia).

The syndromes are often found in individuals subjected to occupational trauma, *i.e.* who use their hands repeatedly as a hammer for pushing, pounding and twisting during their daily work. The constant striking of the hypothenar or thenar eminence hammers the distal ulnar and radial arteries and superficial palmar arch against the underlying carpal bones. This may result in traumatic damage of the vessels with subsequent thrombosis and distal ischaemia.

a. The Hypothenar Hammer Syndrome
Digital ischaemia from traumatic occlusion of the distal ulnar artery has been termed 'the hypothenar hammer syndrome' by Conn Jr. *et al.* (1970). It is a clinical entity characterized by varying degrees

of digital ischaemia as a consequence of chronic traumatic damage of the ulnar artery in the hypothenar.

The main cause of ulnar arterial injury is repetitive blunt trauma to the palm. The injury may result in spasm, thrombosis or formation of an aneurysm in the ulnar artery. Occasionally various combinations of these lesions exist together. Minor repetitive trauma may produce only distal arterial spasm. Thrombosis of the ulnar artery will occur if the intima is damaged, but if the major site of damage of the arterial wall is the tunica media, then a true palmar aneurysm can develop. Arterial spasm may be reversible if the source of irritation is eliminated (Conn Jr. *et al.*, 1970). The other pathological changes are irreversible.

The syndrome usually develops in manual workers whose palms are exposed to constant minor traumata during their daily activities. It has been found in mechanics, lathe operators, metal workers, farmers and others. Occasionally this syndrome may develop in devotees of the ancient arts of karate and judo, and rarely in persons who lean heavily on canes or crutches (Conn Jr. *et al.*, 1970).

The ulnar artery and nerve, when entering the palm, pass through a groove (Guyon's tunnel) bounded medially by the pisiform bone and dorsally by the transverse carpal ligament, and on the volar side by the volar carpal ligament. Within this tunnel the artery bifurcates into deep and superficial branches. The deep branch penetrates the hypothenar muscles and becomes the deep palmar arch. The superficial branch of the artery remains superficial up to the hypothenar muscles; farther distalwards, it penetrates the palmar aponeurosis to form the superficial palmar arch. Over this short distance of approximately 2 cm between the distal margin of Guyon's tunnel and the palmar aponeurosis the artery is vulnerable to acute and chronic trauma, since it lies superficially in the palm, covered only by skin, subcutaneous tissue and the short palmar muscle.

On the dorsal side of the artery are the carpal bones. The artery lies immediately above them. There is no soft tissue between the vessel and the bones to protect it from injury.

The hook of hamate serves as an anvil against which the ulnar artery is hammered. In the majority of cases the superficial palmar branch of the ulnar artery is the main source of blood to the fingers. An incomplete palmar arch or poor anastomoses between the superficial and deep palmar arches apparently predisposes to digital ischaemia when trauma to the hand occurs. Thus, the presence or absence of ischaemic symptoms following occlusion of the ulnar artery or its superficial palmar branch depends upon the completeness of the arches as well as the size and number of collaterals from the terminal branches of the radial artery. An incomplete arch with few collaterals is obviously more vulnerable (Benedict *et al.*, 1974).

Initial symptoms of a damaged ulnar artery are episodes of acute, severe pain and tenderness over the hypothenar eminence.

Some patients noted that the pain radiated to the medial fingers, suggesting possible compression of the ulnar nerve (Paaby and Stadil, 1968).

In ulnar arterial occlusion the clinical symptoms include varying degrees of digital ischaemia, numbness, paraesthesia, stiffness, coldness, blanching, pain on effort and very rarely atrophic ulcerations on the fingertips. The third and fourth fingers are the most frequently involved. The ischaemic symptoms may be precipitated or aggravated by exposure to cold (Raynaud's phenomenon). The most severe signs and symptoms of digital ischaemia are seen in patients who have both ulnar and digital occlusions.

In patients with a true aneurysm in the palm of the hand the ischaemic symptoms of the hand are usually not severe, but symptoms of compression of the ulnar nerve may be present. On physical examination a hypothenar mass may be observed, which may or may not be pulsatile. This syndrome should be considered in patients with a history of chronic palmar trauma to the hand, unilateral Raynaud's phenomenon, ischaemia of the fingers, a pulsatile hypothenar mass and evidence of ulnar arterial occlusion, *i.e.* a positive Allen test (Allen, 1962).

Allen's test is performed by manual compression of the radial and ulnar arteries at the wrist, while the patient forcefully opens and closes his hand a few times. Normally a slight ischaemia of the skin of the palm and fingers will be seen, which disappears quickly when the hand is kept still and one of the forearm arteries is no longer compressed. This will happen only when the released artery is patent. If this artery is occluded, the pallor

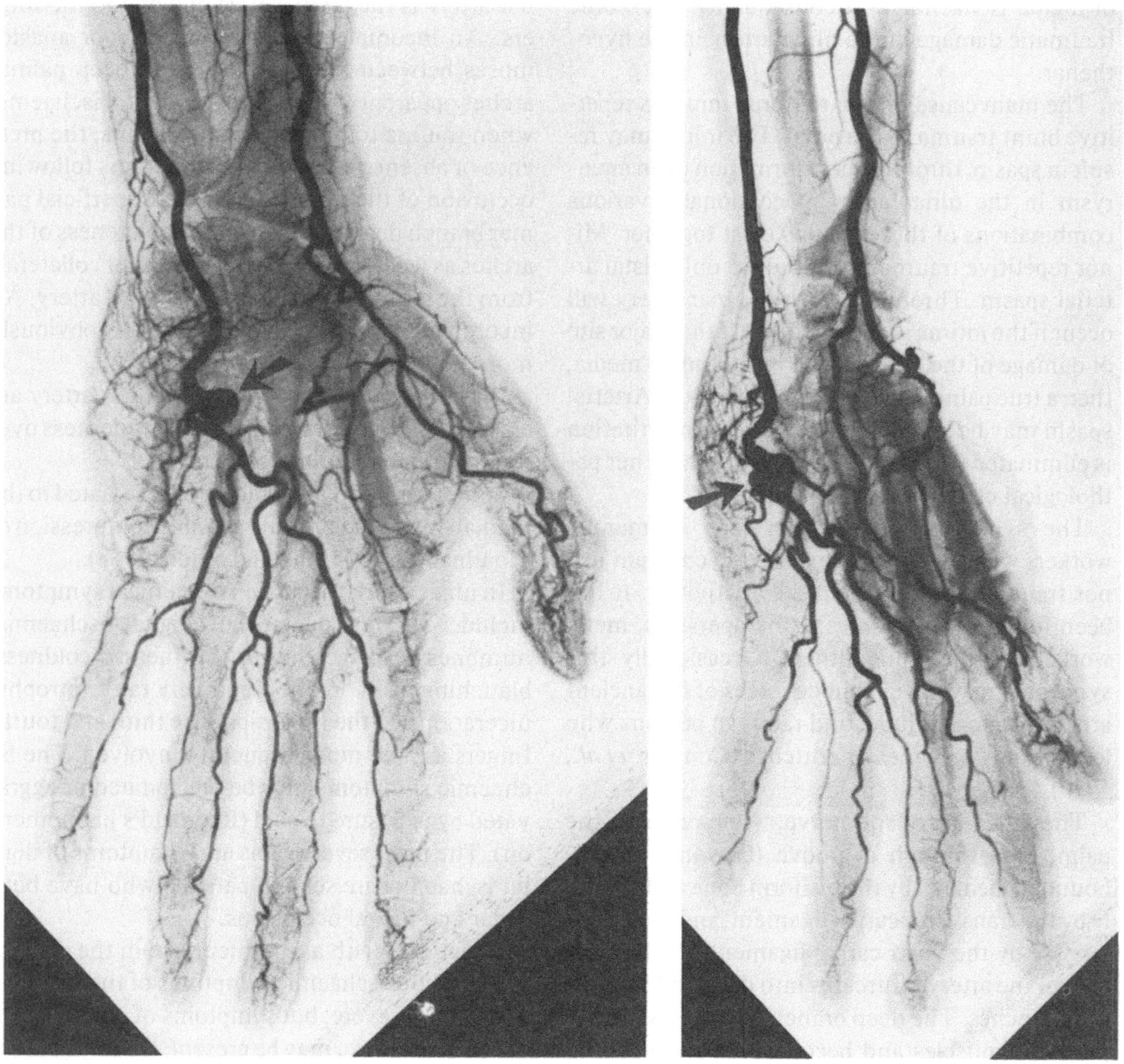

Fig. 106A and B a b
True aneurysm of the ulnar artery at the hypothenar eminence (arrow) in a patient with a history of repeated falls on his left palm.

of the hand will persist as long as compression of the other artery continues. In such cases the test is regarded as positive.

Brachial arteriography, however, is necessary to demonstrate the exact anatomy and pathological changes such as arterial spasm, palmar aneurysm and occlusions of the distal part of the ulnar artery which usually are the most characteristic angiographic findings for this syndrome.

b. The Thenar Hammer Syndrome

Posttraumatic digital ischaemia of the thenar portion of the hand develops after occlusion of the terminal radial artery and the deep palmar arch. Repetitive blunt trauma to the thenar eminence of the palm is less common than that to the hypothenar, because the thenar eminence of the palm is not frequently used as a hammer. One case of thenar hammer syndrome was reported by Wandtke *et al.*, 1976. They referred to this condition as traumatic thenar ischaemia.

The term thenar hammer syndrome has not been used in the literature. In close analogy to the original case described by Conn jr. (1970) termed hypothenar hammer syndrome, we propose that this similar condition should be called the thenar

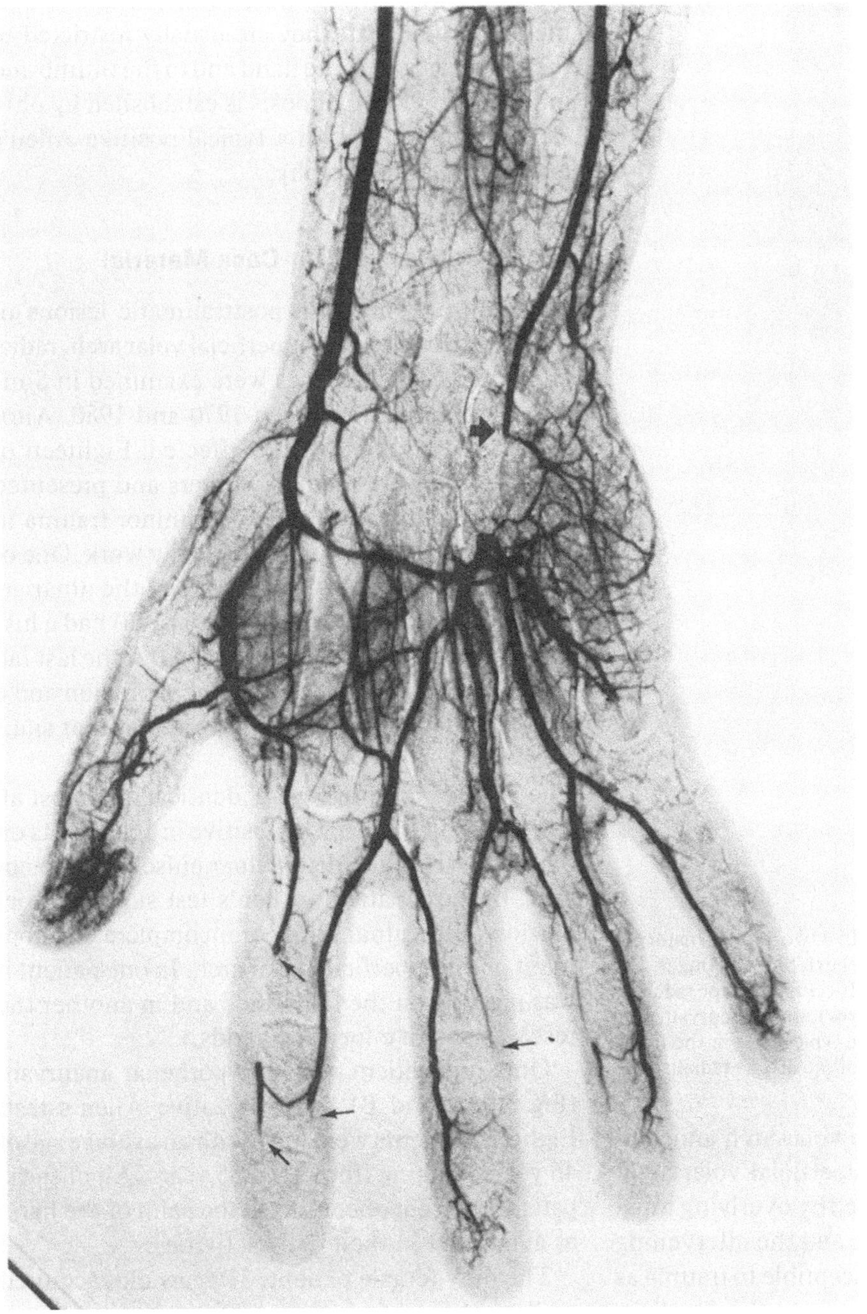

Fig. 107
Hypothenar Hammer Syndrome.
Arteriogram of the right hand of a 42-year-old air hammer operator with persistent numbness, coldness and tingling of the digits of the hand demonstrates complete occlusion of the ulnar artery at typical site (large arrow) and occlusion of several proper digital arteries (small arrows).

hammer syndrome, notwithstanding the fact that the artery is usually occluded at the distal part of the thenar, where it enters the palm between the first and second metacarpal bones.

The aetiology and pathogenesis of this vascular condition are the same as those of the hypothenar hammer syndrome.

The thenar portion of the hand receives its blood supply from the branches of the radial artery. The blood supply to the thumb and index finger arises

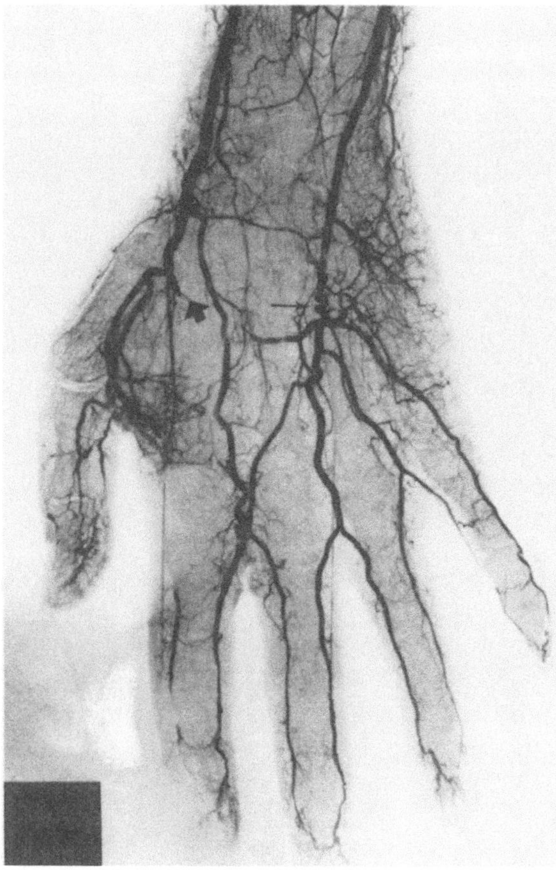

Fig. 108
Thenar Hammer Syndrome.
A 26-year-old healthy bricklayer with a two-month history of coldness and numbness of the tip of the right index finger. The arteriogram of the right hand showed occlusion of the radial artery at the thenar eminence (large arrow), small aneurysms and irregularity of the ulnar artery at the typical site in the hypothenar (small arrow) and occlusion of the arteria radialis indicis.

predominantly from the deep volar arch and supplemental branches of the superficial volar arch. The deep volar arch is protected by overlying musculature, subcutaneous tissue and the intervening first metacarpal bone. It is susceptible to trauma as it crosses the second metacarpal. At this location, it is protected only by the flexor pollicis brevis muscle and by subcutaneous tissue and may easily become compressed against the base of the second metacarpal bone. In patients exposed to chronic repetitive trauma of the palm, occlusion of the deep radial branch is often seen at this site. The proximal deep arch and the termination of the radial artery are protected along part of their course by the first metacarpal bone and the trapezium. Injuries to that segment of the artery are rare.

The clinical signs of the thenar hammer syndrome are the same as those for hypothenar hammer syndrome. But they are usually restricted to the thenar aspect of the hand and to the thumb and index finger. The diagnosis is established by physical examination with a typical positive Allen's test and by arteriography.

7.3.2 Analysis of Our Case Material

Nineteen patients with posttraumatic lesions of the distal ulnar artery, superficial volar arch, radial artery and digital arteries were examined in Sint-Annadal Hospital between 1970 and 1980. Altogether, twenty hands were affected. Eighteen of the patients were manual workers and presented with similar histories of chronic minor trauma to the hands associated with their daily work. One of the patients with a true aneurysm of the ulnar artery in the hypothenar region (Fig. 106) had a history of repeated falls on his palm. After the last fall he developed pain in the hypothenar region and a week later a pulsatile mass appeared at that site.

The physical findings were identical in almost all patients. Allen's test was positive in 16 patients on one side, where the distal ulnar pulse was also absent. In these patients Allen's test suggested occlusion of the ulnar artery or incomplete development of the superficial volar arch. In one patient it was positive on the radial side and in another the test was positive for both hands.

Only one patient with a hypothenar aneurysm (Fig. 106A and B) had a negative Allen's test. Eighteen patients were male with an average age of 46 years, ranging from 31 to 55 years. All of these patients, except one, utilized the palm of the hand as a hammer in their daily activities.

The only female patient, 31 years old, acquired a bilateral traumatic lesion during her work in a cheese shop. She pressed with her palms on a large bimanual knife when cutting cheese. She had the hypothenar hammer syndrome on the right side and a typical thenar hammer syndrome on the left. Severe digital ischaemia was present in both hands (Fig. 109A and B).

In one patient, in addition to an occlusion of the ulnar artery at the typical site, multiple microaneurysmata were found in the distribution area of this vessel, namely in the arteries which supply the fourth and fifth digits (Fig. 110).

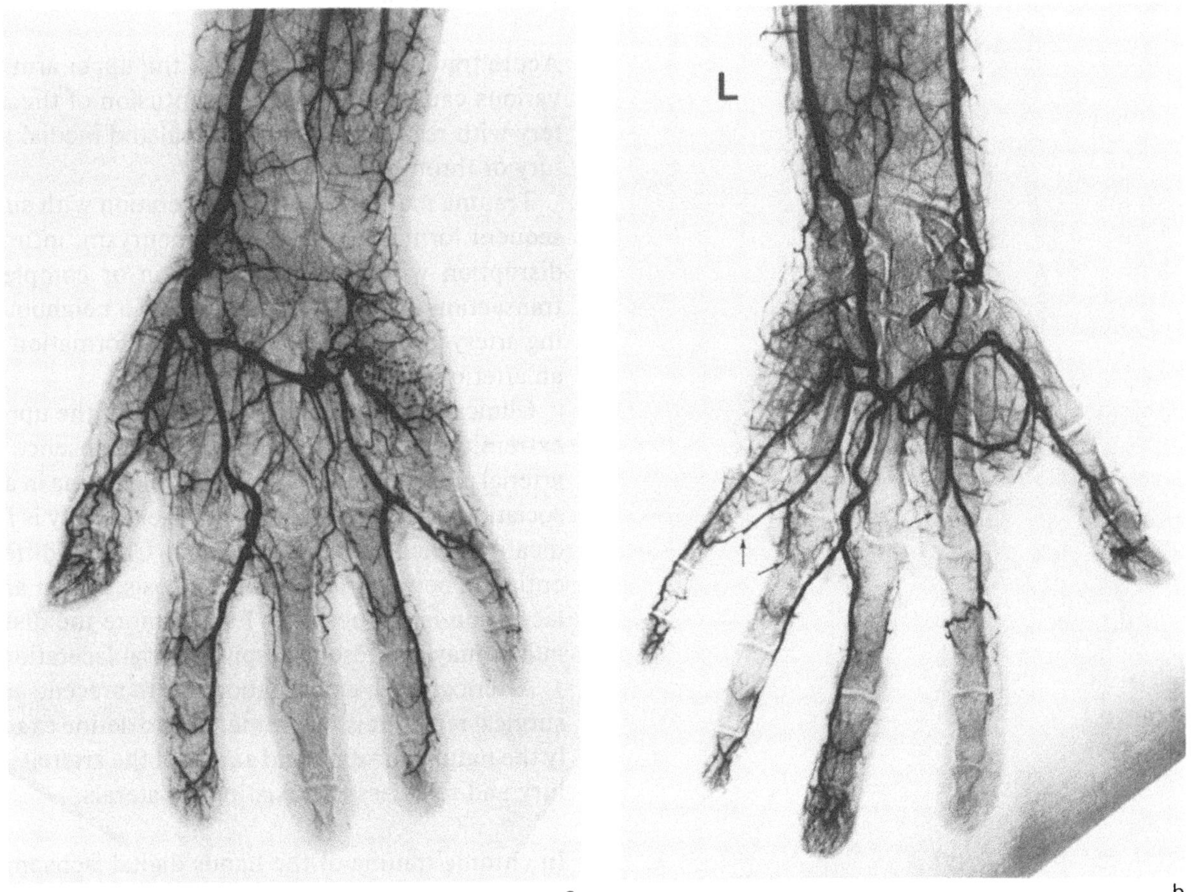

a b

Fig. 109
Right Hypothenar and Left Thenar Hammer Syndrome.
In a 31-year-old woman with complaints of Raynaud's phenomenon and bluish discolouration as well as coldness of the right middle finger for 6 months and left index finger for 3 months.
The patient's work history include 12 years of cutting cheese with a heavy knife held in both hands while exerting a downward pressure with the thenar and hypothenar eminences of the palms. Arteriographic evaluation of the arms and forearms was negative. Arteriography of the right hand showed occlusions of the ulnar artery and several common and proper volar digital arteries. The middle finger is the most severely involved.
The left hand arteriogram showed total occlusion of the radial artery at the thenar eminence (large arrow) and occlusion of several digital arteries (small arrows).

One patient had bilateral ulnar and digital arterial blocks. In all other patients, the dominant hand was the one involved. None of the patients with symptoms of hand ischaemia had any clinical evidence of associated generalized occlusive vascular diseases, such as thromboangiitis obliterans, arteriosclerosis, diabetes or collagen diseases.

In our patients with occlusion of the distal radial artery (thenar hammer syndrome) the most severe and extensive arterial changes were found in the proper digital arteries of the index and middle fingers. These arteries were either occluded or contained multiple stenoses (Fig. 109B). In patients with occlusion of the distal ulnar artery (hypothenar hammer syndrome) the arterial changes were found in almost all fingers, with the exception of the principal artery of the thumb which was not often involved.

The most common sites of occlusion of the proper digital arteries were in the proximity of the first interphalangeal joint (Fig. 107) or, less frequently, near their origin in the web spaces (Fig. 109). In those fingers which were involved by acronecrosis, both proper digital arteries were occluded. The common volar digital arteries were constricted or completely occluded in seven patients.

A large true aneurysm was found in one patient (Fig. 106). Small aneurysms of the ulnar artery

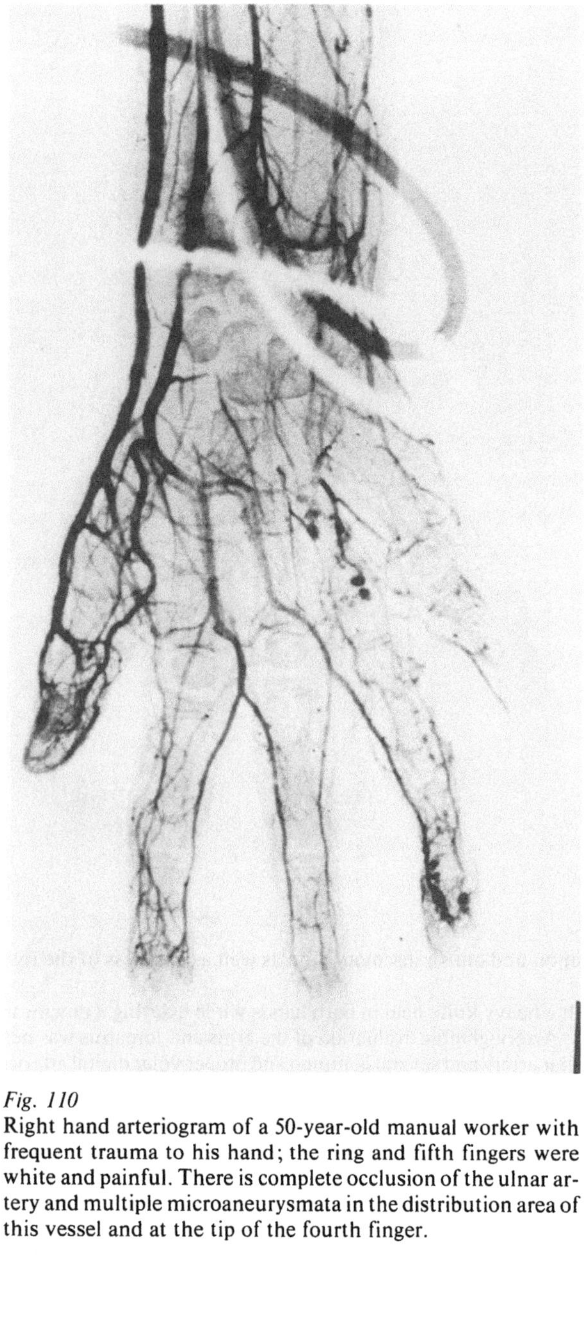

Fig. 110
Right hand arteriogram of a 50-year-old manual worker with frequent trauma to his hand; the ring and fifth fingers were white and painful. There is complete occlusion of the ulnar artery and multiple microaneurysmata in the distribution area of this vessel and at the tip of the fourth finger.

were found in the carpal area in two patients (Figs. 108 and 110). An irregular calibre of the ulnar artery in the hypothenar was observed in one patient (Fig. 108).

In four patients with the hypothenar hammer syndrome the involvement of the digital arteries was minimal, because both palmar arches were complete (Fig. 111).

Additional clinical and angiographic features are added to the descriptions of the illustrations.

7.4 Conclusions

Acute trauma of the arteries of the upper arm of various causes may produce contusion of the artery with resultant spasm, intimal and medial injury or thrombosis.

Trauma may cause arterial laceration with subsequent formation of a pseudoaneurysm, intimal disruption with vascular occlusion or complete transection of the vessel. Trauma of a neighbouring artery and vein may result in the formation of an arteriovenous fistula.

Clinically the traumatic ischaemia of the upper extremities is easily recognizable. The absence of arterial pulsations distal to the site of trauma in association with a cold, pale, painful extremity is indicative of acute arterial occlusion. Clinical differentiation between arterial thrombosis, spasm and laceration is not possible. Furthermore the distal pulses may be present despite arterial laceration.

Arteriographic examination has to precede any surgical repair. It is recommended to define exactly the nature, location and extent of the arterial injury and to assess the existing collaterals.

In chronic trauma of the hands digital ischaemia seldom develops although many individuals use their hands in traumatic circumstances every day. This is probably due to the dual arterial supply to the hands through their superficial and deep palmar arches. The persistent palmar arch intercommunications prevent digital ischaemia if one artery is damaged or occluded. Ischaemia is more likely to develop in individuals with incomplete arterial arches than in those with complete palmar arches.

Fortunately, it is rare for the changes produced by trauma alone to progress to actual loss of a digit, since once the symptoms appear it is usually impossible for the patient to continue the traumatic activity; the clinical manifestations then recede in part, if not completely.

The diagnosis of the hypothenar or thenar hammer syndrome should be suspected in all cases of symptomatic digital ischaemia involving the dominant hand, when there is also a history of repetitive minor blunt trauma to the hands. The presence of thickening, tenderness or a pulsatile mass in the hypothenar or thenar eminence associated with cold, pale or ulcerated fingers makes the diag-

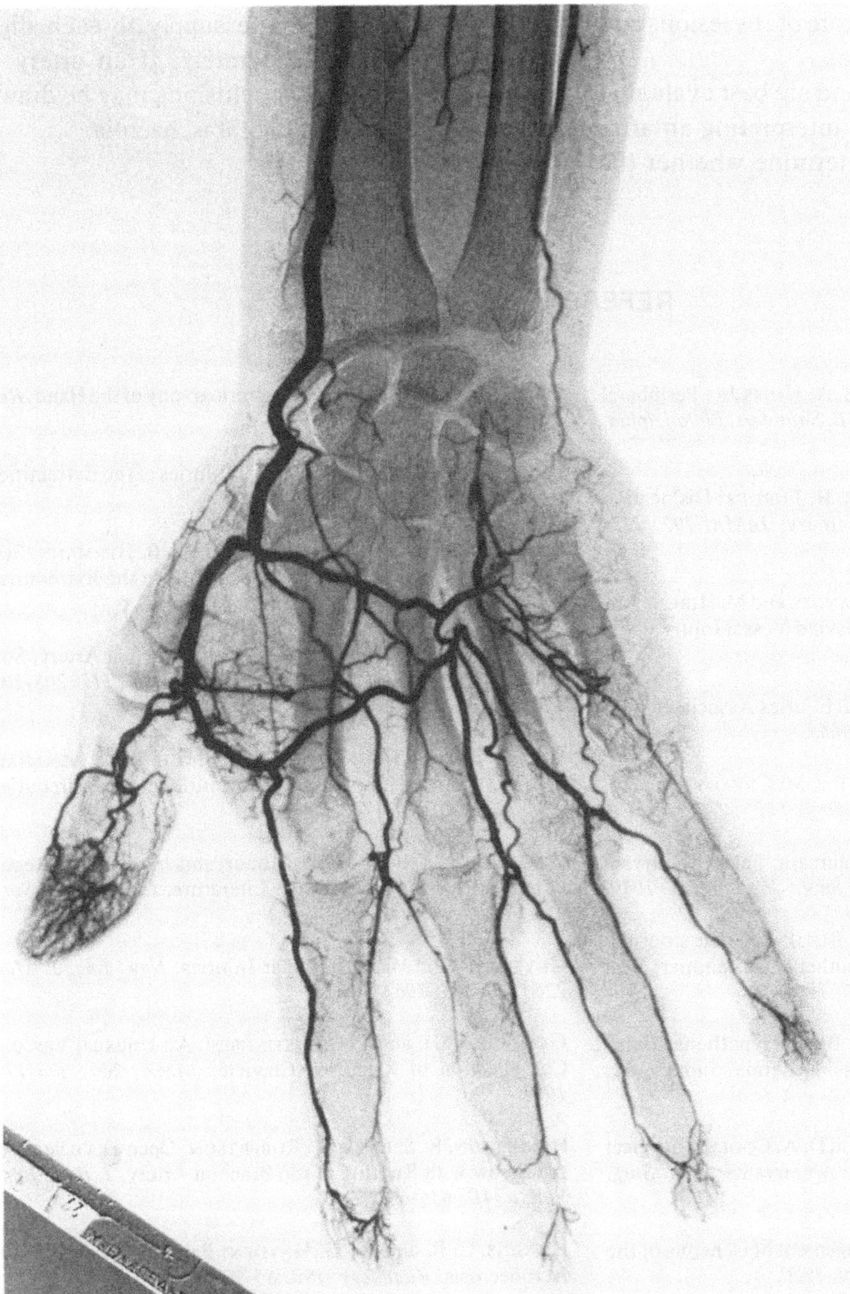

Fig. 111
A 45-year-old right-handed man with a history of repetitive blunt trauma to the palm and mild symptoms of Raynaud's phenomenon.
The arteriograms demonstrated complete occlusion of the ulnar artery at the typical site. Because of both palmar arches were complete, there are no angiographic signs of severe digital ischaemia.

nosis more likely. Angiography serves to verify the diagnosis, show the exact nature of the lesions and localize the sites of occlusions.

The arteriograms of the hand are best evaluated on subtraction films. When interpreting an arteriogram, one should first determine whether the palmar arches are complete or incomplete. If the arches are incomplete, the supply to each digit should be evaluated separately. If an artery is found to be damaged, conclusions may be drawn regarding the cause of digital ischaemia.

REFERENCES

ALLEN, E. V., N. W. BARKER and E. A. HINES Jr.: Peripheral Vascular Diseases. *Ed. 3: 31-32, W. B. Saunders, Philadelphia, 1962.*

AUFRANC, O. E., W. N. JONES and R. H. TURNER: Dislocation of the Elbow with Brachial Artery Injury. *JAMA, 197: 127-129, 1966.*

BAR-ZIV, J., M. EGER, M. FEUCHTWANGER and M. HIRCH: Angiography in the Diagnosis of Subclavian Vessel Injury. *Clin. Radiol. 23: 471-473, 1972.*

BASSET, F. H. and D. SILVER: Arterial Injuries Associated with Fractures. *Arch. Surg. 92: 13-19, 1966.*

BENEDICT, K. T., Jr., W. CHANG and F. J. MCCREADY: The Hypothenar Hammer Syndrome. *Radiology, 111: 57-60, 1974.*

BOWIE, D. C. and A. W. KAY: Traumatic False Aneurysm Simulating Bone Sarcoma. *British J. Surg., 36: 310-331, 1949.*

CAROL, E. J., J. M. H. TORDOIR en J. BUTH: Arteriële stoornissen in de hand bij gebruik van de hypothenar als hammer. *Ned. T. Geneesk., 125, nr. 36: 1444-1450, 1981.*

CONN, J., Jr., J. J. BERGAN and J. L. BELL: Hypothenar Hammer Syndrome: Posttraumatic Digital Ischemia. *Surgery, 68: 1122-1128, 1970.*

CRAWFORD, E. S., M. E. DEBAKEY and D. A. COOLEY: Surgical considerations of Peripheral Arterial Aneurysms. *Arch. Surg. 78: 226-237, 1959.*

DALE, W. A. and L. M. LEWIS: Management of ischemia of the hand and fingers. *Surgery, 67: 62-79, 1970.*

DAVIDSON, K. G.: Closed Injuries of the Aorta and Great Vessels in 'Trauma of the Chest'. *Edited by Williams, W. G. and R. E. Smith, Wright Co. Bristol, 1977.*

DEBAKEY, M. E. and F. A. SIMEONE: Battle Injuries of the Arteries in World War II. *Am. Surg. 123: 534-546, 1946.*

DEBAKEY, M. E.; A. C. BEALL Jr. and D. C. WUKASCH: Recent Developments in Vascular Surgery with Particular Reference to Orthopedics. *Amer. J. Surg. 109: 134-142, 1965.*

FISHER, R. G., F. HADLOCK and Y. BEN-MENACHEM: Laceration of thoracic aorta and brachiocephalic arteries by blunt trauma: Report of 54 cases and review of literature. *Radiol. Clin. N. Amer., 19: 91-110, 1981.*

EKELUND, L. and J. GERLOCK: Arteriography of the Hand. *Rev. S. Am. Rad. 2: 233-237, 1977.*

ENGE, L.: Angiography in Vascular Injuries of the Extremities. *Acta Radiol. 16: 193-199, 1975.*

ENGLEMAN, R. M., J. M. CLEMENTS and J. B. HERMANN: Stab Wounds and Traumatic False Aneurysms in the Extremities. *J. Trauma, 9: 77-87, 1969.*

FRIEDMANN, E.: Simple Rupture of the Brachial Artery, Sustained in Elbow Dislocation. *Am. J. Med. Assn., 117: 208-209, 1961.*

GILL, S. S., F. C. EGGLESTON, C. M. SINGH, K. A. ABRAHAM, S. KUMAR and L. H. LOBO: Arterial Injuries of the Extremities. *J. Trauma, 16: 766-772, 1976.*

GREEN, D. P.: True and False Aneurysms in the Hand. Report of two cases and Review of the Literature. *J. Bone Joint Surg. 55A: 120-128, 1973.*

GRYSKA, P. F.: Major Vascular Injuries. *New. Eng. J. Med. 226: 381-385, 1962.*

GUILFOIL, P. H. and T. CHRISTIANSEN: An Unusual Vascular Complication of Fractured Clavicle. *JAMA, 200: 178-179, 1967.*

HENDERSON, R. S. and I. M. ROBERTSON: Open Dislocation of the Elbow with Rupture of the Brachial Artery. *J. Bone Joint. Surg., 34B: 636-637, 1952.*

HIGGINS, C. B. and W. G. HAYDEN: Palmar arteriography in Acronecrosis. *Radiology, 199: 85-90, 1976.*

JACKSON, J. A.: Simple Anterior Dislocation of the Elbow Joint with Rupture of the Brachial Artery. Case Report. *Am. J.Surg. 47: 479-483, 1940.*

JOHNSON, G. W. and J. H. LOWRY: Rupture of the axillary artery Complicating Anterior Dislocation of the Shoulder. *J. Bone Joint. Surg. 44-B: 116-118, 1962.*

KILBURN, P., J. G. SWEENEY and F. F. SILK: Three cases of compound posterior dislocation of the elbow with rupture of the brachial artery. *J. Bone and Joint Surg., 44: 119-121, 1962.*

KLEINERT, H. E., G. C. BURGET, J. A. MORGAN, J. E. KUNTZ and E. ATASOY: Aneurysms of the hand. *Arch Surg., 106: 554-557, 1973.*

LANDMAN, G. H. M.: First experiences with a New Installation for Angiography. *Medicamundi, 23: 137-146, 1978.*

LEBORGNE, J.: J. C. LE NEEL, D. MITARD *et al.*: Les lésions de l'artere axillaire et de ses branches consecutive a un traumatisme fermé de l'épaule. *Am. Chir. (Paris) 27: 587-589, 1973.*

LINSCHEID, R. L. and D. K. WHEELER: Elbow Dislocation. *JAMA, 194: 1171-1176, 1965.*

LOVE L. and T. BRAUN: Arteriography in peripheral Vascular Trauma. *Am. J. Roentg. 102: 431-432, 1968.*

LOUIS, D. S. and M. A. SIMON: Traumatic False Aneurysms of the Upper Extremity. *J. Bone Joint Surg. 56A: 176-179, 1974.*

LUMPKIN, M. B., W. D. LOGAN, C. M. COUVES and J. M. HOWARD: Arteriography as an and in the diagnosis and localization of acute arterial injuries. *Am. Surg. 147: 353-358, 1958.*

LUNDE-VALL, J.: The mechanism of Traumatic Rupture of the Aorta. *Acta Rad. Microb. Scand. 62: 34-36, 1966.*

MAKIN, G. S., J. H. HOWARD and R. C. GREEN: Arterial Injuries Complicating Fractures of Dislocations. *Surg. 89: 203-221, 1966.*

MARNHAM, R.: Dislocation of the Elbow with Rupture of the Brachial Artery. *Brit. Journ. Surg., 22: 181-189, 1934.*

MATLOFF, D. B. and J. H. MORTON: Acute Trauma to the Subclavian Arteries. *Am. J. Surg. 115: 675-680, 1968.*

MCDONALD, E. J. Jr., P. C. GOODMAN and D. P. WINESTOCK: The Clinical Indications for Angiography in Trauma to the Extremity. *Radiology, 116: 45-47, 1975.*

MCMULLAN, M. H. and J. D. HARDY: Lesion of the Subclavian Artery. *Am. Surg. 173: 80-86, 1973.*

MOLNAR, W. and W. G. PACE: Traumatic rupture of thoracic aorta. *Radiol. Clin. No. Amer. 4: 403-404, 1966.*

MORRIS, G. C., A. C. BEALL, W. R. ROOF and M. E. DEBAKEY: Surgical Experience with 220 Acute arterial injuries in civilian practice. *Am. J. Surg. 99: 775-781, 1960.*

NARSETE, E. M.: Traumatic Aneurysm of the Radial Artery: A report of three cases. *Am. J. Surg., 108: 424-427, 1964.*

NEER, C. S.: Displaced Proximal Humerus Fractures. *J. Bone Joint Surg. 52A: 1090-1095, 1970.*

PAABY, H. and F. STADIL: Thrombosis of the Ulnar Artery. *Acta Orthop. Scand., 39: 336-345, 1968.*

PATTERSON, D.: Retrosternal Dislocation of the Clavicle. *J. Bone and Joint Surg. 47A: 1525-1526, 1965.*

PIYACHON, C. and S. ARTHACHINTA: Arteriography in Trauma of the Extremities. *Act. Radiol. 119: 580-585, 1973.*

RICH, N. M., J. H. BAUGH and C. W. HUGHES: Acute Arterial Injuries in Vietnam: 1000 cases. *J. Trauma 10: 359-369, 1970.*

RICH, N. M., R. W. HOBSON, B. S. JARSTFER and T. M. GREEN: Subclavian Artery Trauma. *J. Trauma, 13: 485-396, 1973.*

SALETTA, J. D. and R. J. FREEARK: Occult Vascular Injuries of the Extremities. *J. Occup. Med. 12: 304-307, 1970.*

SEELEY, S. F., C. W. HUGHS, F. N. COOK and D. C. ELKIN: Traumatic Arteriovenous Fistulas and Aneurysms in War Wounded. A Study of 101 cases. *Amer. J. Surg. 83: 471-479, 1952.*

SHUCK, J. M., G. E. OMER Jr. and C. E. LEWIS Jr.: Arterial Obstruction due to Intimal Disruption in Extremity Fractures. *J. Trauma, 12: 481-487, 1972.*

SINKLER, W. H. and A. D. SPENCER: The Value or peripheral Arteriography in Assessing acute vascular injuries. *Arch. Surg. 80: 300-302, 1960.*

SLANEY, G. and F. ASHTON: Arterial injuries and their management. *Postgrad. Med. Jour., 47: 257-269, 1971.*

SMITH, R. F.: Arterial Trauma. *Arch. Surg. 86: 825-835, 1963.*

SMYTH, E. H. J.: Major arterial Injury in closed fractures of the neck of the humerus. *J. Bone Joint Surg. 51B: 508-518, 1960.*

SPEAR, H. C. and J. M. JANES: Rupture of the Brachial Artery Accompanying Dislocation of the Elbow or Supracondylar Fracture. *J. Bone Joint. Surg., 33-A: 889-894, 1951.*

SPENSER, F. C. and R. K. TOMPKINS: Management of acute arterial injuries. *Postgrad. Med. Jour., 28: 476-481, 1960.*

SPENCER, A. D.: The reliability of Signs of Peripheral Vascular Injury. *Surg. Gynec. Obst. 114: 490-496, 1962.*

SPITTAL, J. A. Jr.: Aneurysms of the Hand and Wrist. *Med. Clin. N. Amer., 42: 1007-1010, 1958.*

STAPLES, O. S.: Disruption of the Brachial Artery. *J. Bone Surg. 47A: 1525-1526, 1965.*

STONE, W.: A Case of Traumatic Aneurysm. *New Orleans Med. Surg. J. 6: 555-556, 1949.*

THEODORIDES, T. and G. DE KEIZER: Injuries of the Axillary Artery Caused by Fractures of the Neck of the Humerus. *Brit. J. Acc. Surg. 8: 120-123, 1976.*

WANDTKE, J. C., R. M. SPITZER, H. E. OLSSON and E. WELCH: Traumatic Thenar Ischemia. *Am. J. Roentg. 127: 569-571, 1976.*

WENZ, W.: Die Bedeutung der Angiographie für die Traumatologie. In: Angiographie in ihre Leistungen. Arbeits- und Fortbildungstagung 1968, S. 43. Herausgegeben von K. E. LOOSE. *George. Thieme Verlag, Stuttgart 1968.*

WHOLEY, M. H. and J. BOCHER: Angiography in Musculoskeletal Trauma. *Sur. Gynaec. Obst. 18: 730-736, 1967.*

WINEGARDER, F. G., A. G. BAKER Jr., J. F. BASCOM and G. F. JACKSON: Delayed vascular Complications in Vietnam Casualities. *J. Trauma, 10: 867-873, 1970.*

Chapter 8

CONGENITAL VASCULAR LESIONS AND VASCULAR TUMOURS

Literature

The congenital vascular lesions include atresia and congenital stenosis of the subclavian artery, arterial hypoplasia and aplasia and congenital arteriovenous communications.

8.1 Congenital Stenosis, Atresia, Hypoplasia and Aplasia

Congenital stenosis and atresia of the subclavian arteries are usually associated with other anomalies of the heart and aortic arch. The most frequent condition reported in the literature is a congenital atresia of the left subclavian artery associated with a right aortic arch (Antia and Ottesen, 1966; Gerber, 1967) and/or atresia of the left carotid artery (Levine *et al.*, 1966).

A case of congenital atresia of the left subclavian artery associated with the right aortic arch and tetralogy of Fallot has been reported by Skalpe and Semb (1969).

All cases reported were children between 6 and 12 years old, with symptoms of left-sided subclavian steal syndrome and physical and mental retardation. In all of them the diagnosis was confirmed by surgical exploration.

Unilateral and bilateral hypoplasia of the subclavian and axillary arteries are regarded as rare conditions. Hypoplasia of both subclavian arteries is the result of a congenital anomaly, but unilateral and segmental hypoplasia may be associated with neurofibromatosis.

To the best of our knowledge no case of total aplasia of the subclavian or axillary artery has been reported. However, total aplasia of one of the forearm arteries is a known condition. Aplasia of the ulnar artery associated with a high bifurcation of the brachial artery was recently described by Kappert (1976).

A similar condition was found in our case material only once (Fig. 55). Total aplasia of the radial artery was also seen in one of our patients (Fig. 54).

8.2 Arteriovenous Communications

Literature

The most common arteriovenous communications involving the arteries of the upper extremity and their branches are arteriovenous malformations and arteriovenous fistulae.

8.2.1 Arteriovenous Malformations

By definition an arteriovenous malformation is a vascular lesion of congenital origin. Dilated tortuous arteries and veins with arteriovenous shunting are characteristics of these lesions.

An arteriovenous malformation can usually be separated into three distinct components of vascular alteration (Luessenhop *et al.*, 1965):

1. The primary abnormality, *i.e.* the direct artery-to-vein shunt.
2. Secondary enlargement of the feeding arteries; and
3. Secondary enlargement of the draining veins.

On serial angiograms an arteriovenous malformation has a characteristic appearance with one or more enlarged afferent arteries and early filling of one or more tortuous efferent veins.

Angiography requires a rapid injection of contrast medium and exposures taken at short intervals. In rare instances, a malformation does not opacify totally during serial angiography owing to partial thrombosis in the vessels.

Arteriovenous malformations occur more commonly in the head than in the rest of the body. The extracranial arteriovenous malformations in the region of the neck and upper thorax usually receive blood from the branches of the subclavian artery. In general they appear clinically in early adult life.

It is relatively unusual for them to appear during infancy, unless they are superficial and readily detectable.

Arteriovenous malformations may remain undetected until a routine physical examination reveals a pulsatile mass associated with a bruit (Lawson and Newton, 1970). As in other locations, the arteriovenous malformations of the upper extremity may be supplied by several arteries. Large arteriovenous malformations may cause cardiac hypertrophy, or even congestive heart failure. When an arteriovenous malformation is limited to the *hand*, it rarely produces significant central cardiovascular changes (Ennis *et al.*, 1972). The clinical diagnosis is based on the discolouration of the skin and extensive venous varicosity. Local changes include increased temperature and a bruit. X-ray pictures may demonstrate extensive bony involvement. The extent and degree of vascular involvement however is best determined by arteriography (Neviaser and Adams, 1974).

8.2.2 Arteriovenous Fistulae

The second large group of common arteriovenous communications of the upper extremity are the arteriovenous fistulae. These are communications between arteries and veins through which arterial blood enters the veins without traversing a capillary network (Ennis *et al.*, 1972). In contrast to the congenital arteriovenous malformations the arteriovenous fistulae are usually acquired. According to previous reports, congenital arteriovenous fistulae are a great rarity.

The first reports of arteriovenous fistulae of congenital origin were presented by Lealis (1707) and Winslow (1732). William Hunter in 1757 described a patient with a pulsating mass over the temple which had been present since birth. Callander in 1920 recorded 447 cases of arteriovenous fistulae; out of this large series, only three were definitely congenital. In 1932 a large series of 23 congenital arteriovenous fistulae of the extremities seen at the Mayo Clinic was investigated by Horton. In 1940, Ward and Norton reviewed 44 examples in children, including 25 involving the lower limbs and nine involving the upper extremities.

Robertson (1956) reviewed 40 cases of congenital arteriovenous fistulae of the extremities, and described the pathology, clinical features and treatment of this condition.

Szilagyi *et al.* (1965) reported a series of 33 cases and also reviewed the pathogenesis of the condition. Finally excellent reviews of congenital arteriovenous fistulae of the extremities were published by Flanc (1968), Malan (1972) and Hoogendam (1974).

Curtis in 1953 pointed out that the pathogenesis of an arteriovenous fistula lies in the embryonic period. It is a congenital failure of the embryonic differentiation into arteries and veins leading to persistence of the communication between these structures. He suggested that trauma may cause a reopening of the congenital arteriovenous communication and subsequent rapid proliferation of the lesion. This hypothesis was supported by Neviaser and Adams in 1974.

A congenital arteriovenous fistula is usually not evident, because it is painless and very small. According to Curtis a minor trauma may produce a rapid enlargement of this fistula, causing it to become clinically manifest (Curtis, 1953).

Most of the acquired arteriovenous fistulae reported in the literature are the result of a trauma, but they may also occur as a complication after minor or major surgical procedures (Garland *et al.*, 1965).

The majority of posttraumatic arteriovenous fistulae are usually the result of penetrating injuries to the arteries and veins of the upper extremity. This category of arteriovenous fistulae is comprised almost entirely of gunshot wounds. Presumably, the passage of the bullet through the upper thorax or the shoulder can injure two vessels in such a way as to produce an arteriovenous fistula. A fistula after penetration of the subclavian artery and vein is not surprising in view of the anatomical relationship between the subclavian artery and the adjacent subclavian vein. Subclavian arteriovenous fistulae arising from blunt trauma are rare. In recent reports, puncture of the subclavian or axillary artery during direct percutaneous subclavian arteriography has been described as a cause of arteriovenous fistulae.

The second group of fistulae are spontaneous arteriovenous fistulae. The cause of these fistulae is often rupture of a pre-existing arterial aneurysm into the necrotic wall of an adjacent vein. These fistulae are always single.

8.2.3 Clinical Features

The congenital arteriovenous fistulae of the extremities can be classified into two distinct clinical groups:

1. The localized type, in which one or several arteriovenous fistulae are restricted to one particular part of the extremity.
2. The diffuse type, in which multiple arteriovenous fistulae are distributed diffusely throughout the extremity (Robertson, 1956).

The localized type of fistula is the less common; it is found most often in a peripheral part of an extremity and in the upper rather than the lower part of the limb. The patients in this group usually become symptomatic in the period between 20 and 30 years of age as the result of complications such as ischaemic ulceration of a digit, recurrent haemorrhages or dilatation of superficial veins. On examination the characteristic features of an arteriovenous fistula are present, namely local warmth, dilated superficial veins, a pulsatile swelling with a palpable thrill, a machinery murmur and often evidence of peripheral ischaemia (Flanc, 1968) or even an ischaemic gangrene (Malan, 1972).

The diffuse type of involvement of the whole extremity is seen more frequently. It is mainly the lower limb that is affected. The diffuse arteriovenous anastomoses are very small, their diameter rarely exceeds 220-250 microns (Malan, 1972). As a rule the patients with these abnormalities present with gigantism of a limb and, since this is due to hypertrophy of the bones and soft tissues during the growth period, the symptoms develop at an earlier age, usually during the first decade. In 18 of the 23 cases reported by Horton in 1932 the bones of the involved extremity were longer than those of the other extremity. It is in this 'diffuse' group that systemic cardiovascular effects are common. Although in the majority of cases a clinical diagnosis of congenital fistula can be made, angiography is of great value in confirming the diagnosis, particularly of large solitary fistulae, and demonstrating the extent of the lesion (Szilagyi *et al.*, 1965). A postoperative angiogram provides evidence of the thoroughness of any surgical treatment undertaken (Malan, 1972).

Angiographic examination of small multiple arteriovenous fistulae diffusely distributed throughout an extremity is useless. These arteriovenous anastomoses are usually associated with some syndromes and are clinically easily recognizable (Terpstra *et al.*, 1977).

8.2.4 Haemangioma

The most common vascular tumour of the upper extremity is the cavernous haemangioma. It usually occurs in the palm and digits, but other locations in the arm are also possible. The tumour is composed of mature capillaries and thin-walled vascular spaces (Helwig, 1955). It can be either a painful or a painless lesion.

Clinically the diagnosis can be quite obvious if the tumour is located superficially. Less obvious are those situated deep in the subcutaneous soft tissue. Large subcutaneous haemangiomas may cause pressure changes in the underlying bones and are usually painful (Neviaser and Adams, 1974).

Radiological diagnosis is made by angiography, although irregular calcifications in the tumour may be seen on plain films. These phleboliths do not occur in every haemangioma.

On arteriograms the appearance of haemangioma of the hand is essentially the same as elsewhere in the body. Since it is a highly vascular lesion it is usually visualized completely.

In the arterial phase the enlarged feeding arteries and immediate opacification of the vascular spaces of the tumour are seen. On later serial films the early venous filling is demonstrated. The most

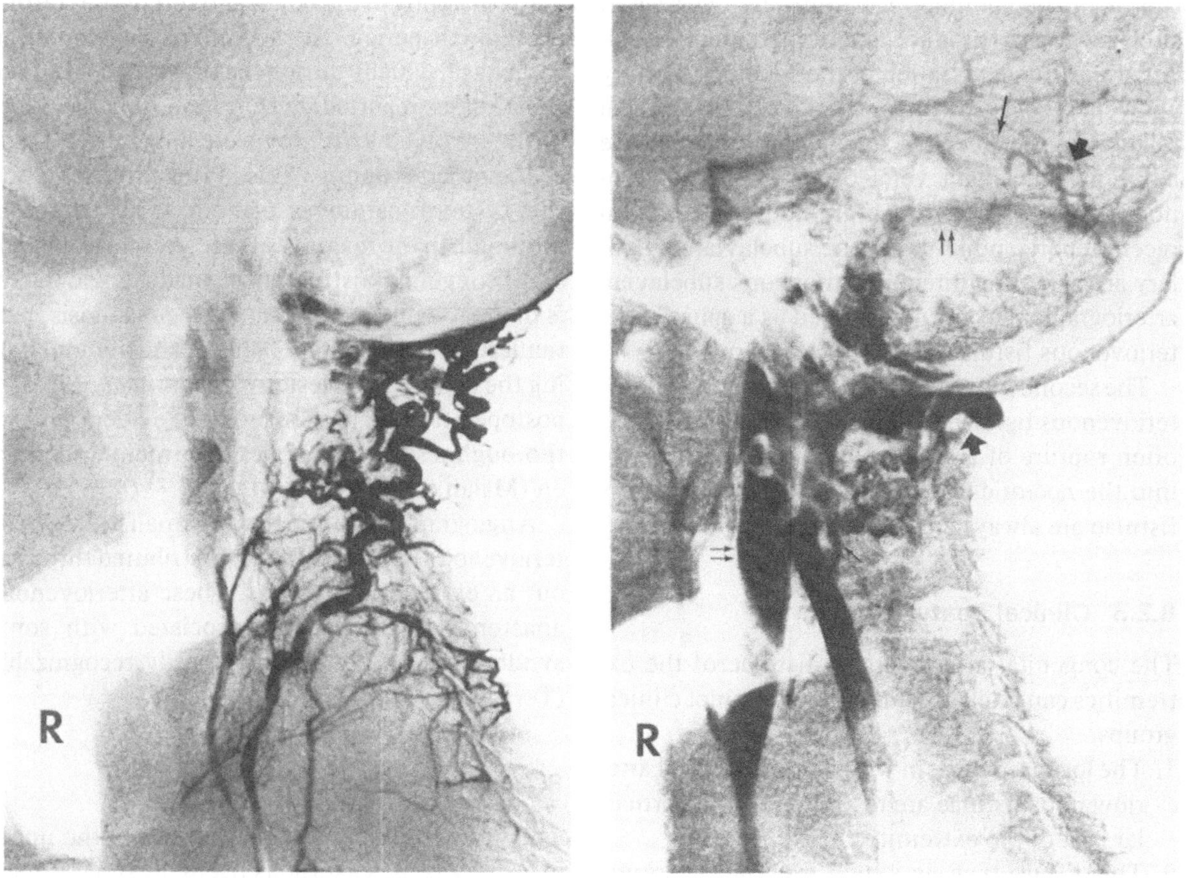

Fig. 112A and B a b
Congenital arteriovenous malformation in the right suboccipital region.
A. Selective injection into the right thyrocervical trunk shows that markedly enlarged muscular branches and ascending cervical branch supply the arteriovenous malformation.
B. The right vertebral arteriogram shows an enlarged vertebral artery with very hypertrophic muscular branches along the second and third segments of this artery. The muscular branches supply mainly the extracranial part of the malformation (solid large arrow). Note that a second small arteriovenous malformation is localized intracranially in the posterior fossa (solid large arrow). This small arteriovenous malformation is supplied mainly by the hemispheric branches of the superior cerebellar artery (small arrow).
There is also early venous drainage into the right lateral sinus and good opacification of the right jugular vein in the arterial phase (double arrows).

typical angiographic sign of cavernous hemangioma is its dilated vascular spaces which retain contrast medium of arterial density until the end of the venous phase (Fig. 114).

8.2.5 Report of Our Cases

Case 1

A 22-year-old woman had complained of bilateral tinnitus for four months. The tinnitus was associated with a bruit in the neck, which was audible to the patient.

Significant physical findings included a pulsatile mass in the right suboccipital region of the neck with a soft murmur which was not affected by carotid compression. The blood pressure was equal on both sides. Cardiac abnormalities were not present.

Selective angiography of the right thyrocervical trunk, as well as the vertebral and both carotid arteries was performed using the transfemoral route. It revealed a large arteriovenous malformation extending along the right side of the neck, localized partly intracranially in the right posterior fossa but mainly extracranially in the right suboccipital region (Fig. 112).

Both the vertebral and the external carotid arteries supplied the malformation in the right suboc-

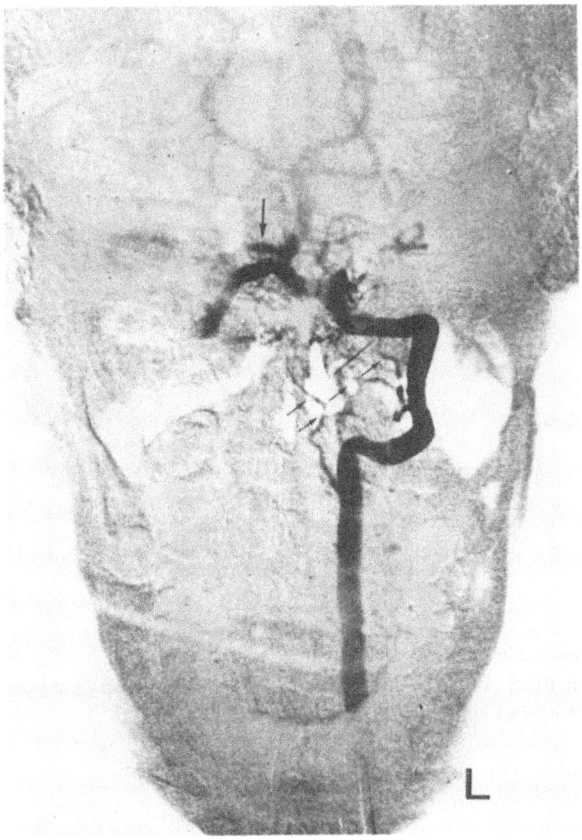

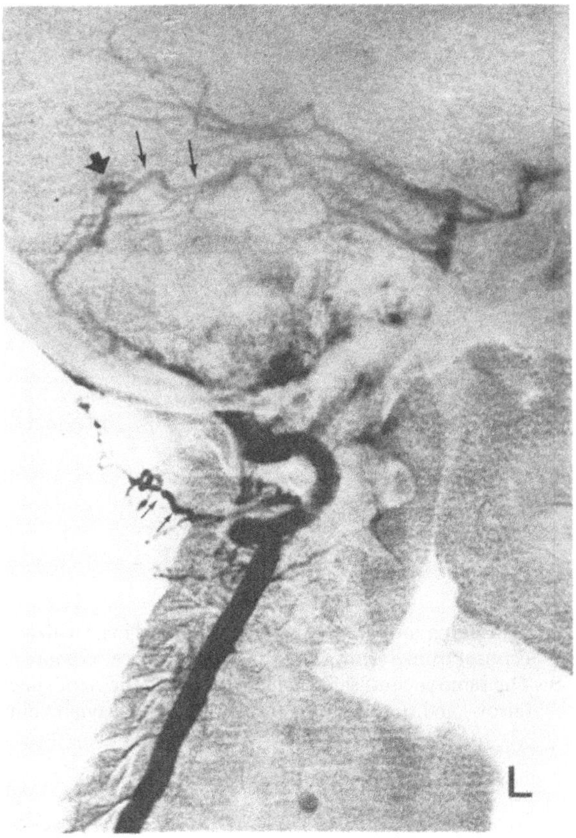

Fig. 112 C and D

C. Left Vertebral Angiogram (same patient as in Fig. 112 A and B).
Frontal projection demonstrates slightly dilated muscular branches arising from the third segment of the vertebral artery (small arrows) which crossed the midline and supplied the vascular malformation in the right suboccipital region. Note the hypertrophic inferior anterior cerebellar artery (large arrow) which supplies the intracranial portion of the malformation.

D. Lateral projection shows the second small intracranial arteriovenous malformation (solid arrow) supplied by the branches of the right superior cerebellar artery (long arrows). The muscular branches from the third segment of the vertebral artery which supply the extracranial suboccipital malformation on the opposite side are also clearly demonstrated (small arrows).

cipital region. The right thyrocervical trunk was the main source of arterial blood supply to the vascular anomaly. The intracranial portion of the malformation and a second small arteriovenous malformation in the right hemisphere of the cerebellum were supplied exclusively by the branches of the vertebrobasilar system (Fig. 112 A, B, C, D).

Case 2

A 22-year-old male was admitted for investigation of a thrill and a systolic murmur in the right midclavicular region.

The history revealed no trauma in the past. On physical examination, a thrill was palpable and arterial pulsations were visible in the superior midclavicular region. On auscultation a constant bruit with systolic accentuation was audible in the supraclavicular region radiating to the high midsternal area. Clinically, no other abnormalities were present.

Aortography and selective arteriography of the right subclavian artery showed a large arteriovenous fistula between a hypertrophic descending branch of the right thyrocervical trunk and the subclavian vein (Fig. 113).

Since there was no trauma in the patient's history we considered this arteriovenous fistula to be congenital.

Case 3

A 34-year-old man had noted slight swelling and colour changes in the web between the first and

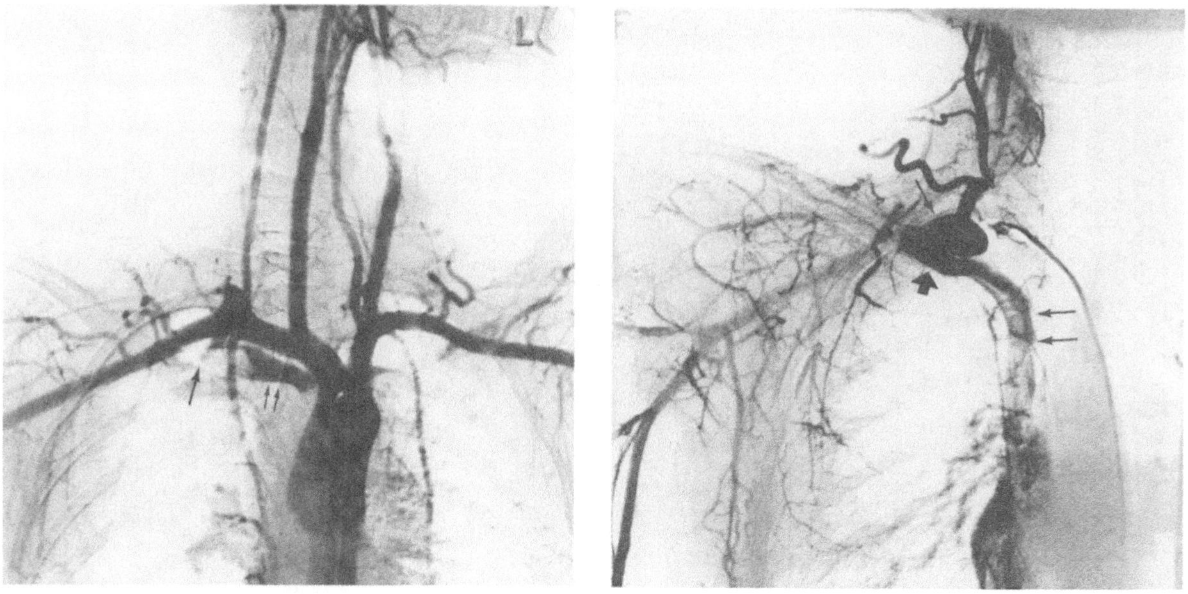

a b

Fig. 113

A. Aortic arch aortogram of a sixteen-year-old male with an arteriovenous fistula between a descending branch of the right thyro-cervical trunk (arrow) and the subclavian vein (double arrows).

B. The same patient, selective injection into the right subclavain artery; the late film shows hypertrophic thyrocervical branch (arrow) and simultaneous filling of the subclavian vein (large arrow) and superior vena cava (double arrows).

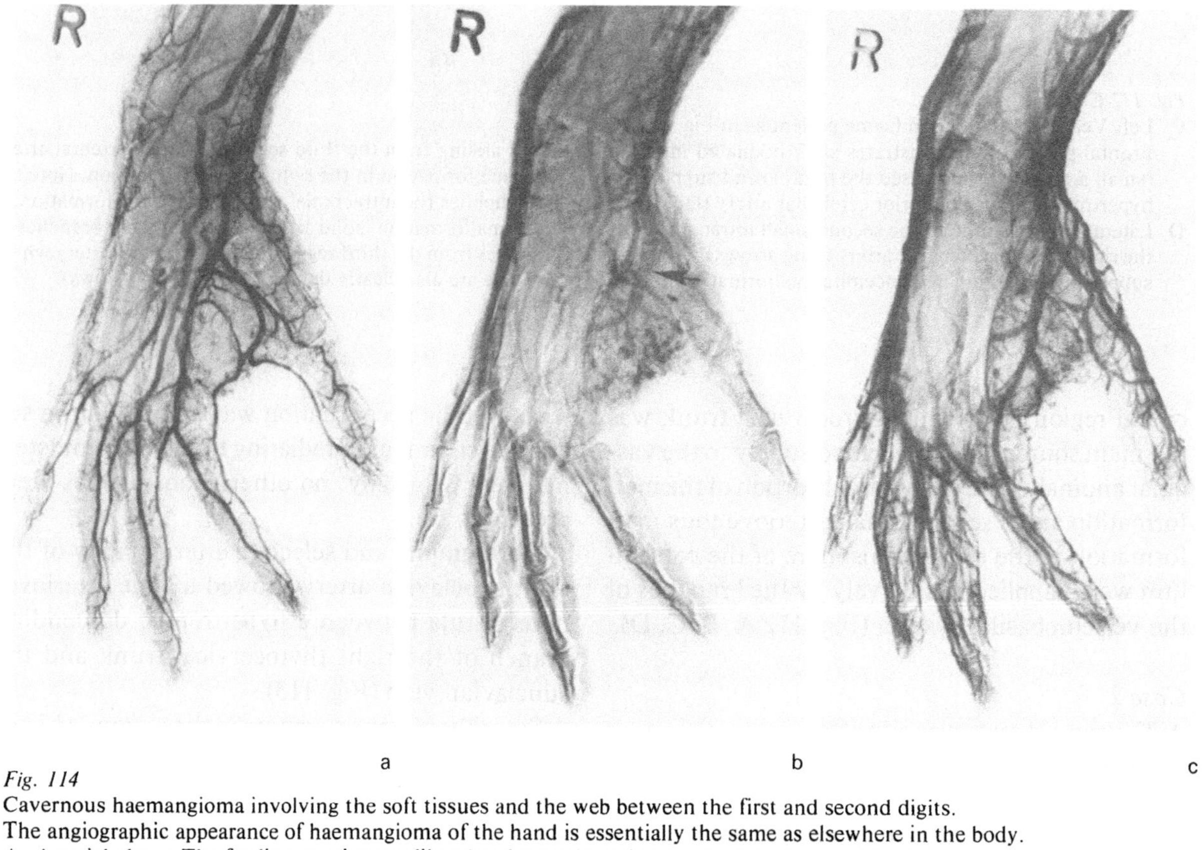

a b c

Fig. 114

Cavernous haemangioma involving the soft tissues and the web between the first and second digits.

The angiographic appearance of haemangioma of the hand is essentially the same as elsewhere in the body.

A. Arterial phase. The feeding arteries are dilated and some branches are stretched around the tumour.

B. Capillary phase. The accumulation of contrast medium within the tumour is more pronounced. There is early filling of the draining veins (arrow). The dilated vascular spaces in the haemangioma retain contrast medium of arterial density.

C. Venous phase. The veins draining the haemagioma are slightly dilated.

second digits of his right hand since age 16. He had no complaints, the swelling was painless even on compression. During the last two years he noted a slight enlargement of the mass and engorgement of the vessels around the mass and in the palm. These venous varicosities were the reason for medical consultation. On examination including angiography a cavernous haemangioma was diagnosed and confirmed during surgery (Fig. 114).

8.3 Conclusions

The arteriovenous malformations are in general asymptomatic. If they are large enough and localized superficially they can be detected easily. The subcutaneous malformations located deep in the soft tissues often manifest as a pulsatile mass associated with local colour changes such as discolouration of the skin and venous varicosity. Other clinical signs usually encountered are increased local temperature and bruit.

Arteriovenous fistulae of congenital origin are usually small and asymptomatic. They can be diffusely distributed throughout an extremity and are associated usually with other abnormalities as well as hypertrophy of the involved limb. The acquired arteriovenous fistulae are mainly posttraumatic or occur as a complication of a surgical procedure. In rare cases they can develop following the rupture of an arterial aneurysm through the necrotic wall of an adjacent vein. On physical examination a local pulsatile swelling with a palpable thrill and evidence of peripheral ischaemia may be found. In large arteriovenous fistulae a systolic murmur is always present.

The third group of vascular lesions in the arm are haemangiomas. The cavernous haemangioma is the most common vascular neoplasm of the upper extremity.

Early and exact diagnosis of all of these vascular lesions depends to a great extent on angiography. It is the most suitable procedure for delination of the lesion, definition of its exact location and extension, identification of the feeding arteries and demonstration of recurrence after excision or irradiation therapy.

REFERENCES

ANTIA, A. U. and O. E. OTTESEN: Collateral circulation in subclavian stenosis or atresia. *Amer. J. Cardiol., 18: 599-604, 1966.*

CALLANDER, C. L.: Arteriovenous fistulae. *Ann. Surg., 7: 428-452, 1920.*

CHOU, S. N. and L. A. FRENCH: Arteriovenous fistula of vertebral vessels in the neck. *J. Neurosurg., 22: 77-80, 1965.*

CURTIS, R. M.: Congenital Arteriovenous Fistulae of the Hand. *J. Bone Joint. Surg., 35A: 917-929, 1953.*

ENNIS, J. T., E. M. BATESON and N. J. MOULE: Uncommon Arteriovenous fistulae. *Clin. Radiol. 23: 392-397, 1972.*

FLANC, C.: Congenital Arteriovenous Fistulas of the Extremities. *Aust. N. Zel. J. Surg., 37: 222-232, 1968.*

GARLAND, H., J. T. LAMB and J. PEARCE: Iatrogenic vertebral arteriovenous fistulae. *Brit. Med. Jour. 5432: 429-430, 1965.*

GERBER, N.: Congenital Atresia of the Subclavian Artery. *Med. J. Dis. Child., 113: 709-713, 1967.*

HELWIG, E. B.: 'Juvenile hemangioma' in Seminar on the Skin Neoplasms and Dermatoses. *Amer. Soc. Clinic. Pathol., pp 74-77, Washington, 1955.*

HOOGENDAM, I. J.: Aangeboren vaatmisvormingen in de extremiteiten. *Proefschrift, Groningen, 1974.*

HORTON, B. T.: Hemihypertrophy of extremities associated with congenital arteriovenous fistula. *J. Amer. Med. Ass. 98: 373, 1932.*

HUNTER, W.: Cyted by C. FLANC (1968).

KAPPERT, A.: Lehrbuch und Atlas der Angiologie. *Verlag H. Huber, Bern, Stuttgart, Wien, 3: 285, 1976.*

LAWSON, T. and T. NEWTON: Congenital Cervical Arteriovenous Malformations. *Radiology, 97: 565-570, 1970.*

LEALIS, L.: 'De partibus semen confic'. *Leyden, 1707. (Cited by Malan, 1979.)*

LEVINE, S., L. S. SARFAS and A. RUSINKO: Right Aortic Arch with Subclavian Steal Syndrome (Atresia of Left Common Carotid and Left Subclavian Arteries). *Amer. J. Surg., 3: 632-637, 1966.*

LUESSENHOP, A. J., R. KACHMANN Jr., W. SHEVLIN and A. A. FERRORO: Clinical evaluation of the arteficial embolization in the management of large cerebral arteriovenous malformations. *J. Neurosurg., 23: 400-417, 1965.*

MALAN, E.: History and different clinical aspects of arteriovenous communications. *J. Cardiovasc. Surg. 35:491-494, 1972.*

NEVIASER, R. J. and J. P. ADAMS: Vascular Lesions in the Hand. *Clin. Orthop. Research, 100: 111-119, 1974.*

ROBERTSON, D. J.: Congenital Arteriovenous fistulae of the extremities. *Ann. Roy. Coll. Surg. Engl. 18: 73-80, 1956.*

SKALPE, I. O. and G. S. SEMB: Collateral Circulation in Subclavian Atresia. Report of A Case with Right Arch and Tetralogy of Fallot. *Scand. J. Cardiovascul. Surg., 3: 207-210, 1969.*

SZILAGYI, D. E., J. P. ELLIOTT, F. J. DERUSSO and R. F. SMITH: Peripheral Congenital Arteriovenous fistula. *Surgery, 57: 61-81, 1965.*

TERPSTRA, J. L., H. J. P. BEERSTECKER, M. N. VAN DER HEYDE and L. TH. F. L. STUBBÉ: Gecombineerde vasculaire misvormingen in het boek 'Arteriële en veneuze pathologie'. *9: 217-219, 1977.*

WARD, C. E. and B. T. NORTON: Arteriovenous fistulae in the Extremities of children. *J. Pediatr., 16: 746-752, 1940.*

WINSLOW, J. B.: Exposition anatomique de le structure du corpus humain. *Paris, 1732.*

Chapter 9

THE THORACIC OUTLET COMPRESSION SYNDROME

9.1 Introduction

The term thoracic outlet compression syndrome was recommended by Rob and Standeven in 1958. It is a general term for a number of neurovascular symptoms which are attributed to compression of the brachial plexus, subclavian artery or subclavian vein in the anatomical areas of the scalene triangle, costoclavicular space and minor pectoral muscle space. Numerous terms have been used in the literature to connect these symptoms with one of the potential pressure points, such as:

Scalenus Anticus Syndrome
Costoclavicular Syndrome
Cervical Rib Syndrome
Cervical-brachial Compression Syndrome
First Thoracic Rib Syndrome
Hyperabduction Syndrome
Pectoralis Minor Syndrome

These syndromes are often extremely difficult to separate clinically. The incidence of neurovascular compression at the thoracic outlet is not known. It is predominantly seen in adults with a sex ratio of four females to one male (Parry, 1979). The symptoms generally appear after the third decade of life.

Left-sided lesions are more common (Adler *et al.*, 1973).

The pathophysiology of this syndrome rests upon the fact that as the brachial plexus and subclavian artery and vein leave the neck and chest on their way to the upper extremity, they run together through three tunnels.

The first tunnel is the interscalene triangle, which consists of the anterior and middle scalene muscles; the base of the triangle is formed by the first rib.

The brachial plexus and subclavian artery pass between these two muscles; the subclavian vein passes over the first rib in front of the anterior scalene muscle (Fig. 115).

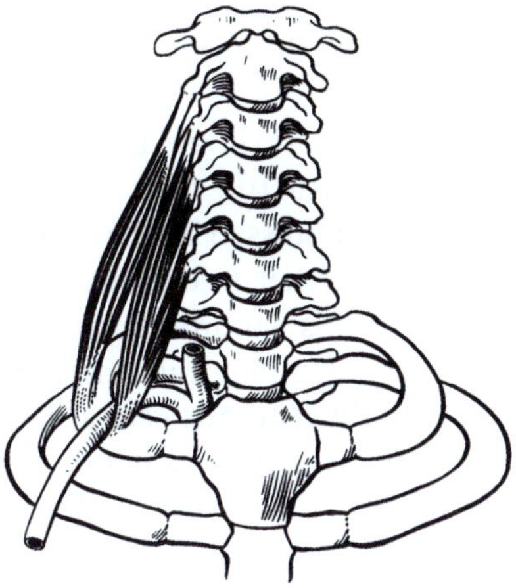

Fig. 115
The normal pattern of insertion of the anterior and middle scalene muscles. The subclavian artery passes through the scalene triangle posterior to the anterior scalene muscle.

The second tunnel is the costoclavicular space. The roof of this tunnel consists of the clavicle and the subclavius muscle; the floor of the first rib. Through this space pass the brachial plexus and the subclavian artery and vein.

The third tunnel is in the axilla between the smaller pectoral muscle and the lateral thoracic

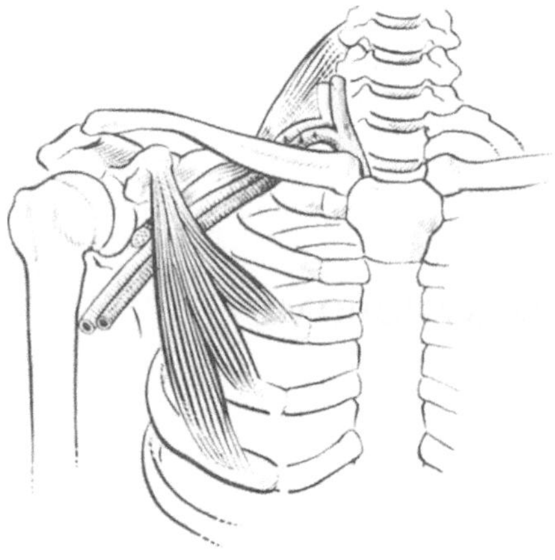

Fig. 116
Costoclavicular space and pectoralis minor tunnel.

wall. This is the so-called pectoralis minor tunnel (Fig. 116).

During muscular contractions the brachial plexus, subclavian artery and subclavian vein can be compressed. When compression gives rise to symptoms, the term compression syndrome is used.

The force and duration of the compression and its location will probably determine the incidence and nature of the symptoms. It should be emphasized that any of the three structures, *i.e.* vein, artery and nerve, may be compressed by these bony ligamentous structures – either selectively or in combination. Therefore, this syndrome can produce vascular symptoms, neurological symptoms or a combination of both (Delaurentis *et al.*, 1974). Neurological symptoms are more frequently encountered than vascular (Nelson and Davis, 1969).

The above-mentioned tunnels are basically three anatomical sites of potential compression of the neurovascular structures as they pass from the thoracic outlet to the upper limb. The head of humerus, however, has also been mentioned in the literature as a cause of compression of the axillary artery when the arm is in an extremely provocative position (Lord and Rosati, 1958; Dijkstra and Westra, 1978). In the cases reported abduction of the arm to 100 degrees resulted in total obstruction of the axillary artery by the head of humerus.

9.1.1 Historical Background

The first patient described in medical literature with exostosis of the first rib, gangrenous fingers and absence of radial pulse was reported by Hilton in 1853. He recognized the compression of the subclavian artery by this exostosis, but incorrectly attributed the digital gangrene to compression of the ulnar nerve. The patient was not treated surgically and auto-amputation of his digits followed.

In 1861 Coote reported on a patient with pressure on the subclavian vessels and the brachial nerve by an exostosis localized on a cervical rib. His patient had an absent radial pulse and a poststenotic aneurysmal dilatation of the subclavian artery on the same side. After resection of the cervical rib, the radial pulse returned. Considering this surgical treatment it can be said that vascular complications of the thoracic outlet syndrome have attracted surgical interest for more than a century.

In 1869 Poland reported on a fusiform or tubular aneurysm of the right subclavian artery associated with a cervical rib. He treated the aneurysm by digital compression on the proximal side of the artery for 96 hours. Physical examination after treatment suggested that the aneurysm had thrombosed. In 1909 Halsted became interested in the problem of poststenotic aneurysms because an aneurysm suddenly developed in one of his patients with a resected cervical rib. In 1916 he was able to confirm his ideas about the origin of poststenotic aneurysms by producing poststenotic dilatation of the aorta in experimental animals. He demonstrated that in dogs after constriction of the aorta via an encircling metal band, the vessel showed dilatation distal to the band.

Halsted ascribed this phenomenon partially to physical changes in the blood flow. In 1913 Todd postulated that vascular changes, in particular poststenotic dilatations occurring in patients with a cervical rib, are not mechanical in origin but are trophic in character and are caused by paralysis of sympathetic fibres passing to the vessels. This theory was also advocated by Telford and Stafford in 1937. Eleven years later (1948) Telford and Mottershead suggested that the aetiology of the poststenotic aneurysm may lie in paralysis of the vasomotor nerves, which degenerate as the result of repeated contusion. Secondary dilatation and stretching of the denervated middle coat (muscularis layer) would extend distalwards from the site of injury to the point where the next nerve comes in. It has also been suggested that the poststenotic aneurysm may be caused by trophic changes and weakness of the arterial wall subsequent to damage of the nutrient vessels of the arterial wall (vasa vasorum). In uncomplicated aneurysms, however, Telford and Mottershead (1948) found no microscopic evidence to support this theory; the arterial wall of the poststenotic aneurysm was uninjured.

Holman demonstrated in 1954 that poststenotic dilatation may be caused by structural fatigue of the arterial wall secondary to vibrations originating in the turbulent flow.

9.2 Anomalies Predisposing to the Thoracic Outlet Compression Syndrome

The vast majority of patients with a thoracic outlet compression syndrome have congenital anomalies in the scalene triangle or skeletal abnormalities of the thoracic outlet.

When Eden reviewed the syndrome in 1939 only one out of 42 cases had no bony abnormality. Cervical rib is by far the most common abnormality, and it is usually a complete cervical rib articulating with the first rib (Raphael *et al.*, 1974). This rib is often found bilaterally, and may or may not articulate with the first thoracic rib. Compression of the artery is produced by the prominence formed by the joint between the cervical rib and first rib or by the strong fibrous band which extends from the tip of a nonarticulating rib to the first thoracic rib. Not all cervical ribs, which are seen on 0.16 to 0.5 percent of all chest roentgenograms, give rise to this syndrome. Extremely short cervical ribs without fibrous junction to the first rib are not able to produce arterial compression (Rainer *et al.*, 1968).

Other common skeletal abnormalities found in patients with this syndrome are a prominent transverse process on C7, a congenitally anomalous first rib fused with the second rib or connected to the second rib by synarthrosis, a bifid first rib, exostosis and tumour of the first rib, elevation of the first rib, a first rib with a broad middle or ventral portion, and cervicothoracic scoliosis. In examining 40,000 chest X-rays Etter (1944) found the incidence of synostosis of the first and second ribs to be 0.19% and the incidence of scoliosis to be 0.31%.

Important compressing mechanisms in the thoracic outlet syndrome are acquired clavicular deformities such as a tumour or callus formation due to fracture, which may narrow the costoclavicular space and cause compression of the neurovascular structures passing between the clavicle and the first rib. Although fracture of the clavicle is readily recognizable, fracture of a first rib following a severe upper extremity strain or injury is more common than formerly believed, but often remains unrecognized on routine chest films.

Other compressing mechanisms which have been described as causing this syndrome are poor posture and inadequate musculature of the shoulder girdle, especially with the sagging shoulders frequently seen in women, pendulous breasts, muscular hypertrophy, hypertrophic costocoracoid ligament and whiplash injuries (Selman *et al.*, 1969; Tomsick *et al.*, 1974).

Neurovascular compression in the scalene triangle can be caused by a variety of abnormalities. The anterior and middle scalene muscles may become thickened and fibrotic following a flexion-extension injury of the neck. This hypertrophy produces narrowing of the base of the triangle, which normally measures 1.2 to 2.5 cm. Other congenital anomalies such as a broad anterior scalene insertion (normal 0.4 to 2.5 cm), an aberrant vessel of the thyrocervical trunk, a hypertrophic omohyoid muscle or the coexistence of a smallest scalene muscle are occasionally associated with this narrowing.

The smallest scalene muscle, or scalenus minimus is also called the muscle of Albinus. It is a

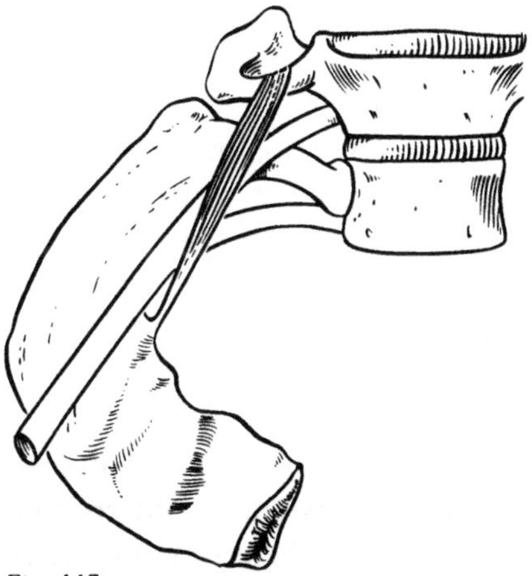

Fig. 117
Smallest scalene muscle (scalenus minimus or muscle of Albinus) passes anterior to the first thoracic nerve root.

small band of muscle or a fibrous band arising from the transverse process of the seventh cervical vertebra and ending as a slender rounded tendon attached to a small spur on the inner margin of the first rib at a point between the two scalene muscles (Fig. 117). At autopsy it is found in 34 percent of the cases (Telford and Mottershead, 1948). The tendon of the smallest scalene muscle passes between the subclavian artery and the brachial plexus. Fibrosis or contractions of the scalene muscles can produce a certain elevation of the first rib, stretching the structures passing over it.

Patients in whom a thoracic outlet compression syndrome has been diagnosed can be divided into two groups:

1. Patients with static (continuous) arterial or venous compression and permanent vascular changes, and
2. Those whose symptoms are attributable to *dynamic*, intermittent arterial or venous compression without permanent vascular changes.

The second group of patients shows no signs of compression when they are resting in the recumbent or sitting position. In provocative positions of the arm, compression appears with the typical signs such as diminished or absent radial pulse and symptoms of ischaemic diffuse pain, numbness, fatigue and colour change (Cox *et al.*, 1974).

The symptoms and signs of dynamic venous compression do not occur directly after elevation of the arm above the head but if the arm remains longer in this provocative position, a slight or moderate swelling may be observed and a bluish or reddish-blue discolouration of the skin of the peripheral parts of the arm may be seen. The patients may then complain of pain in the shoulder and axilla (Greenstone *et al.*, 1971).

Constant arterial compression may lead to secondary arterial injury or disease in the form of:

a. Fusiform or aneurysmal dilatation
b. Local atheroma
c. Thrombosis of the artery
d. Peripheral arterial embolization.

The most vulnerable part of the subclavian artery is its second portion. Constant or intermittent compression of this part of the artery may cause one or more of the above-mentioned abnormalities (Parry, 1979). An aneurysmal poststenotic dilatation demonstrable when the arm is in a neutral position always indicates a haemodynamically significant lesion. A thrombus may have formed in the lumen of the artery and may, if it extends distalwards and proximalwards, lead to complete occlusion of the lumen. Emboli may dislodge and become impacted distally, producing symptoms of secondary Raynaud's phenomenon or they may cause occlusion of one forearm or palmar artery, giving rise to ischaemic attacks in the fingers and the hand. This condition is called *asphyxia manus et digitorum*. Recurrent micro-embolization in the circulation to the fingers may lead to total occlusion of the digital arteries, causing complete ischaemia of the finger (Fig. 118).

This condition was termed *digitus moriens or dying digit* by Lemmens in 1977. It is a very painful condition, characterized by bluish, livid discolouration of the finger. When both proper digital arteries remain occluded the possibilities for collateral circulation are so small that the end result will be necrosis and auto-amputation of the fingertip (Lemmens, 1979).

The third area of potential compression of the neurovascular fascicle is the point where the vessels enter into the axilla. At this point the axillary artery and vein pass together with the median nerve through a common tunnel between the pectoralis minor tendon and the lateral thoracic wall. This is the so-called pectoralis minor tunnel (Fig. 116). Since the vein accompanies the artery in this space compression will affect both vessels. Bony callus, tumours, or haematomas can cause narrowing of this tight space which may result in static compression of the vessels or even thrombosis of the vein. In young muscular individuals an extreme position of hyperabduction of the scapulohumeral joint can give rise to compression of the axillary artery and vein by the pectoralis minor tendon. This physiological compression usually does not cause any symptoms (Lord and Rosaty, 1958).

A pathological dynamic compression of the axillary artery and vein, however, will always manifest with symptoms. The pressure effect should be demonstrable in any position causing hyperabduction of the scapulohumeral joint and stress on the pectoralis minor tendon.

In this position the axillary artery and vein are compressed together. Arterial compression at this

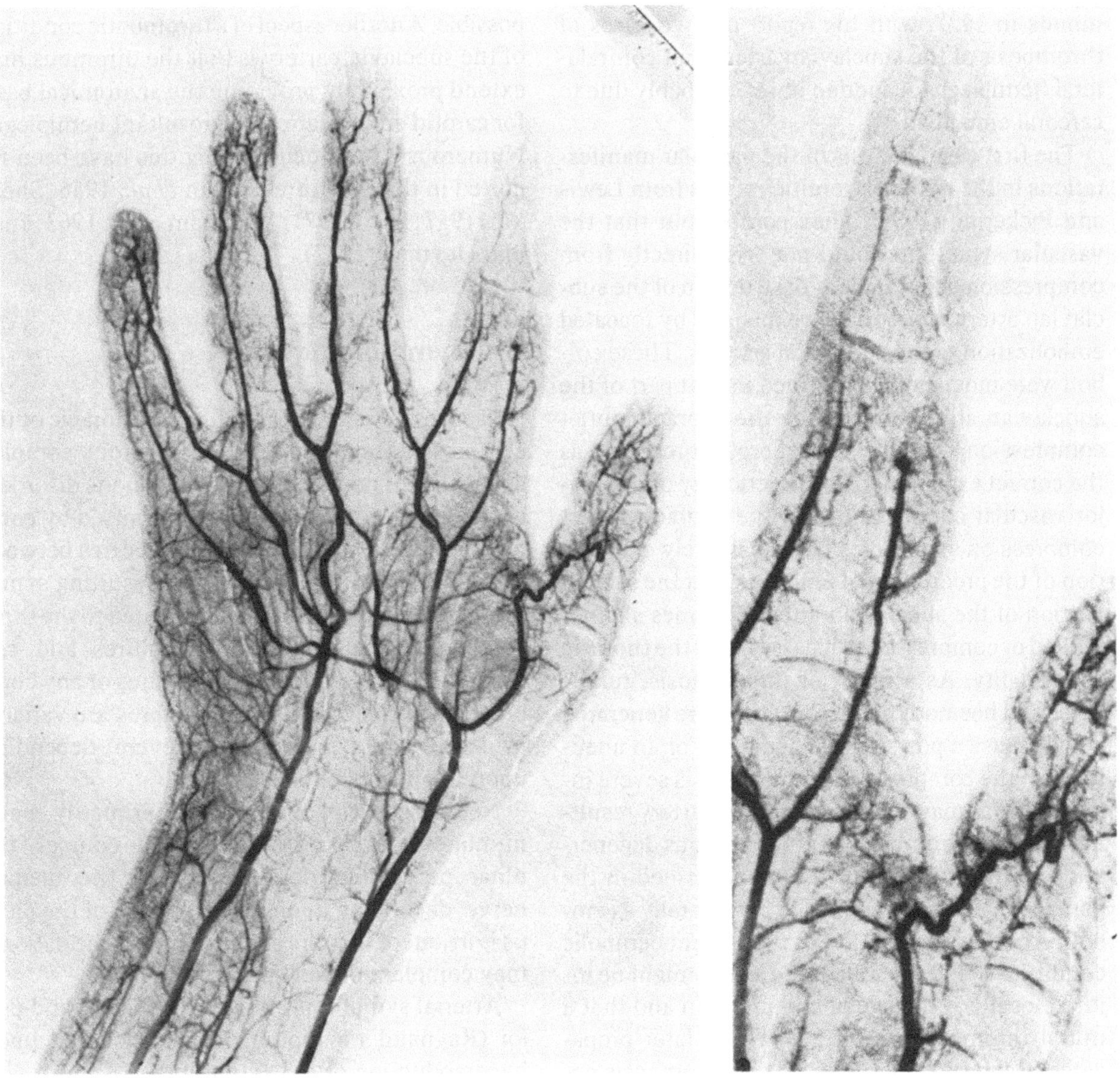

a b

Fig. 118
Digitus Moriens.
A. Occlusion of both proper digital arteries of the index finger with no evidence of collaterals distal to the occlusions.
B. Magnified angiographic pattern of dying digit.

point produces symptoms attributable to impairment of arterial flow. Venous compression or even thrombosis does not cause significant symptoms because of the existence of collateral venous pathways.

The phlebograms of patients with complete obstruction of the axillary vein will demonstrate abundant venous collaterals and obvious preferential flow through the cephalic vein. The axillary and very often the basilic veins are not opacified. Once again, because of the existence of many collaterals the symptoms arising from this condition do not appear severe, except when phlebitis exists (Drewes, 1979). If the compression of the axillary artery and vein is accompanied by constant symptoms the term pectoralis minor syndrome will be used (Roy, 1972; Lord and Stone, 1956).

9.3 Aetiology of Vascular Changes

The first clear suggestion of the thromboembolic

origin of the vascular symptoms was made by Symonds in 1927, with his report on two cases of thrombosis of the subclavian artery and contralateral hemiplegia of sudden onset, probably due to cerebral embolism.

The first clear analysis of the vascular manifestations in the upper extremities stems from Lewis and Pickering (1934). They pointed out that the vascular symptoms could not arise directly from compression or permanent obstruction of the subclavian artery, but could be explained by repeated embolization to the peripheral arteries. These emboli were most probably formed in that part of the subclavian artery affected by the thoracic outlet compression. This theory is at present regarded as the correct explanation of the aetiology of the major vascular complications of the thoracic outlet compression syndrome. The most likely explanation of the production of emboli is that the second portion of the subclavian artery becomes slightly kinked or compressed as it passes over the thoracic abnormality. As a result of this stenosis, turbulence and haemodynamic vibrations are generated which cause a poststenotic dilatation or an aneurysm. If the compression of the artery is severe intimal lesions may occur in the dilated artery resulting in mural thrombosis or atheromatous degeneration of the arterial wall. Thrombi formed in the damaged vessel can propagate peripherally as emboli. Another explanation of the thromboembolic condition is that the wall of the artery might be injured locally at the site of compression and that a mural thrombus has formed which later propagates (Raphael *et al.*, 1974). If the thrombosis occludes the subclavian artery completely and no distal embolization occurs, the most likely result will be a viable extremity with some degree of claudication. If, however, the thrombosis obstructs the vessel completely it may produce emboli that will occlude distal arteries, particularly the digital arteries. In such instances the only symptoms may be transient pain and paraesthesia with coolness of the digits and the hand, Raynaud's phenomenon or ulcerations on the fingertips. This can ultimately result in severe ischaemia leading to loss of the limb, unless adequate therapy is applied (Wickham *et al.*, 1963; Haimovici and Caplan, 1966).

Baird and Lajos in 1964 showed that embolization of the arm only results in severe ischaemia if the brachial artery is occluded above the elbow collaterals, because that makes revascularization impossible. Another aspect of a thrombotic condition of the subclavian artery is that the thrombus may extend proximally providing the anatomical basis for carotid embolization and resultant hemiplegia. Numerous cases documenting this have been reported in the literature (Schein *et al.*, 1956; Shenkin, 1957; Lord, 1971; Wickham *et al.*, 1963; Judy and Heyman, 1972).

9.4 Symptomatology

Nelson and Davis (1969) define the thoracic outlet compression syndrome as a symptom complex consisting of neural, arterial and venous disorders of the upper extremity which are caused by compression of the neurovascular structures between the clavicle and the first rib. The resulting symptoms are directly and obviously related to the three compressed neurovascular structures and can originate from any of these structures or any combination of the three. The symptoms are variable in degree; mild, moderate or severe, depending upon the degree of compression.

Neurological symptoms are primarily pain, numbness and paraesthesia along the course of the ulnar nerve and, less frequently, the median nerve, depending upon which portion of the plexus is irritated. In more advanced cases the patients may complain of weakness of the hand.

Arterial symptoms consist of coolness and pallor (Raynaud's symptoms), usually noted upon hyperabduction of the extremity.

Symptoms of venous compression are swelling with a resultant feeling of tightness in the hand and colour changes such as cyanosis or reddish-blue discolouration of the skin. In all three categories the complaints may be elicited by various hyperabduction manoeuvres related to the individual's work or other activities such as combing hair or sleeping with the arm over the head (Greenstone *et al.*, 1971).

9.5 Physical Examination

The findings on physical examination are defined by the particular anatomical structure that is compressed, *i.e.* the nerve, artery or vein. Isolated neurological, arterial or venous findings are rarely seen, usually two or all three are present together.

The clinical examination consists of inspection, palpation and auscultation of the upper thoracic and neck region. This part of the examination is best performed from behind with the patient sitting (Dunant, 1979).

The inspection comprises body build, posture, position and symmetry of the shoulder girdle, presence and filling of collateral veins, changes in skin colour, muscular atrophy, presence of wounds or necrosis of the fingertips.

Palpation of the neck may reveal an anomalous structure such as a cervical rib, exostosis, callus, tumour or lymph node. The muscular tonus of the shoulder girdle, arm and hand has to be checked too. In patients with thoracic outlet compression syndrome light percussion or pressure over the brachial plexus and downward traction of the arm can produce symptoms (Dunant, 1979). Pain produced by supraclavicular pressure is almost a pathognomonic sign of this syndrome (Greenstone *et al.*, 1971). Pain is usually distributed along the medial side of the arm (Padberg, 1979). In positive cases careful neurological examination will reveal hyperaesthesia, generally following the course of the ulnar nerve. In more advanced cases weakness and muscular atrophy of the arm and hand can be observed (Padberg, 1964).

The arterial signs on physical examination are coolness of the extremity, pallor when the arm is hyperabducted and diminished pulse in this position, usually associated with a supra- or infraclavicular bruit. In the event of peripheral embolic complications, wounds and necrosis of the fingertips are present.

To detect a murmur auscultation has to be performed at three locations:

- in the supraclavicular region
- in the midclavicular region, and
- in the infraclavicular region, below the lateral third of the clavicle (Dunant, 1979).

When venous compression exists oedema, cyanosis and engorgement of the superficial veins may be observed. If complete obstruction of the vein exists enlarged venous collaterals can be seen on the medial side of the upper arm, over the pectoral muscle and on the lateral side of the neck, often with a prominent jugular vein. When thrombosis and inflammation of the veins occur, all the symptoms of acute phlebitis are present. It will be self-evident that some of these signs and symptoms may not be clear when the patient is examined with the arm in a relaxed and neutral position. Therefore a variety of provocative tests have been described for the clinical examination of patients with a suspected thoracic outlet compression syndrome.

Adson test: deep inspiration with the neck slightly hyperextended and the head turned toward the affected side.

Modified adson test: deep inspiration, the neck slightly hyperextended and the head turned toward the unaffected side.

The hyperabduction manoeuvre, sidewards elevation (abduction) of the arm beyond 90 degrees.

The simple abduction test: 90 degree abduction and rotation of the arm in the external direction.

If any of these manoeuvres causes a reduction in the amplitude of the radial pulse, the test is positive. Simultaneous auscultation of the supra- or infraclavicular spaces during these tests can reveal a bruit in a number of the positive cases and often this will correspond with the diminished radial pulse felt by the observer. These diagnostic tests are not completely pathognomonic and should not be overemphasized, because extreme hyperabduction may occasionally result in a diminished radial pulse in normal individuals (Selman *et al.*, 1969) Conn Jr. (1974) published the false-positive results of these tests performed experimentally on asymptomatic healthy individuals. He found alterations of the radial pulse with the Adson test in 38 percent, with the hyperabduction manoeuvre in 68 percent and with the simple abduction test in 54 percent of the normal population.

If the tests are not performed with great care they may have no effect on patients with thoracic outlet compression. In some instances the arm has to be kept in the provocative position for several minutes before the signs and symptoms develop. If the tests are positive and the patient's symptoms can be reproduced, this can be interpreted as a strong indication for the existence of the thoracic outlet compression syndrome.

Selective subclavian arteriography and measurement of the ulnar nerve conduction time are also regarded as reliable procedures for the diagnosis of a thoracic outlet compression syndrome.

The ulnar nerve conduction time is measured by recording the conduction velocity of an electrical stimulus applied to the ulnar part of the brachial plexus in the neck. The conduction time across the thoracic outlet is reduced in the event of compression of the nerves (Urschal *et al.*, 1979).

9.6 Roentgenological Examinations for the Thoracic Outlet Compression Syndrome and Radiodiagnosis

Routine X-ray studies should include chest films as well as films of the upper thoracic aperture, cervical spine and shoulder. The chest film for example may reveal a superior sulcus (Pancoast) tumour invading the brachial plexus, mimicking outlet compression. Radiographs of the upper thoracic aperture and neck can show a cervical rib, an elongated C7 transverse process and deformities of the clavicle or the first rib such as callus formation, tumour, exostosis or congenital malformation. Presence of these abnormalities helps to confirm the diagnosis, but they are not definitively diagnostic (Conn Jr., 1974).

Radiographs of the cervical spine are important for definition of cervical vertebral pathology such as arthritis, arthrosis or fractures. Cervical arthritis and radiculitis produce symptoms similar to those of the thoracic outlet compression syndrome and have to be differentiated. Not infrequently the two conditions exist together as a result of neck trauma in the past (Mulder *et al.*, 1973). In the differential diagnosis consideration must be given to a herniated cervical dise, cervical spondylosis and spondylarthrosis, neuritis of the brachial plexus, Pancoast's tumours, carpal tunnel syndrome, deltoid bursitis and tendonitis. All of these conditions may produce symptoms of the upper extremities that are almost identical in type and distribution pattern to those of the thoracic outlet compression syndrome.

While some of these conditions can be diagnosed by clinical and roentgenographic examinations, the diagnosis of the syndrome of neurovascular compression is often established by exclusion of the other entities (Falconer, Weddel, 1943; Winsor, 1966). The restricted reliability of the diagnostic tests and clinical symptoms explains the search for examinations with a higher level of sensitivity and specificity. In recent years arteriography and venography have been introduced for the preoperative evaluation of symptomatic patients.

Today various opinions have been expressed in the literature concerning the usefulness of arteriography and phlebography for the diagnosis of this syndrome. A number of experts in this field are of the opinion that arteriograms and venograms are of limited value and not always necessary (Greenstone *et al.*, 1971, Conn Jr., 1974). Others have demonstrated that arteriography and venography are useful adjuncts for the diagnosis of thoracic outlet syndrome, in particular for demonstration of multiple lesions (Lang, 1965, 1969 and 1972; Winsor, 1966; Heymann, 1972).

Achterberg and Jansen van Wigmont (1974) made a retrospective study and came to the conclusion that arteriography is not useful for the evaluation of dynamic compression since less than half of the diagnosed compressions presented with brachialgia. They concluded that arteriography is indicated only if an intrinsic vascular disorder is suspected, such as arteritis, thrombosis, etc.

The opinion of the vascular team of the St. Annadal Hospital is that functional arteriography and phlebography should be performed for all patients in whom the vascular signs and symptoms predominate. Arteriography enables us to localize and identify single or multiple lesions and to differentiate extrinsic compression from intrinsic disease.

Although total arterial occlusion is rare in patients with thoracic outlet compression, the correct diagnosis is best achieved by angiography. Large collateral arteries around the shoulder sometimes preserve distal pulses. Thus, on physical examination apparently normal pulses may be palpated notwithstanding complete subclavian artery occlusion. Furthermore, the flow pattern may change as the arm is manipulated through the various abduction manoeuvres and Doppler examination may not show the expected damping of the flow distal to the obstruction. Functional angiography is the best method for detecting an arterial occlusion and differentiating patients with permanent occlusion from those with intermittent obstruction. Our results will be discussed below.

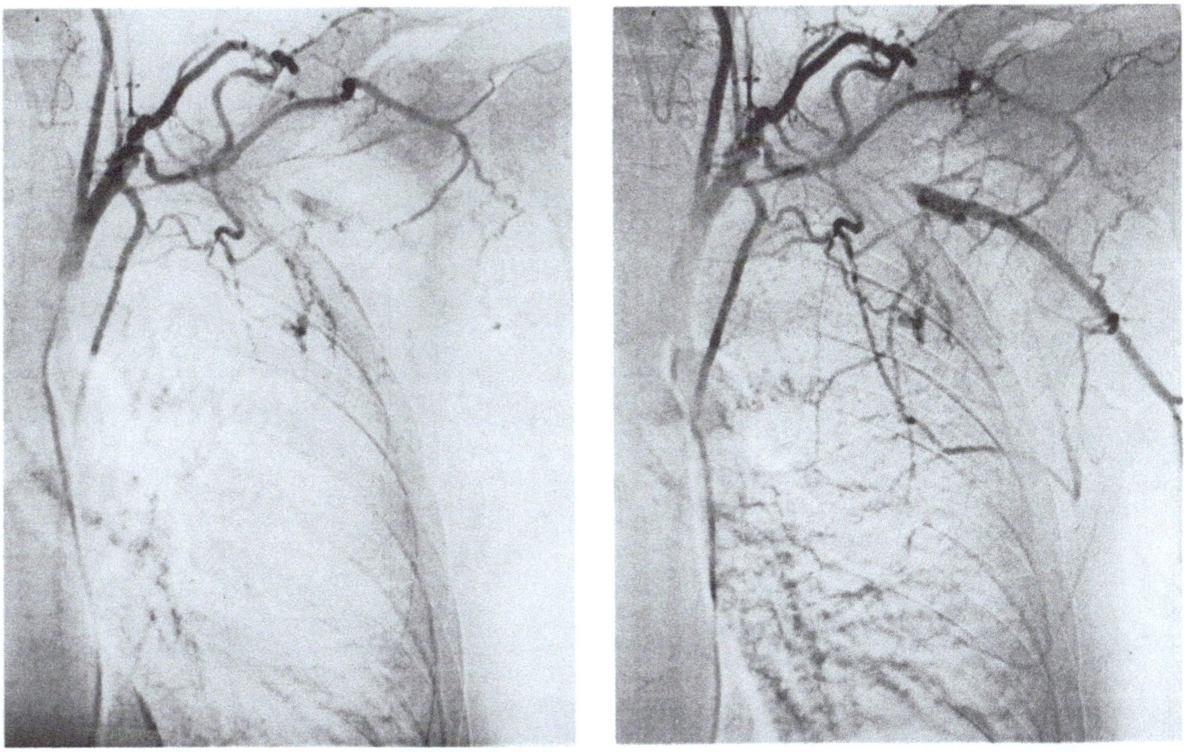

Fig. 119 a b

A. Early arterial phase of the left subclavian arteriogram shows a total occlusion of the subclavian artery, as a complication of the thoracic outlet compression syndrome.

B. Late arterial phase shows filling of the axillary artery through collaterals.

(Reproduced from J. M. Greep *et al.*, Pain in Shoulder and Arm, chapter 3. Martinus Nijhoff, The Hague, Boston, London, 1979.)

9.7 Our Investigation

In the course of the past ten years the thoracic outlet compression syndrome was frequently encountered in our hospital. 269 patients with clinical signs of this syndrome were submitted for angiography.

9.7.1 Arteriography: Technical Aspects

Transfemoral catheterization of the subclavian arteries is the favoured method since antegrade flow of contrast medium is maintained, simulating conditions of normal blood flow. The technique of selective catheterization of the left and right subclavian arteries is described in Chapter 3 (3.4).

To permit a free movement of the patient and to insure normal muscle tone, the examination should be carried out under local anaesthesia. According to some authors the definitive assessment and diagnosis of thoracic outlet compression syndromes necessitate examinations in several positions. In our opinion, two series of roentgenograms are sufficient in most cases. On very rare occasions a third series is necessary. The first series of radiographs of the thoracic outlet is taken with the arm in the neutral position. The patient is placed supine on the examination table, assuming a relaxed position with the arm along the thoracic wall. This series is primarily intended for identification of permanent vascular lesions such as obstruction, thrombosis, aneurysmal dilatation or local atheroma (Figs. 119, 120, 121).

The second study is intended to demonstrate the arterial compression. This series of roentgenograms should be taken with the arm in a provocative position. The determination of the final position of the arm should be made under fluoroscopy, using small injections of contrast medium for each provocative position of the arm.

During the second series the arm has to remain in the chosen position. If the position of the arm is

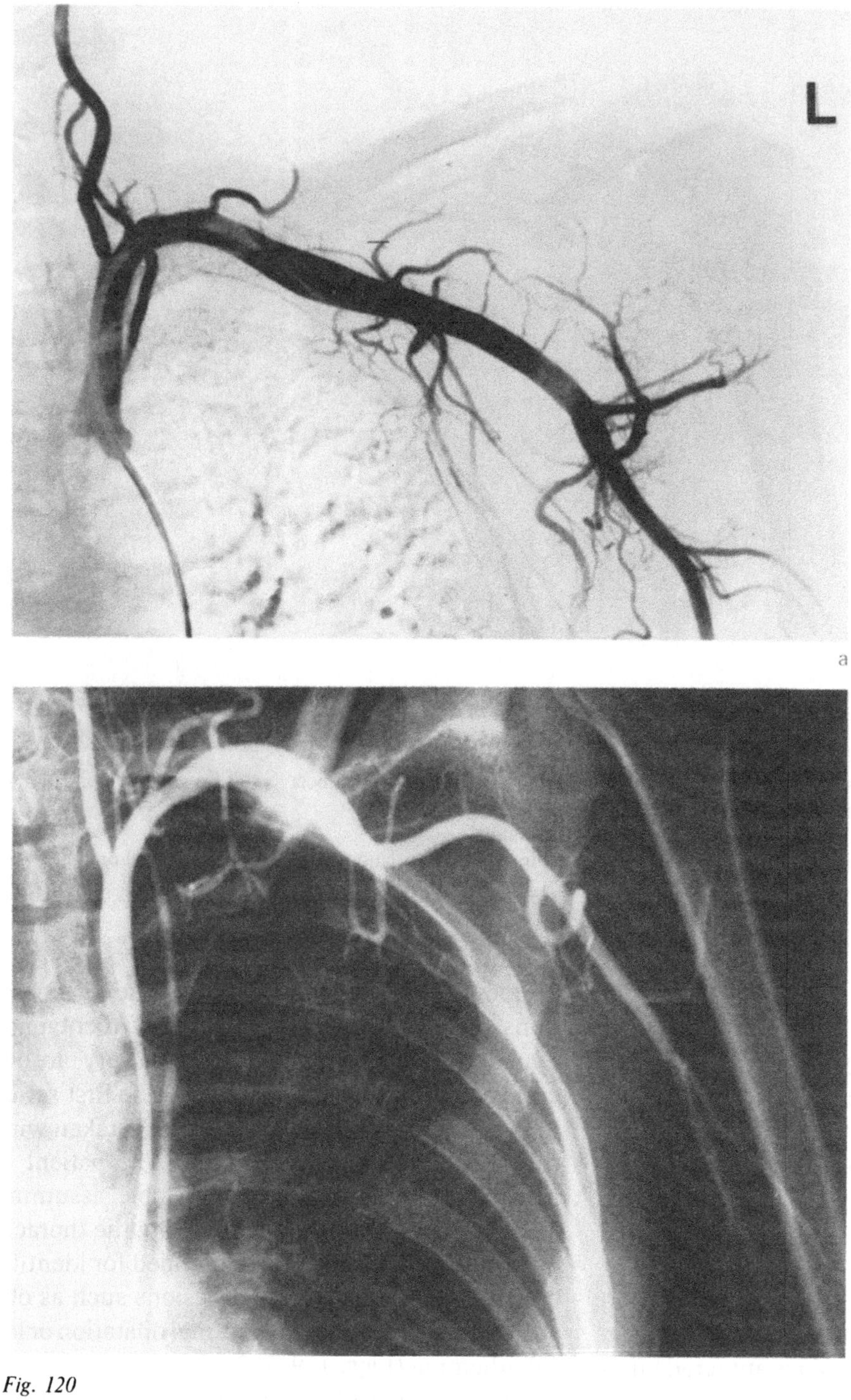

Fig. 120
Selective arteriograms of the left subclavian artery (arm in neutral position) in two different patients with poststenotic (aneurysmal) dilatation of the subclavian arteries.
A. Slight dilatation of the left subclavian artery at the scalene triangle.
B. Severe poststenotic dilatation of the subclavian artery caused by static compression by a rudimentary cervical rib.

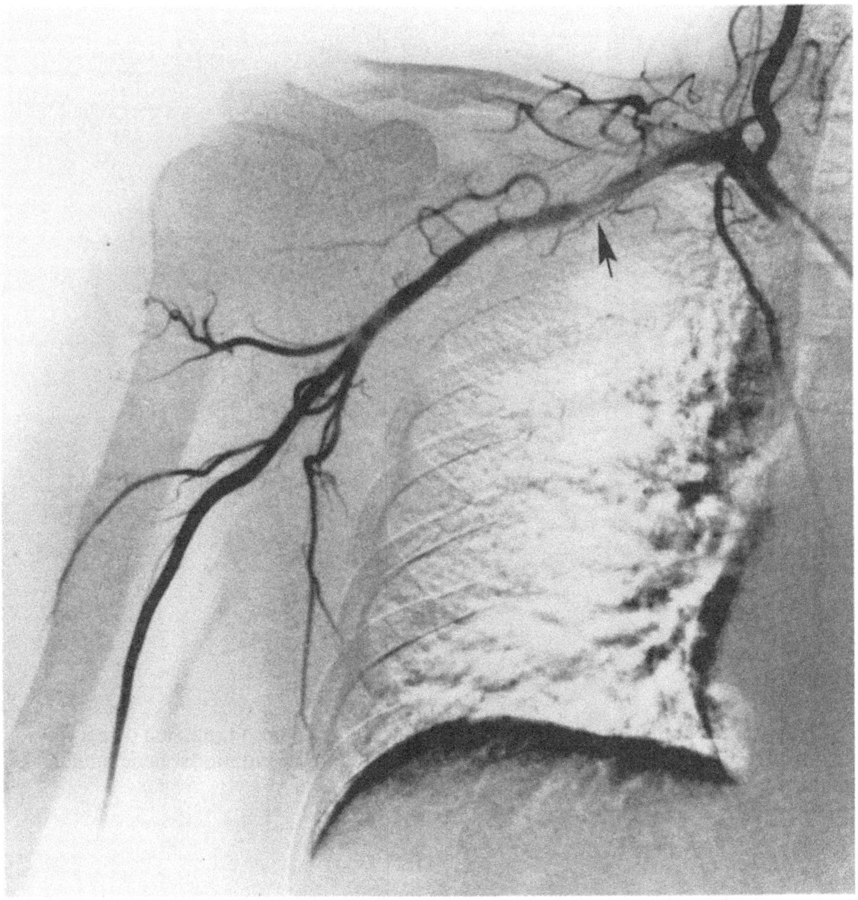

Fig. 121
Local atheroma in the wall of the right subclavian artery (arrow) in young subject. A complication of the thoracic outlet compression syndrome.

determined in this way, multiple series of roentgenograms as recommended by some authors can be avoided.

In some individuals the compression phenomenon is seen in all positions. In such cases arteriography should be performed in the position which causes maximal symptoms and physical discomfort. To discover microemboli in the peripheral arteries, which might stem from that part of the subclavian artery involved by the thoracic outlet compression, every subclavian arteriogram should be completed with an additional brachial angiogram. Also if compression at the thoracic outlet cannot be demonstrated brachial angiography should be performed, since there is a strong association between the thoracic outlet syndrome and distal emboli.

We believe that a complete angiographic investigation of the arm is indicated in every case presenting with the symptoms and signs of thoracic outlet compression syndrome or Raynaud's phenomenon in order to establish or exclude a source of embolization at the thoracic outlet. Whenever the subclavian arteriogram demonstrates occlusive disease, atheroma or intramural thrombus in the artery at the thoracic outlet, brachial catheterization should not be used for the examination of the arteries of the forearm and hand. In such instances the direct brachial artery puncture or cutdown technique for brachial arteriography is usually preferred.

To avoid any risk of iatrogenic embolization of the distal arteries of the arm, the brachial artery should not be catheterized until the arteriograms of the proximal subclavian and axillary arteries have been studied.

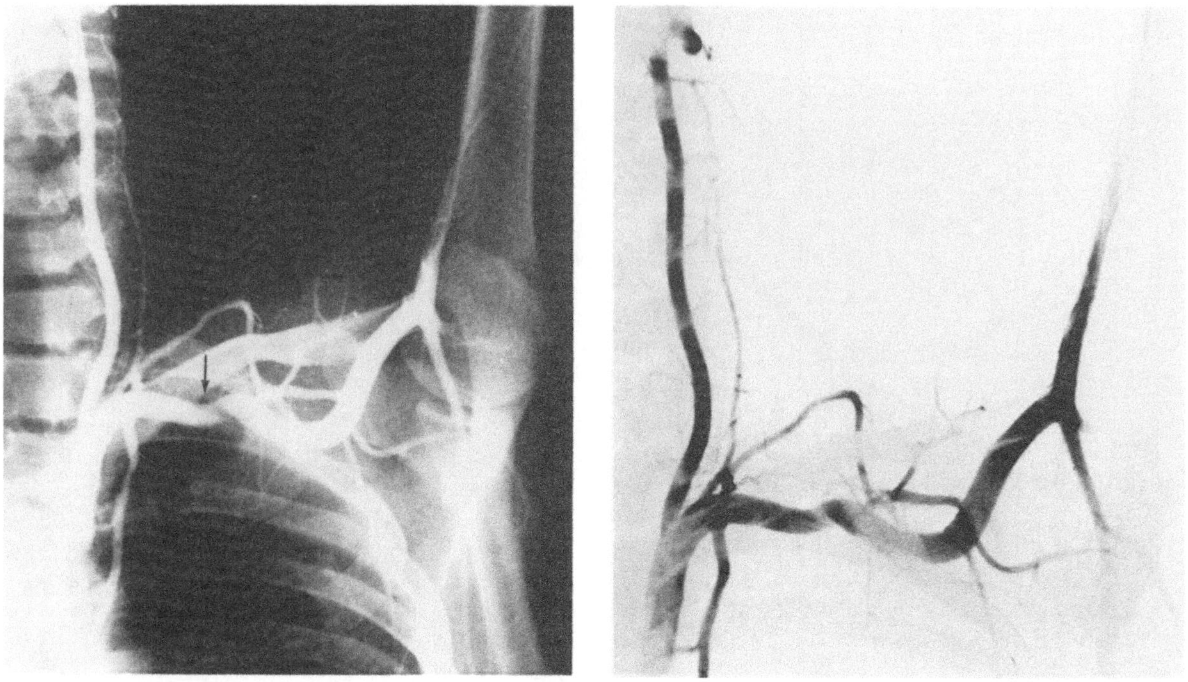

a b

Fig. 122

A. Left selective arteriogram taken with arm in hyperabductive positon demonstrates an oblique compression defect traversing the subclavian artery (arrow). This angiographic pattern of compression is attributed to the anterior scalene tendon.

B. The same case when the subtraction technique is applied.

9.7.2 Phlebography: Technical Aspects

Although arteriographic assessment usually identifies the causative lesion, phlebography is advocated as an adjuvant examination since the somewhat different pathway of the subclavian vein can show different pressure effects and thus facilitate differentiation of some of these entities. Phlebography of the upper extremity is indicated if there is a history of intermittent or persistent oedema of the hand or arm or if a prominent venous pattern is present over the arm, shoulder and chest. Venous occlusion may be complete or intermittent; if demonstrated only upon changes of posture intermittent subclavian obstruction can be diagnosed (Conn Jr., 1974).

Functional phlebography of the upper extremity is carried out with the patient supine. It is best done by injection of contrast medium through a short puncture needle into a superficial vein on the medial side of the antecubital fossa. We usually employ the so-called 'Butterfly' needles with a length of 22.2 mm.

These needles are supplied with polythene tubing 305 mm long and are very convenient for intravenous injection when the arm is in different positions. Appropriate placement of the needle in a medial antecubital vein results in the distribution of contrast medium into both the cephalic and basilic groups as well as the filling of the axillary and subclavian veins via these pathways. Injection of contrast medium into a vein on the lateral side of the antecubital fossa, however, may result in filling of the cephalic and subclavian veins only without filling of the axillary vein. Such phlebograms, which do not visualize the axillary vein, are insufficient because they cannot exclude occlusion or compression of the axillary vein by the tendon of the minor pectoral muscle.

The relatively slow flow in the veins permits a low film frequency. The exposures are usually taken first with the arm in the relaxed abducted position and then in the hyperabducted and externally rotated position. The required dose is usually about 20-30 ml per injection; if a detailed examination of a thrombotic case is necessary a large dose may provide better information about the anatomy of the central parts of the venous system.

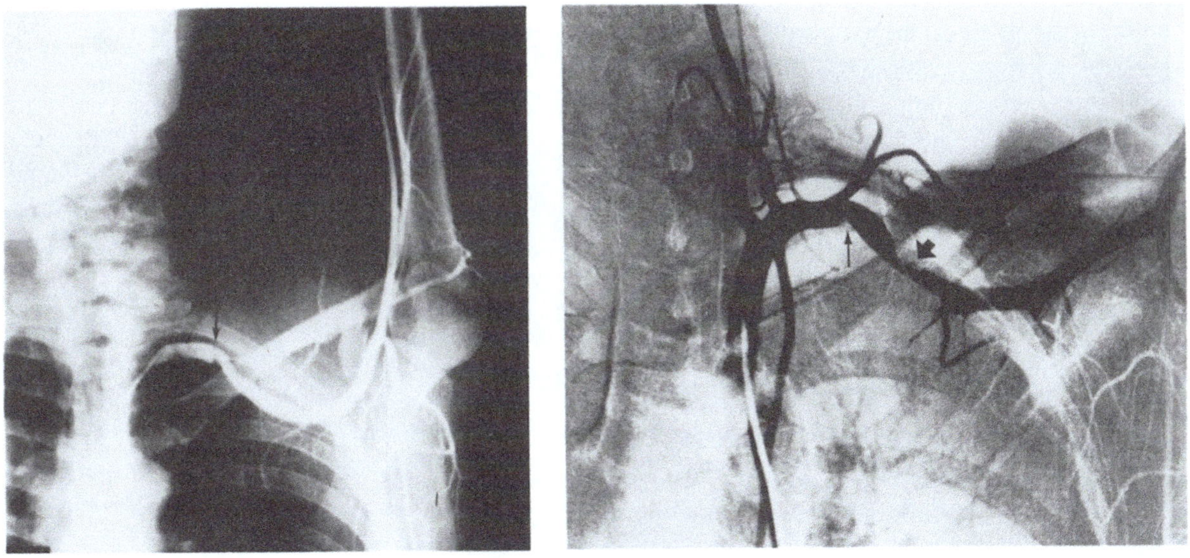

Fig. 123 a b

Left subclavian arteriograms (arm in provocative position) of two different patients.

A. Small band-like defect at the most proximal part of the subclavian artery (arrow) characteristic of compression by fibrous band or smallest scalene muscle.

B. Double compression of the subclavian artery. A fibrous band compression (small arrow) and costoclavicular compression (large arrow).

9.7.3 Angiographic Signs of Compression at Different Points of the Thoracic Outlet and Radiological Diagnosis

The subclavian artery can be subjected to extrinsic compression at three points as it passes through the thoracic outlet. The first potential site of compression is located between the anterior and middle scalene muscles and over the superior rim of the first rib. The subclavian vein passes in front of the anterior scalene muscle and cannot be compressed in this area.

Depending on the predominant cause of the arterial compression at this point, different characteristic compression effects will show up on the arteriograms. The most frequent pattern at this point is an oblique compression defect, that can be attributed to compression of the vessel by the anterior scalene tendon (Fig. 122). A small band-like defect at the most proximal part of the second subclavian segment is characteristic of compression by fibrous bands, originating either from a cervical rib or the transverse process of the seventh cervical vertebra and inserting near the tuberculum of the first rib, at a point between the two scalene muscles (Fig. 123). In some instances this band is the smallest scalene muscle or muscle of Albinus. The degree of compression at this point depends on the size of the scalene tunnel. Progressive narrowing of the scalene tunnel can be caused by different stress positions and is reflected on arteriograms as an increasing compression of the subclavian artery, culminating in a complete cutoff of the vessel at its point of exit from the scalene tunnel (Fig. 124A).

Complications of permanent or intermittent compression of the artery at this point can be a poststenotic dilatation or fusiform aneurysm of the artery (Fig. 120). If a poststenotic dilatation of the subclavian artery is demonstrable when the arm is in a neutral position, it always indicates a haemodynamically significant lesion.

In the event of such objective arteriographic findings at the scalene triangle a phlebogram which does not show compression of the subclavian vein must be present to support the diagnosis of the anterior scalene syndrome.

The second point of extrinsic compression of the subclavian artery is the costoclavicular space. At this point the vessels are compressed by the inferior ridge of the clavicle, the subclavius muscle and the medial superior margin of the first rib. On

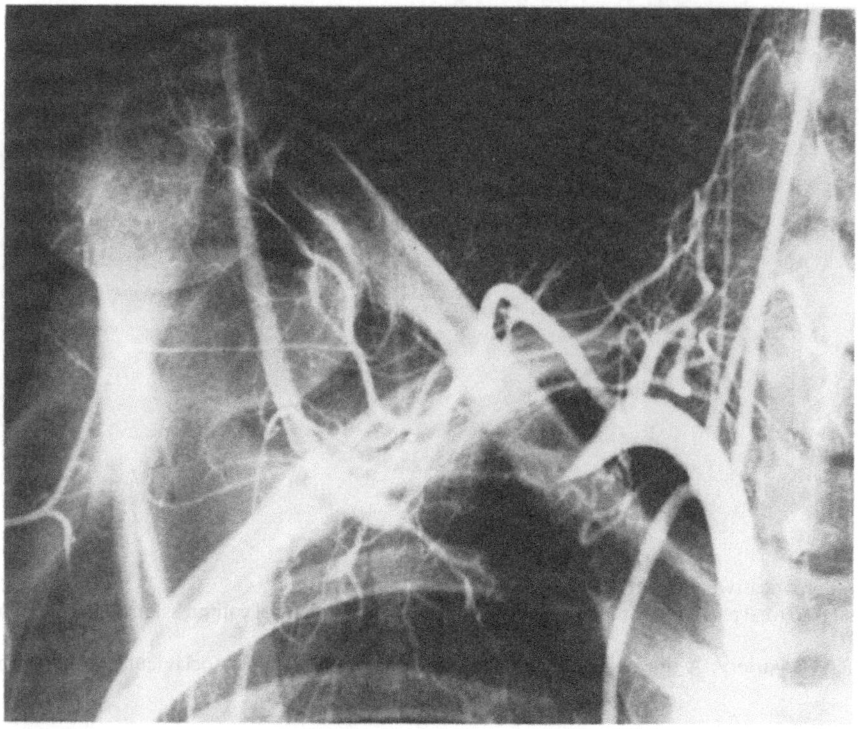

a

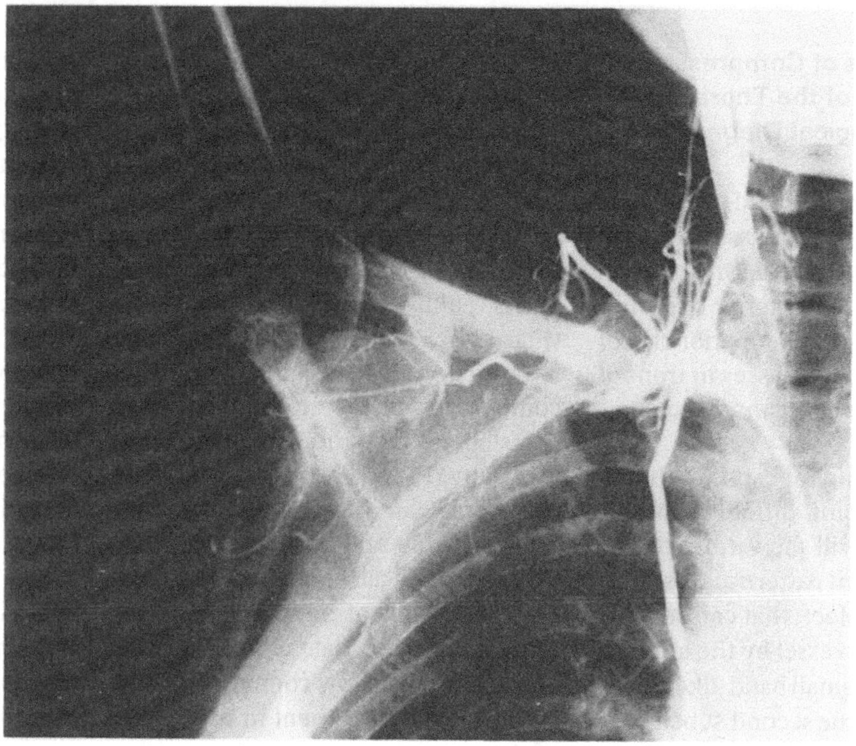

b

Fig. 124

Right subclavian arteriograms of two patients taken with arm in position of extreme hyper-abduction.

A. Severe compression of the subclavian artery at the scalene tunnel resulting in a complete cutoff of the vessel. Note that compression appears medial to the first rib.

B. Complete 'cutoff' of the subclavian artery in the costoclavicular space. This compression always appears at the medial border of the first rib.

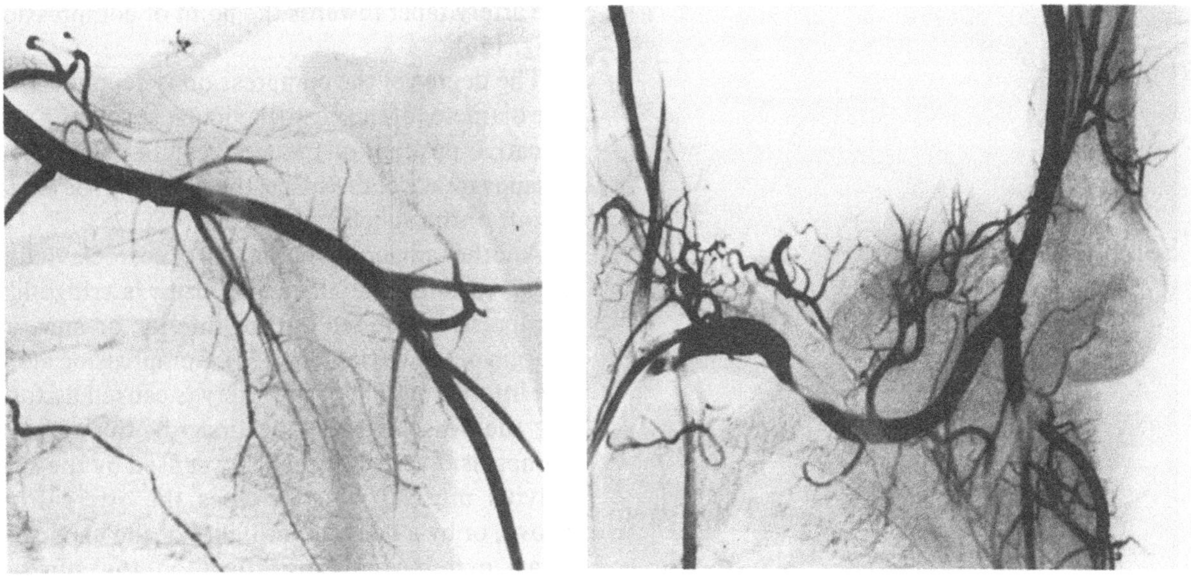

a b

Fig. 125
Dynamic, inconstant arterial compression.
A. Normal left subclavian arteriogram taken with arm in neutral position.
B. Severe costoclavicular compression of the subclavian artery at characteristic site during hyperabduction-external rotation test.

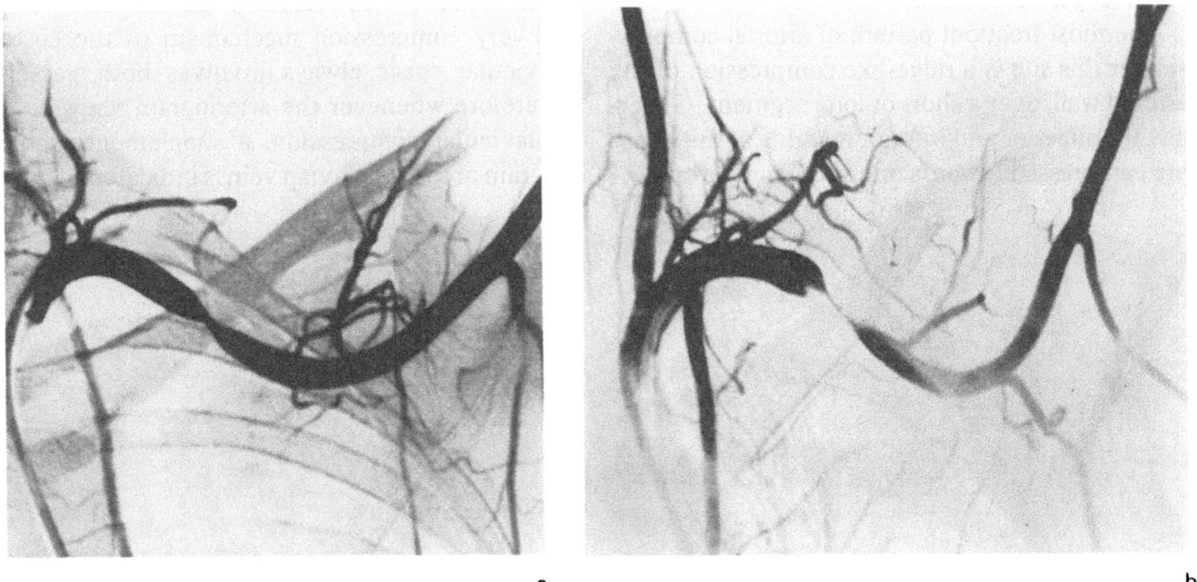

a b

Fig. 126
A ridge-like compression of the subclavian artery over a short segment (A) and a long segment (B).
The superior and the inferior walls of the arteries are compressed towards one another. The ends of the arteries are tapered towards the compressed points. Both compressions appeared at the crossing of the clavicle and the medial margin of the first rib, a typical site of costoclavicular compression.

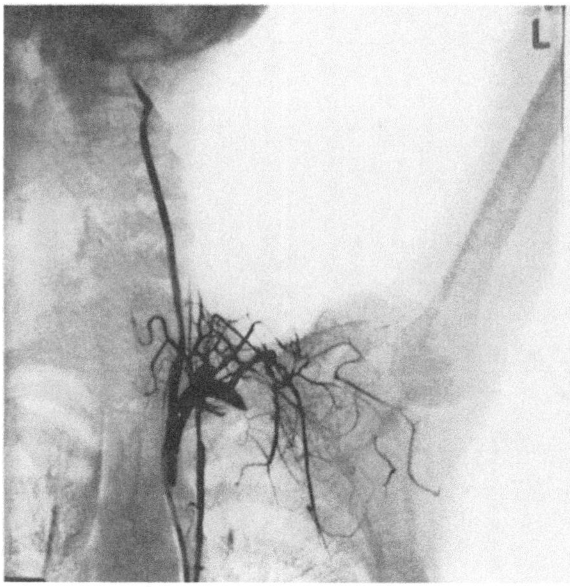

Fig. 127
Left subclavian arteriogram of arm in provocative position demonstrates severe compression in the costoclavicular space resulting in complete 'cutoff' of the vessel.

angiograms the compression occurs exactly at this point (Figs. 124B, 125B).

The most frequent pattern of arterial compression at this site is a ridge-like compression of the arterial wall, over a short or long segment. Generally the superior and inferior margins of the artery are compressed towards one another. The ends of the artery taper towards the point of compression (Fig. 126).

The degree of the compression is dependent on the diameter of the costoclavicular space. If a provocative position of the arm results in complete disappearance of the space, the result will be a total cutoff of the subclavian artery (Fig. 127).

Another angiographic pattern of costoclavicular compression of the subclavian artery is a ridge-like compression limited to the inferior or superior margin of the vessel (Fig. 128). Compression along the inferior margin of the artery is caused by forcing the vessel against the first rib; the superior compression effect is probably caused by the subclavius muscle, which crosses the artery from above, or by a bony abnormality of the clavicle.

An extreme pressure effect on the superior aspect of a large segment of the subclavian artery usually indicates an abnormality of the clavicle, such as callus formation or tumour, causing an important reduction in the costoclavicular space. Since the subclavian vein parallels the artery in this segment, a compression of the subclavian vein will always be present (Figs. 129, 130, 131).

Every compression mechanism in the costoclavicular space always involves both vessels. Therefore whenever the arteriogram shows costoclavicular compression, a supplemental phlebogram of the subclavian vein is indicated. If these

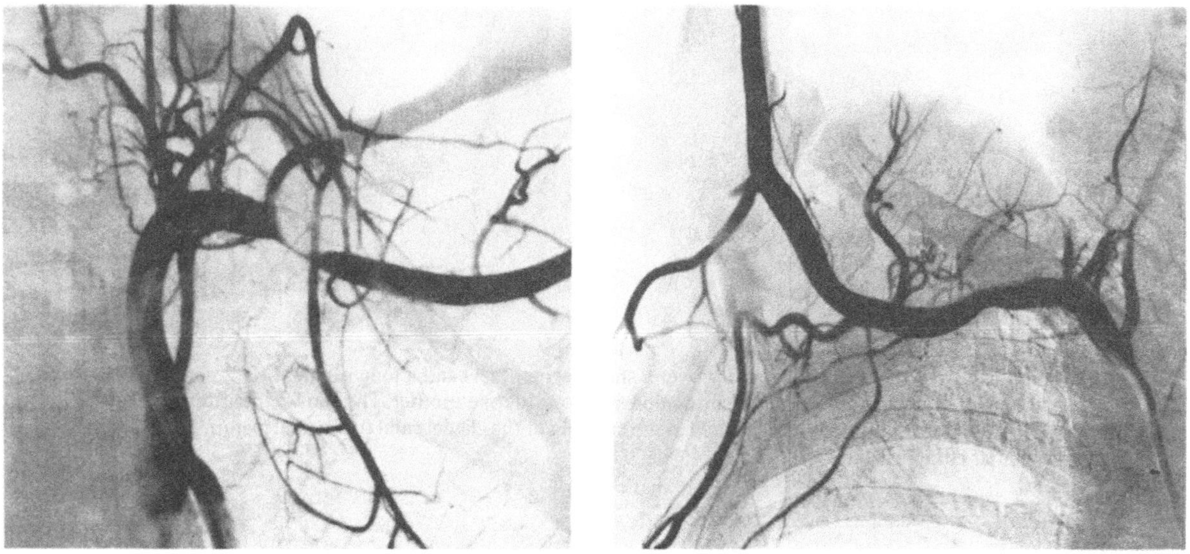

a b

Fig. 128
Ridge-like costoclavicular compressions.
A. Compression only along the superior margin of the left subclavian artery.
B. Ridge-like compression along the inferior margin of the right subclavian artery.

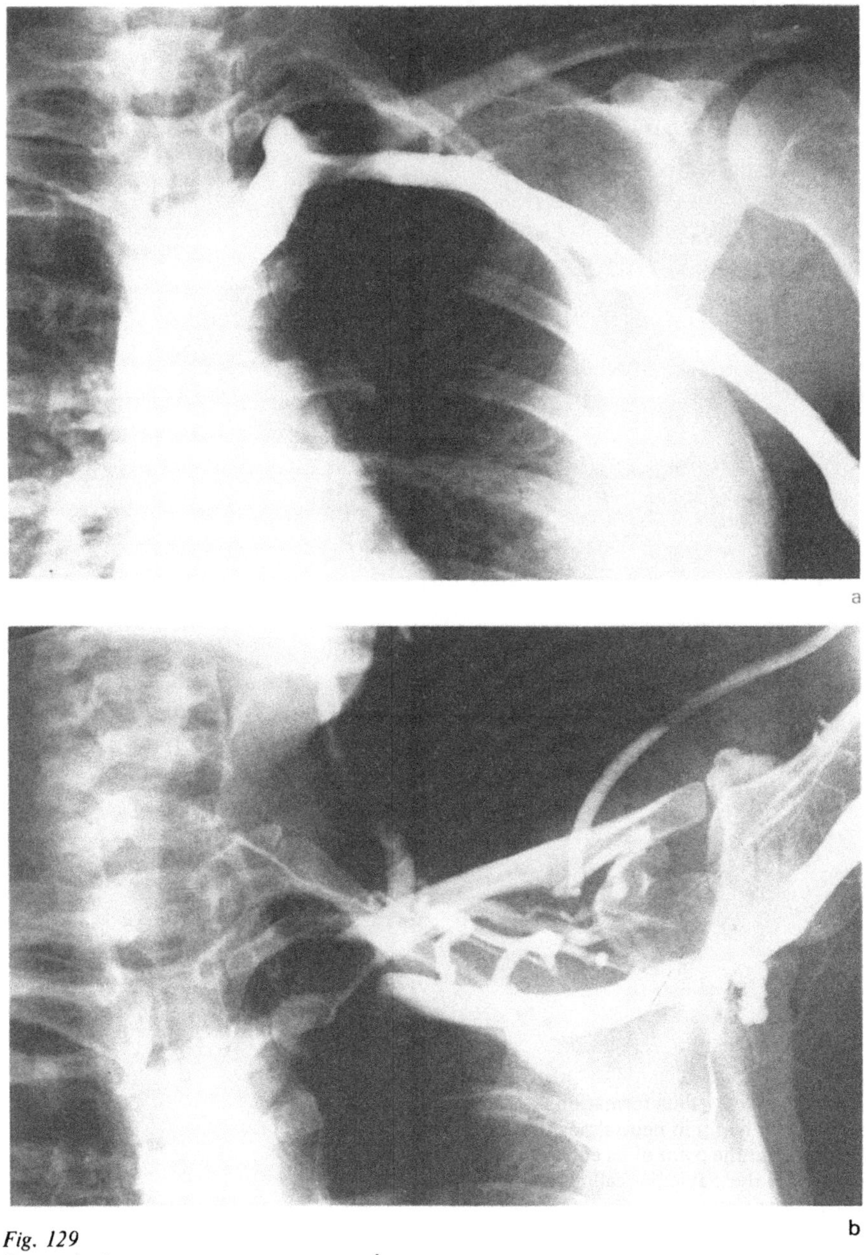

Fig. 129
Dynamic, inconstant venous compression.
A. Normal left subclavian phlebogram taken with arm in neutral position.
B. Complete costoclavicular compression of the subclavian vein during abduction external rotation test.

phlebograms are taken with the arm in the same provocative position as for the arteriograms, they will always demonstrate a significant compression or a total venous obstruction. The compression of the vein is generally more pronounced than that of the artery, because of the thin wall of the vessel and the low intravascular pressure. Thus, only when both vessels are compressed at this point is the diagnosis of costoclavicular compression syndrome justifiable.

The third site of potential compression is the pectoralis minor tunnel. Since the axillary vein runs parallel to the artery in this space compression will affect both vessels. Due to the lateral position of this tunnel and the characteristic appearance of a compression inferior to the coracoid pro-

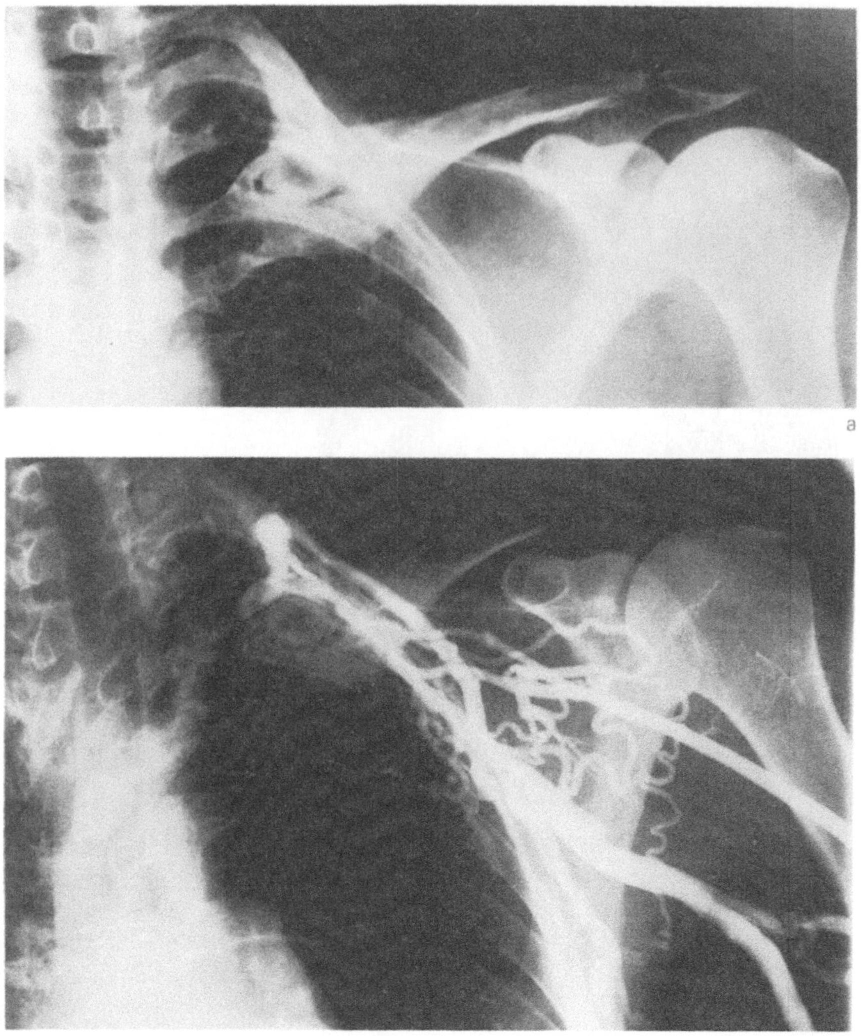

a

b

Fig. 130
Static (constant) venous compression.
A. 'Old' fracture of the left clavicle with massive callus formation.
B. Phlebogram of the left subclavian vein with arm in neutral position demonstrates constant compression of the subclavian vein at the point of its entrance into the costoclavicular space by the inferior component of the clavicular callus. A preferential collateral flow through the cephalic vein therefore exists.

cess, the radiological diagnosis of pectoralis minor compression will never be a problem (Fig. 132).

The fourth site of potential compression is the head of humerus. At this site in some individuals the axillary artery and vein may be compressed separately or in combination in some provocative positions of the arm. Compression of both vessels (artery and vein) is not always present however. According to the observations of other authors (Lord and Stone, 1956; Dijkstra and Westra, 1978) arterial compression is often accompanied by compression of the basilic vein. Once we saw isolated compression of the axillary vein by the head of humerus when the arm was abducted 90 degrees in a patient with deep venous thrombosis of the upper extremity (Fig. 133B).

Because the compression of the vessels caused by the humerus head appears at a characteristic site, the radiological diagnosis is always obvious.

9.8 Case Material

During the period 1970-1980 two hundred and six-

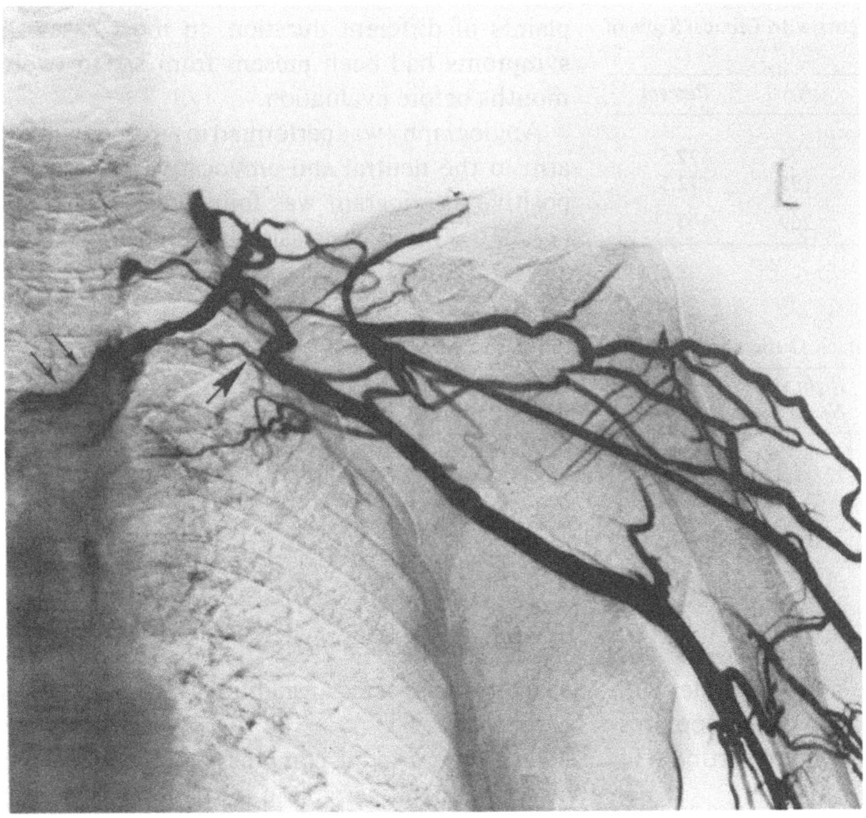

Fig. 131
Phlebogram of the left arm in patient with a cervical rib demonstrates complete thrombosis of the subclavian vein at its point of entrance into the costoclavicular space (arrow). Filling of the left innominate vein (double arrows) through marked collaterals.

TABLE XXIII

Age of Patients with Complaints of Thoracic Outlet Compression.

Years	*Females*		*Males*		*Both sexes together*		
	Nr.	*%*	*Nr.*	*%*	*Nr.*	*%*	
0-20	7	2.6	1	0.4	8	3.0	
21-30	21	7.8	7	2.6	28	10.4	
31-40	48	17.8	36	13.4	84	31.2	62%
41-50	42	15.6	40	14.9	82	30.5	
51-60	26	9.7	27	10.0	53	19.7	
> 60	7	2.6	7	2.6	14	5.2	
Total	151	56.1	118	43.9	269	100	

TABLE XXIV

Age of Female Patients with TOCS.

Years	*Number*	*Percent*
0-20	7	4.6
21-30	21	13.9
31-40	48	31.8
41-50	42	27.8
51-60	26	17.3
> 60	7	4.6
Total	151	100

TABLE XXV

Age of Male Patients with TOCS.

Years	*Number*	*Percent*
0-20	1	0.9
21-30	7	5.9
31-40	36	30.5
41-50	40	33.9
51-60	27	22.9
> 60	7	5.9
Total	118	100

TABLE XXVI

Angiographic Findings in 269 Patients with Clinical Signs of Thoracic Outlet Compression.

	Nr.	*Percent*
Negative arteriograms (compression not visible)	74	27.5
Positive arteriograms	195	72.5
Total	269	100

TABLE XXVII

Arteriographic Findings at the Thoracic Outlet in 195 Patients with Positive Arteriograms.

Lesion	*Right side*		*Left side*		*Both sides*		*Total*	
	Nr.	*%*	*Nr.*	*%*	*Nr.*	*%*	*Nr.*	*%*
Dynamic compression of the subclavian artery	22	11.3	77	39.5	67	34.3	166	85.1
Poststenotic dilatation of the subclavian artery	7	3.6	12	6.1	5	2.7	24	12.3
Complete occlusion of the subclavian artery	1	0.5	3	1.5	1	0.5	5	2.6
Total	30	15.4	92	47.1	73	37.5	195	100

ty-nine patients, 151 female and 118 male, with the clinical diagnosis of thoracic outlet compression syndrome were referred to our department for angiographic investigation.

The age of the patients varied from 18 to 74 years old. Sixty-two percent of the patients were between thirty and fifty years old (Tables XXIII, XXIV, XXV).

All of the patients were symptomatic, with complaints of different duration. In most cases the symptoms had been present from six to twelve months before evaluation.

Angiography was performed in all cases with the arm in the neutral and provocative positions. A positive arteriogram was found for 195 patients (72.5%). When compression in the costoclavicular space was suspected an additional phlebogram was carried out.

Dynamic arterial compression at the thoracic outlet was demonstrable in 166 patients (85%) with a sex ratio of 1.3 females to one male. Left-sided lesions appeared in 77 cases (46%), bilateral compression in 67 patients (40%) and isolated compression on the right side in only 22 cases (13%) (see Table XXVIII). Other results of the angiographic examinations are summarized in Table XXVII.

The complications of the thoracic outlet compression syndromes, namely complete occlusion of the subclavian artery or poststenotic aneurysmal dilatation of the subclavian artery, were found in 29 patients (15%). Peripheral occlusions of the digital arteries due to microemboli in patients with dynamic compression were found in 21% and in patients with poststenotic dilatation of the subclavian artery in 71% of the cases.

TABLE XXVIII

Incidence of Site of Dynamic Compression at the Thoracic Outlet in 166 Patients.

Site of compression at the thoracic outlet	*Females*		*Males*		*Total number*	
	Nr.	*%*	*Nr.*	*%*	*Nr.*	*%*
Right	9	5.4	13	7.8	22	13.2
Left	42	25.3	35	21.0	77	46.4
Both sides	43	25.9	24	14.5	67	40.4
Total	94	56.6	72	43.4	166	100

TABLE XXIX

Incidence of Occlusions in the Circulation of the Hand in Patients with Poststenotic Dilatation and Dynamic Compression of the Subclavian Arteries.

Site	*Poststenotic Dilatation*	*Peripheral occlusions*		*Dynamic compression*	*Peripheral occlusions*	
	Nr.	*Nr.*	*%*	*Nr.*	*Nr.*	*%*
Right	7	5	71.4	22	5	22.7
Left	12	8	66.7	77	16	20.8
Both sides	5	4	80.0	67	13	19.4
Total	24	17	70.8	166	34	20.9

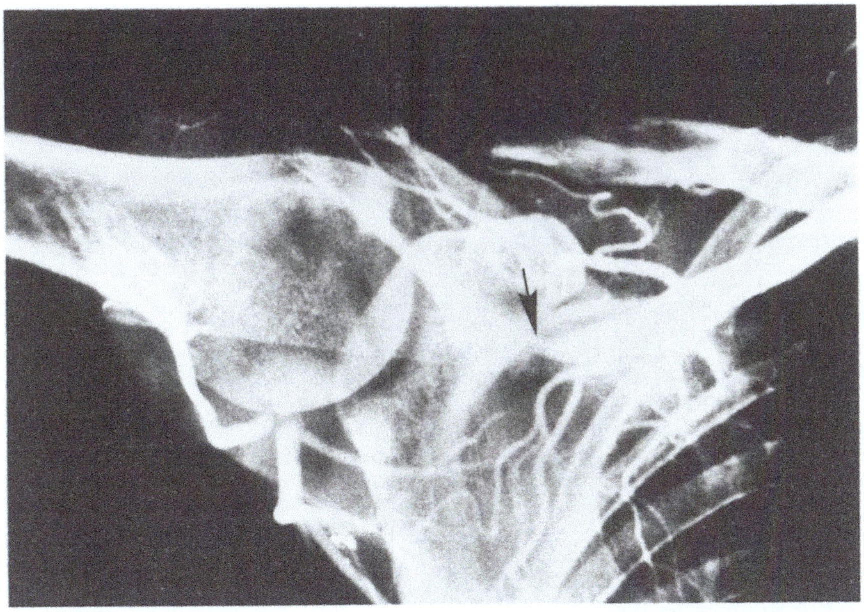

a

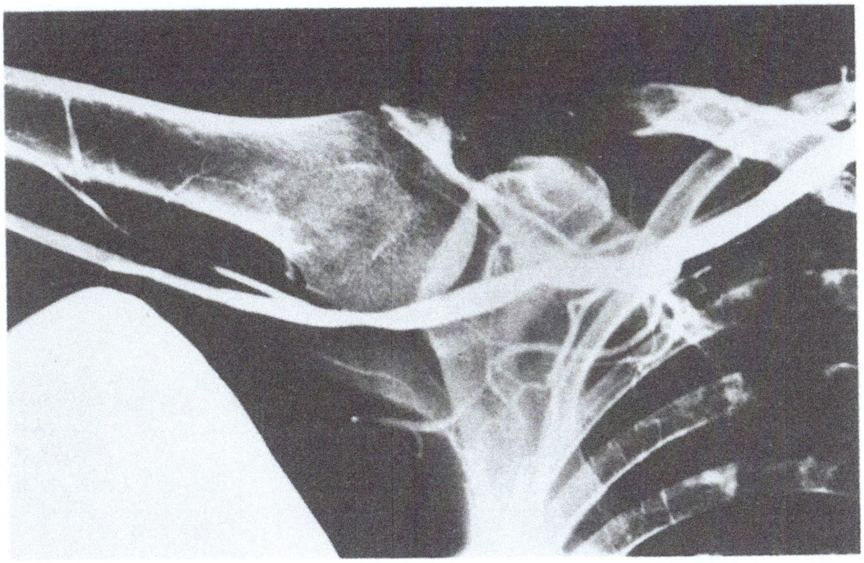

b

Fig. 132

A. Right subclavian arteriogram (arm in the provocative position) shows complete obstruction of the axillary artery caused by the tendon of the minor pectoral muscle (arrow).

B. Repeated arteriogram after surgical tenotomy of the minor pectoral muscle demonstrates that a slight compression of the artery still exists at the characteristic site (inferior to the coracoid process). Note also a minimal compression of the axillary artery by the head of humerus. (Courtesy of Prof. Dr. D. Westra and Dr. P. F. Dijkstra, Department of Radiology, Wilhelmina Hospital, Amsterdam.)

Reproduced from Radiologica Clinica, vol. 47, p. 425 (1978), with permission of S. Karger AG, Basel (april 30, 1981).

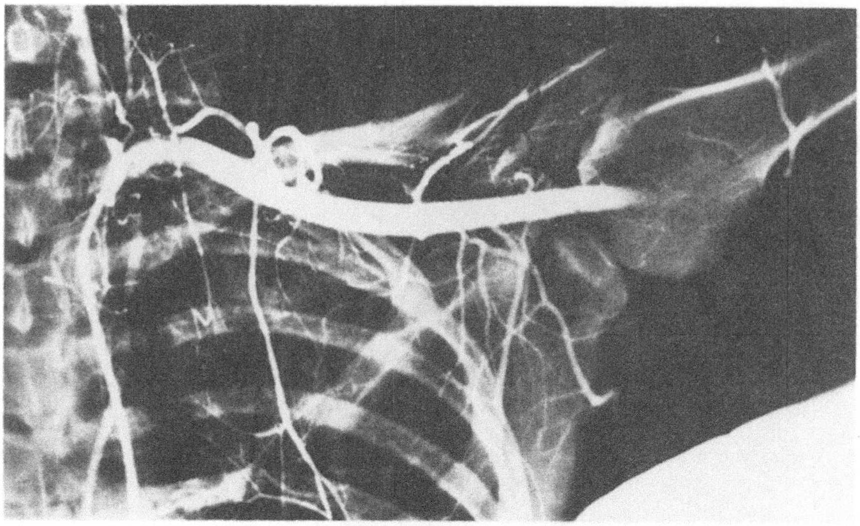

a

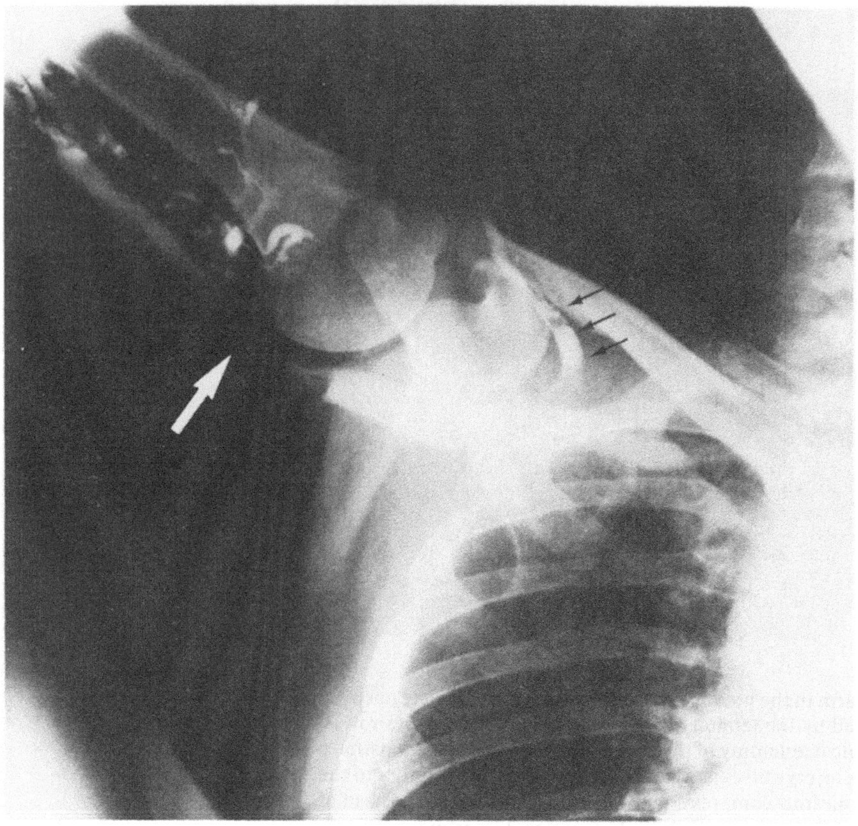

Fig. 133 b

Vascular Compressions of the Head of Humerus.

A. Left subclavian arteriogram of arm in 100 degree abduction demonstrates complete obstruction of the axillary artery caused by the head of humerus. (Courtesy of Prof. Dr. D. Westra and Dr. P. F. Dijkstra, Department of Radiology, Wilhelmina Hospital, Amsterdam.)
Reproduced from Radiologica Clinica, vol. 47, p. 426 (1978), with permission of S. Karger AG, Basel (april 30, 1981).

B. Right subclavian phlebogram demonstrates severe compression of the axillary vein by the head of humerus (white arrow). There is preferential flow in the cephalic vein (black arrows).

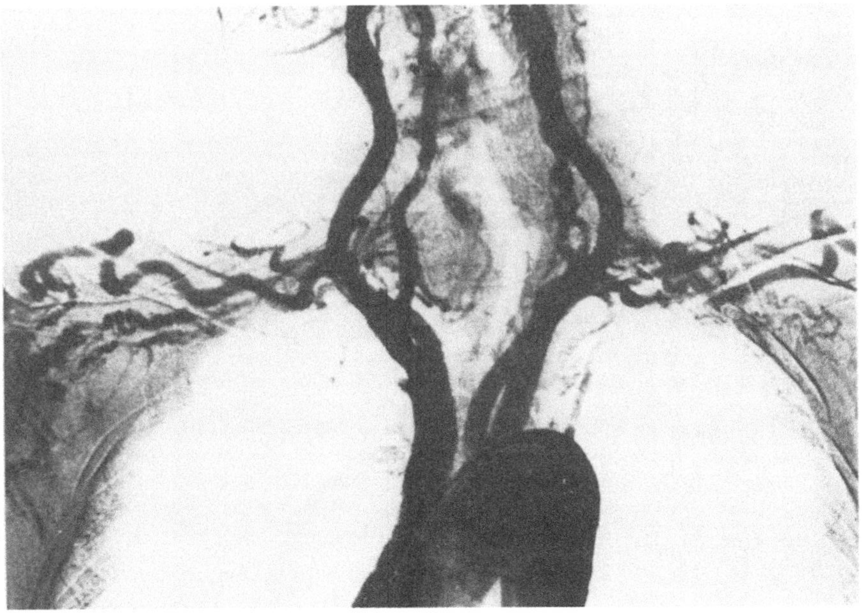

Fig. 134
Aortic arch aortogram of patient with bilateral cervical ribs demonstrates complete occlusion of both subclavian arteries at the thoracic outlet. There is extensive antegrade collateral circulation in the shoulders, especially through the transverse cervical and transverse scapular arteries. The blood supply to the brachial artery is maintained.

The exact data for these findings are given in Table XXIX.

Thrombosis of the vessel with complete occlusion at the level of the entrapment between the first rib and clavicle was seen in five patients (2.6%). In one patient with two cervical ribs both subclavian arteries were occluded (Fig. 134). Extensive collateral circulation was present on both sides and resulted in complete filling of the axillary arteries. The patient had normal radial pulses on palpation but the arterial blood pressure was decreased.

In four other cases occlusion of the subclavian artery was unilateral; in one patient the occlusion appeared on the right side and in the remaining three on the left (Table XXVII). In all five patients

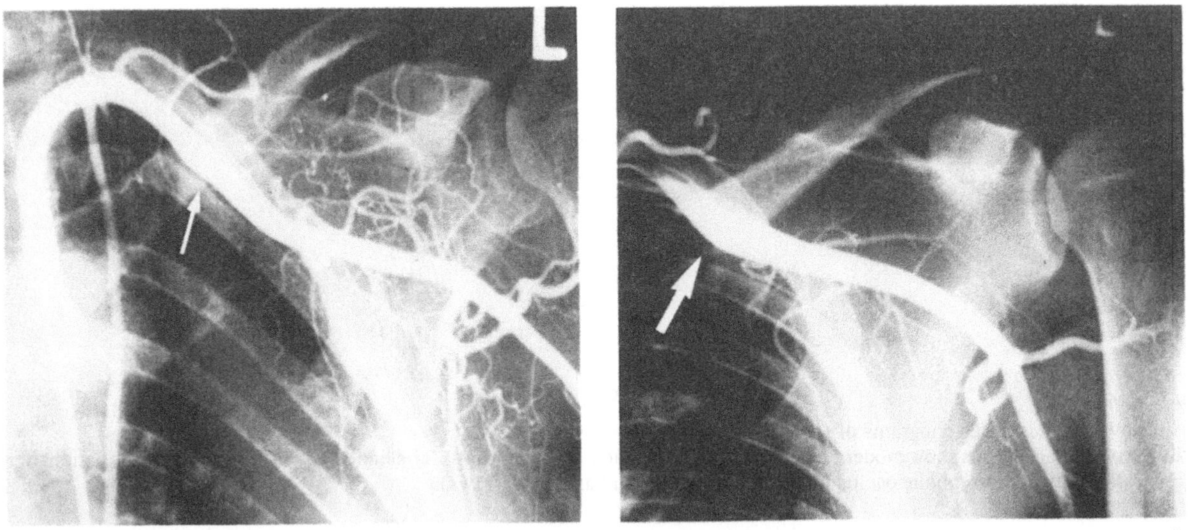

Fig. 135 a b
Left subclavian arteriograms show dilatation of the subclavian arteries at typical sites. Slight dilatation (A); moderate dilatation (B) (arrows).

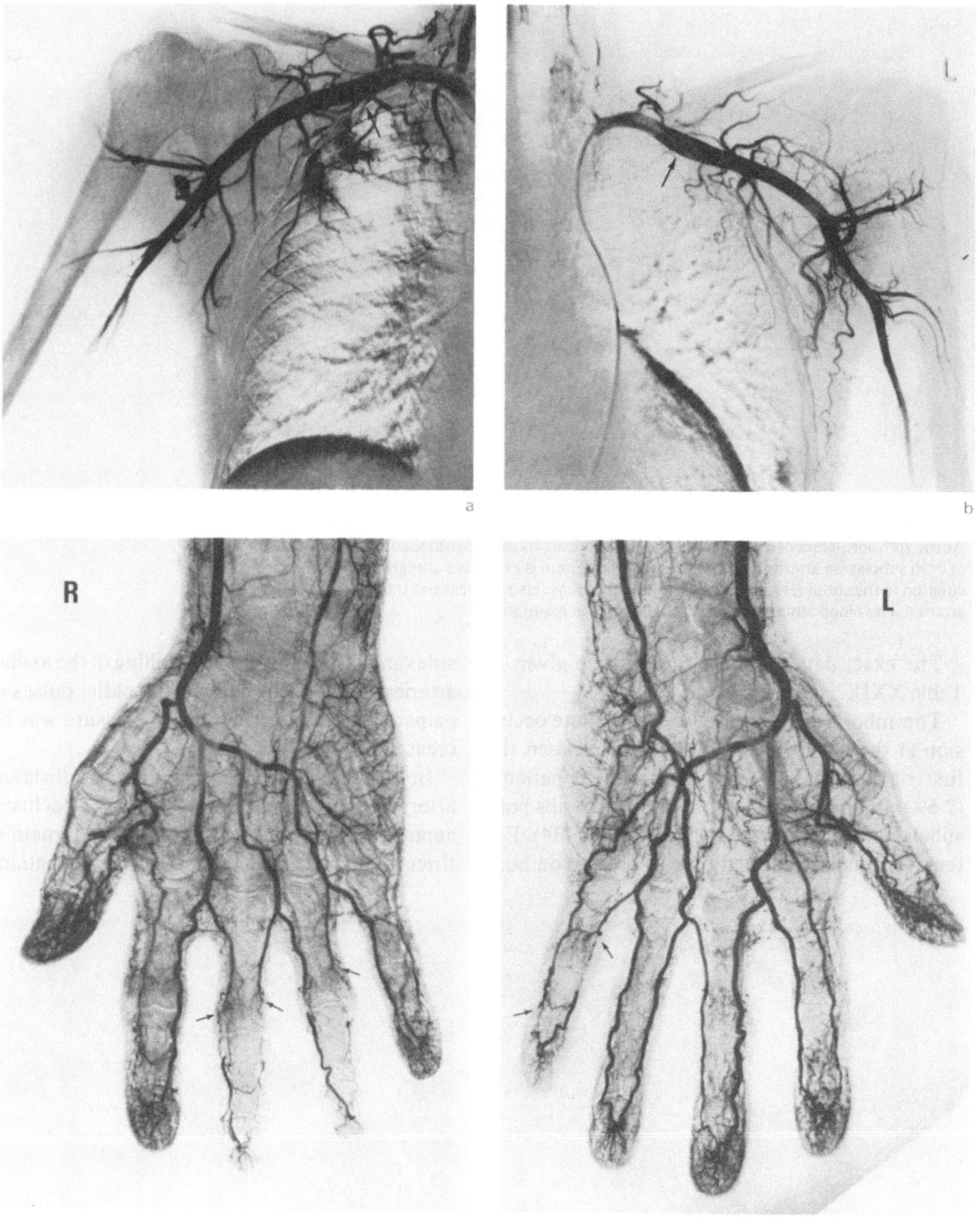

Fig. 136

Subclavian and hand arteriograms of same patient.

Both subclavian arteries show moderate dilatation at the thoracic outlet (arrows). The hand arteriograms of the same patient demonstrate multiple postembolic occlusions of the proper digital arteries (arrows).

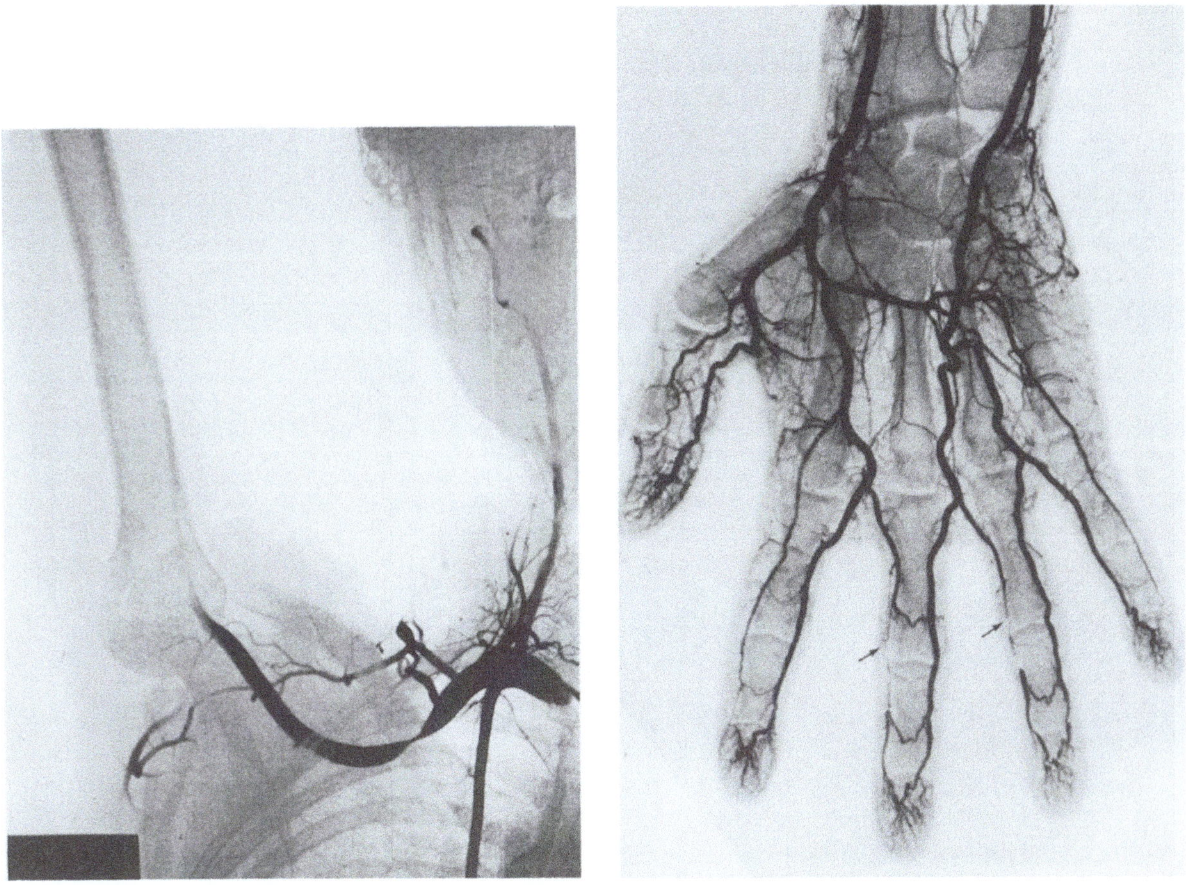

Fig. 137A and B a b
Severe dynamic costoclavicular compression of the right subclavian artery.
Hand arteriogram of the same patient shows occlusions of the proper digital arteries on the radial side of the third and the fourth fingers (arrows). Hypertrophic collaterals distal to the occlusions are present.

occlusion of peripheral digital arteries was found, most probably due to microemboli. Usually marked collaterals existed in the area of the occlusions. The second complication of a thoracic outlet compression syndrome, poststenotic (aneurysmal) dilatation of the subclavian artery, was seen in 24 cases (12.3%), in five patients bilaterally (2.7%), in seven on the right side (3.6%), and in 12 cases on the left side (6.1%) (see Table XXVII).

Slight or moderate dilatation of the subclavian arteries was most common (Fig. 135). Out of these 24 cases with poststenotic dilatation of the subclavian artery, seventeen had occlusions of the small peripheral vessels on the ipsilateral side (Table XXIX). These occlusions of the peripheral arteries were most probably due to microemboli originating from the entrapped part of the artery (Fig. 136).

An analysis of arteriograms of the forearm and hands of patients with dynamic compression of the subclavian artery shows occlusions of the small peripheral arteries of the digits and the palm in 34 cases (20.9%) (Table XXIX).

The youthful age of these patients and the absence of other pathological conditions of the vessels suggest that these occlusions were also caused by small emboli dislodged from the entrapped part of the subclavian artery (Fig. 137). The fact that 17 patients with poststenotic dilatation of the subclavian artery and 34 patients with dynamic compression of the subclavian artery had embolic peripheral occlusions clearly demonstrates the importance of brachial angiography under these conditions. Angiographic studies of patients who are found to have the compression syndrome must include not only the subclavian and axillary vessels but also the vasculature of the forearm and hand.

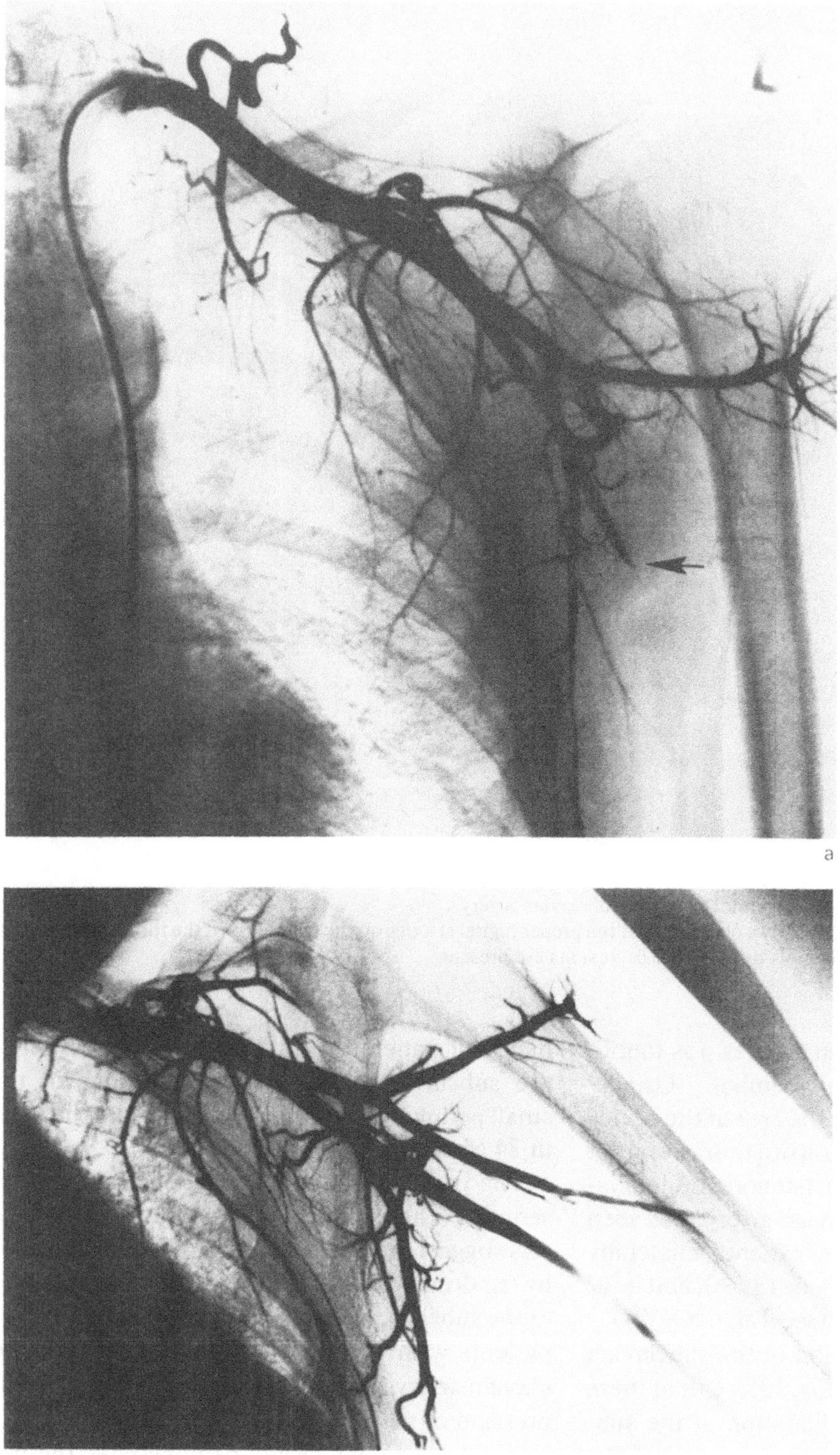

a

b

Fig. 138

A. Complete occlusion of the proximal brachial artery (arrow) due to muscular contraction with arm in extreme adducted position mimicks an occlusive arterial disease.

B. Repeat arteriogram of the same individual after relaxation of the arm. The brachial artery shows a normal calibre and patency.

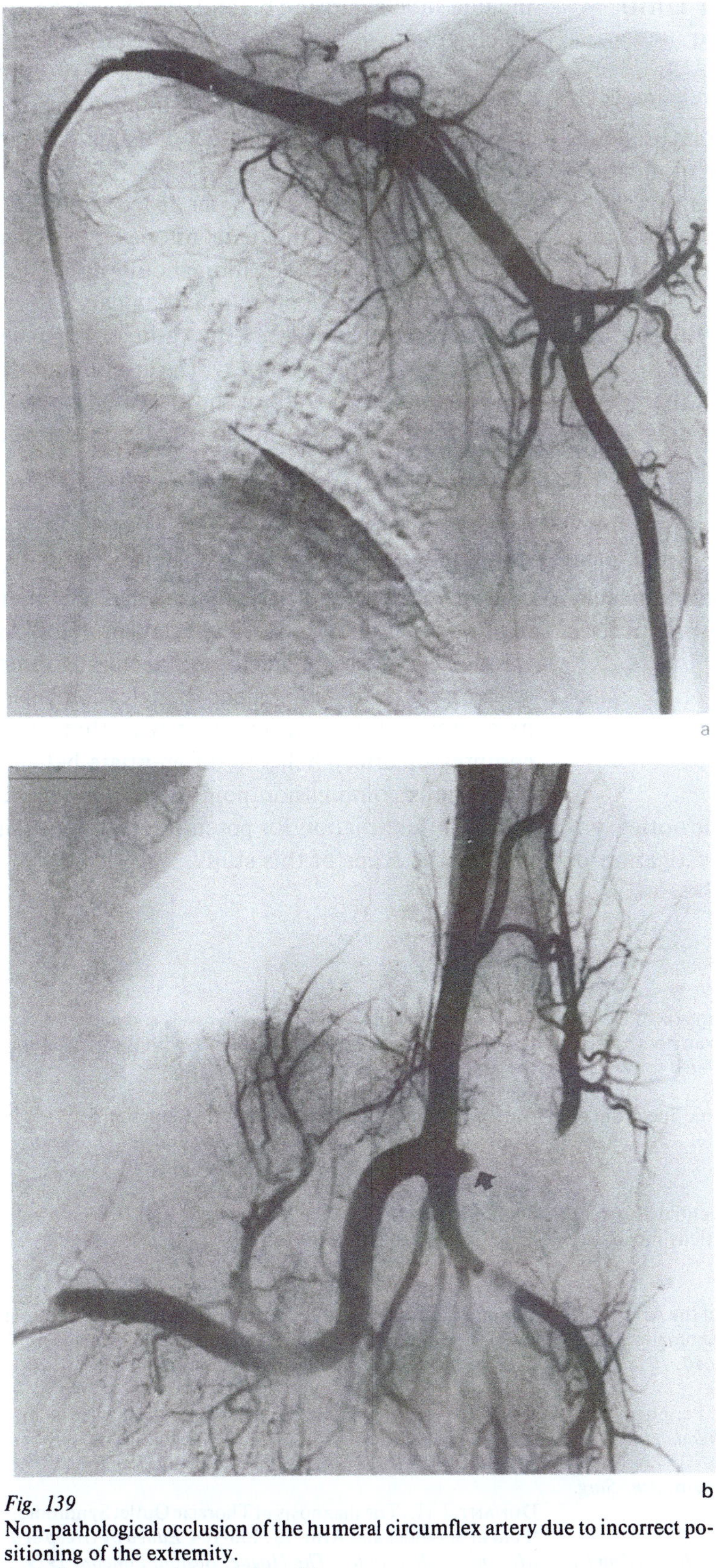

a

b

Fig. 139
Non-pathological occlusion of the humeral circumflex artery due to incorrect positioning of the extremity.

A. Left upper arm in neutral position.
B. Extreme hyperabduction of the same extremity. Complete occlusion of the humeral circumflex artery (arrow), because of severe compression by the head of humerus.

9.9 Non-Pathological Occlusions of the Arteries of the Upper Limb due to Incorrect Positioning of the Extremity

Compression of the brachial artery or its branches may occur due to forceful contraction of the muscles or in certain provocative positions, as seen in Figures 138 and 139. This apparently pathological angiographic pattern can be seen particularly in very muscular subjects. It usually occurs in the axilla when the patient holds his arm tightly adducted against the thoracic wall (Fig. 138).

It is therefore important to instruct the patient to relax his arm before injecting the contrast medium. In some extremely provocative positions of the upper arm the humeral circumflex artery may be compressed by the head of humerus (Fig. 139). This should not be interpreted as a pathological condition. We believe that similar conditions may occur with other arteries in extremely provocative positions of the extremities.

9.10 Conclusions

For the diagnosis of a vascular thoracic outlet syndrome a complete angiographic investigation of the arm is mandatory. The investigation should include subclavian and brachial arteriography and phlebography of the upper arm. The arteriograms can help to localize and identify single or multiple lesions, differentiate extrinsic compression from intra-arterial lesions and detect or exclude microemboli in the peripheral vessels.

To avoid any risk of catheter dislodgement of a thrombotic mass in the distal arteries of the arm, brachial artery catheterization should not be performed until the subclavian and axillary arteries have been studied. Before the catheter is pushed into the distal brachial artery, the arteriograms of the proximal arteries should be inspected carefully for the presence of a thrombotic mass or any other intra-arterial abnormality.

For the establishment of the cause of the compression at the thoracic outlet the location and the angiographic pattern of the compression are indispensible. Phlebography is advocated as a complementary examination. The subclavian vein runs through the costoclavicular and pectoralis minor spaces but outside the scalene triangle; comparing its anatomy during provocation with that of the compressed artery helps to differentiate between the various compression points. The importance of this differentiation for potential treatment falls outside the scope of this study.

REFERENCES

ACHTERBERG, J. R. and J. W. JANSEN van WIGMONT: De betekenis van arteriografie voor de diagnostiek van het thoracic outlet syndroom. *Ned. T. Geneesk. 118: 1550-1554, 1974.*

ADLER, J. and I. HOOSHMANS: The Angiographic Spectrum of the Thoracic Outlet Syndrome. *Clinica Radiol., 24: 35-42, 1973.*

ADSON, A. W.: Cervical ribs: Symptoms, differential diagnosis for section of the insertion of the scalenus anticus muscle. *J. Int. Coll. Surg. 16: 546, 1951.*

ADSON, A. W. and E. V. ALLEN: Thrombosis of the Arteries of the Right Upper Extremity Resulting from Anomalous First Rib. *Proc. Staff. Meet. Mayo. Clin., 13: 637-640, 1938.*

ALLEN, E. V., N. W. BARKER and E. A. HINES: Peripheral vascular diseases. *Ed. 3: 201-224, Saunders Co. Philadelphia 1962.*

BAIRD R. J. and T. Z. LAJOS: Emboli to the Arm. *Am. Surg. 160: 905, 1964.*

CONN, J. Jr.: Thoracic Outlet Syndromes. *Surg. Clin. N. Amer., 54: 155-164, 1974.*

COOTE, H: Pressure on the axillary vessels and nerve by an exostosis from a cervical rib. Interference with the circulation of the arm. *Med. Times Gaz., 2: 108, 1861.*

COX W. A. and R. H. BUXER: First rib Resection for Thoracic Outlet Compression Syndrome. *Amer. Family. Physician, 9: 140: 146, 1974.*

DELAURENTIS D. A., C. C. WOLFERTH and P. FRIEDMANN: Thoracic Outlet Syndrome. *Angiology, 25: 548-553, 1974.*

DIJKSTRA, P. F. and D. WESTRA: Angiographic Features of Compression of the Axillary Artery by the Musculus pectoralis minor and the Head of the Humerus in the Thoracic Outlet Compression Syndrome. *Radiol. Clin. 47: 423-427, 1978.*

DREWES, J.: Thrombosis of the axillary-subclavian vein, in 'Pain in shoulder and Arm', 10: 111-128. *Edited by Greep et al., Martinus Nijhoff Publ., The Hague, Boston, London, 1979.*

DUNANT, J. H.: The diagnosis of Thoracic Outlet Syndrome, in 'Pain in Shoulder and Arm' 13: 153-164. *Edited by Greep et al., Martinus Nijhoff Publ., The Hague, Boston, London, 1979.*

EDEN, K. C.: The vascular complications of cervical ribs and first thoracic rib abnormalities. *Brit. J. Surg. 27: 111-139, 1939.*

ETTER, L. E.: Osseous abnormalities of the thoracic cage seen in fourty thousand consecutive chest photoroentgenograms. *Am. J. Roentg. 51: 359-363, 1944.*

FALCONER, M. A. and WEDDEL: Costoclavicular Compression of the Subclavian Artery and Vein: Relation to the scalenus anticus syndrome. *Lancet, 2: 539-543, 1943.*

GREENSTONE, S. M., T. B. MASSELL, E. C. HARINGMAN and H. A. RAPHAEL: The Thoracic Outlet Compression Syndrome – A reappraisal. *Vascular Surg. 5: 121-125, 1971.*

HAIMOVICI, H. and L. H. CAPLAN: Arterial thrombosis complicating the Thoracic Outlet Syndrome: Arteriographic Considerations. *Radiology, 87: 457-459, 1966.*

HALSTED, W. S.: An experimental study of circumscribed dilation of an artery immediately distal to a partially occluding band and its bearing on the dilation of the subclavian artery observed in certain cases of cervical rib. *J. Exp. Med. 24: 271-1916.*

HILTON, J.: On rest and pain. *2nd. ed. William Wood and Company, New York, 1879.*

HOLMAN, E. F.: The obscure physiology of poststenotic dilatation. Its relation to the development of aneurysms. *J. Thorac. Surg. 28: 109-1954.*

JANEVSKI, B.: Angiography of the Upper Extremity, in 'Pain in Shoulder and Arm' 3: 25-48. *Edited by Greep et al., Martinus Nijhoff Publ., The Hague, Boston, London, 1979.*

JUDY, K. and R. L. HEYMAN: Vascular complications of Thoracic Outlet Syndrome. *Am. J. Surg. 123: 521-531, 1972.*

LANG, E. K.: Arteriography and Venography in the Assessment of thoracic outlet syndromes. *South. Med. J. 65: 129-136, 1972.*

LANG, E. K.: Arteriographic Diagnosis of Neurovascular Syndromes. *J.L.S. Med. Soc., 121: 196-198, 1969.*

LANG, E. K.: Arteriographic Diagnosis of the Thoracic Outlet Syndromes. *Radiology, 84: 292-303, 1965.*

LEMMENS, H. A. J.: Raynaud-Phänomen-Asphyxia manus et digitorum; Digitus mortuus sive Digitus Moriens. *VASA, Band 6: 295-299, 1977.*

LEMMENS, H. A. J.: Costoclavicular compression and dying digits, in 'Pain in Shoulder and Arm: 19: 217-219. *Edited by Greep et al., Martinus Nijhoff Publ., The Hague, Boston, London, 1979.*

LEWIS, T. and G. W. PICKERING: Observations upon maladies in which the blood supply to the digits causes intermittently or permanently and upon bilateral gangrene of the digits: Observations relevant to so-called Raynaud's disease. *Clin. Sci. 1: 327, 1934.*

LORD, J. Jr.: Thoracic Outlet Syndrome, current management. *Am. Surg. 173: 700, 1971.*

LORD, J. W. and L. M. ROSATI: Neurovascular Compression syndromes of the upper extremity. *Ciba Clinical symposia, 10, 35, 1958.*

LORD, J. W. and P. W. STONE: Pectoralis minor anatomy and anterior scalenotomy with special reference to the hyperabduction syndrome and 'effort thrombosis' of the subclavian vein. *Circulation 13: 537, 1956.*

MATHES, S. J. and A. A. SALAM: Subclavian artery aneurysm; sequela of thoracic outlet syndrome. *Surgery, 76: 506-510, 1974.*

MULDER, D. S., F. A. H. GREENWOOD and C. E. BROOKS: Posttraumatic Thoracic Outlet Syndrome. *Jour. Trauma, 13: 706-715, 1973.*

NAFFZIGER, H. C.: The scalenus Syndrome. *Surg. Gynec. and Obst. 64: 119-1937.*

NELSON, R. M. and R. W. DAVIS: Thoracic Outlet Compression Syndrome. *Am. Thoracic Surg. 8: 437-451, 1969.*

PADBERG, G.: Brachialgia. *Psychiat. Neurol. Neurochir. (Amst.) 67: 406, 1964.*

PADBERG, G: Brachialgia – a differential diagnosis, in 'Pain in Shoulder and Arm' 5: 63-72. *Edited by Greep et al., Martinus Nijhoff Publ., The Hague, Boston, London, 1979.*

PARRY, E.: Diagnosis and management of arterial lesions in relations of the outlet compression syndrome, in 'Pain in Shoulder and Arm' 18: 211-215. *Edited by Greep et al., Martinus Nijhoff Publ., The Hague, Boston, London, 1979.*

POLAND, A.: On a case of fusiform and tubular aneurysm of the subclavian artery and its successful treatment by indirect digital compression. *Medico-Chir. Trans. 52: 288, 1869.*

RAINER, W. G., W. VIGOR and J. P. NEWBY: Surgical treatment of thoracic outlet compression. *Am. J. Surg. 116: 704-707, 1968.*

RAPHAEL, M. J., F. F. R. KH. MOAZZEZ and D. N. OFFEN: Vascular Manifestations of thoracic outlet compression. Angiographic Appearances, *Angiology, 25(4): 237-248, 1974.*

ROB, C. G. and A. STANDEVEN: Arterial Occlusion complicating thoracic outlet compression syndrome. *Brit. M. J. 2: 709, 1958.*

ROOS, D. B. and J. C. OWENS: Thoracic Outlet Syndrome. *Arch. Surg. 93: 71, 1966.*

SADLER, T. R., W. G. RAINER and G. TWOMBLEY: Thoracic Outlet Compression. Application of Positioned Arteriographic and Nerve Conduction Studies. *Am. J. Surg. 130: 704-706, 1975.*

SCHEIN, C. J., H. HAIMOVICI and H. YOUNG: Arterial Thrombosis associated with cervical ribs and surgical considerations. *Surgery, 40: 428, 1956.*

SELMAN, M. W., W. A. MCALPINE and H. M. FOSTER: The Thoracic Outlet Syndrome. *The Ob. State Med. J. Sep. 908-911, 1969.*

SHENKIN, H. A.: Cervical rib and thrombosis of the SCA. *J.A.M.A., 165: 335, 1957.*

SYMONDS, C. P.: Two cases of thrombosis of subclavian artery with homo-lateral hemiplegia of sudden onset, probably embolic. *Brain, 50: 259, 1927.*

TELFORD, E. D. and S. MOTTERSHEAD: Pressure at the Cervicobrachial junction. *Jour. Bone and Joint. Surg. 30: 249-265, 1948.*

TELFORD, E. D. and J. S. B. STAFFORD: The vascular complications of cervical rib. *Brit. J. Surg. 18: 557, 1937.*

TODD, T. W.: The arterial lesion in case of 'cervical rib'. *Jour. Anat. and Physiol. 47: 250- 1913.*

TOMSICK, T. A., R. A. AHISTRAND and T. M. KISSEL: Thoracic Outlet Syndrome associated with rib fusion and cervicothoracic Scoliosis. *J. Can. Ass. Rad. 25: 211-213, 1974.*

URSCHEL, H. C., M. A. RAZZUK, E. M. KRUSEN and J. W. CALDWELL: The Technique of measuring conduction velocity for thoracic outlet syndrome, in 'Pain in Shoulder and Arm' 14: 165-172. *Edited by Greep et al., Martinus Nijhoff publ., The Hague, Boston, London, 1979.*

URSCHEL, H. C. jr., D. L. PAULSEN and J. J. MCNAMARA: Thoracic Outlet Syndrome. *Am. Thoracic Surg. 6: 1, 1968.*

URSCHEL, H. C. jr. and M. A. RAZZUK: Management of the Thoracic Outlet Syndrome. *N. Engl. J. Med. 286: 1140-1143, 1972.*

WICKHAM, J. E. A. and P. MARTIN: Aneurysm of the SCA in association with cervical abnormality. *Brit. J. Surg. 50: 205, 1963.*

WINSOR, T. and R. BROW: Costoclavicular syndrome; Diagnosis and treatment. *J.A.M.A., 196: 697-699, 1966.*

Chapter 10

ARTERIAL OCCLUSIVE DISEASES OF THE UPPER EXTREMITY

10.1 Arteriosclerosis

Review of Literature

The term arteriosclerosis is used in different senses by different authors. At the present time arteriosclerosis is used as a collective term for different types of degenerative disorders of the vascular wall which cause hardening of the arterial wall and reduce the functional capacity of the arteries. According to the pathological changes there are four main types of arteriosclerosis, which differ markedly in microscopic appearance and, to some degree, in distribution (Schornagel, 1967, Boyd, 1970).

1. Mönckeberg's medial sclerosis, affecting mainly smaller muscular arteries. The pathological process in this kind of arteriosclerosis is characterized by degeneration of the muscle fibres of the tunica media and deposition of calcium in the arterial wall. The calcified vessels are hard and tortuous but the lumen is not narrowed.

2. Arteriolosclerosis, or diffuse arteriolar sclerosis. It is a degenerative collagenous thickening of the intima of the smaller arteries causing a marked narrowing of the lumen. In the extremities, in later life, this form of arteriosclerosis may lead to peripheral gangrene.

3. Senile arteriosclerosis is the result of the physiological process of ageing of the arteries. The arterial changes in this form of arteriosclerosis include degeneration of muscular and elastic elements and the appearance of connective tissue with simultaneous deposition of calcium salts in the wall. This results in a less flexible, more sclerotic arterial wall. Senile arteriosclerosis depends directly upon the age of the patient.

4. Atherosclerosis or atheromatosis is a nodular form of arteriosclerosis which affects, in particular, the aorta and the cerebral and coronary arteries. The medium-sized arteries of the muscular type are not as susceptible to this disease. Atherosclerosis is the only form of arteriosclerosis which includes a predisposition to thrombosis. It may be seen early in life, secondary to other diseases, or even as a primary process.

The cause and pathogenesis of atherosclerosis are still unknown. According to the definition of the World Health Organization, atheromatosis is a variable combination of changes in the intima of the arteries, consisting of the focal accumulation of lipids, carbohydrates complexis, blood and blood products, fibrous tissue and calcium deposits, and is associated with medial changes.

The pathological process is characterized by a focal degeneration of the intima and the inner fibres of the tunica media where cholesterol and lime salts are deposited (Moossy, 1970). The heavy lime salts accumulate not only in the fatty material deposited in the subendothelial layer of the intima but also in the degenerated and fragmented muscle fibres of the tunica media. If they are deposited only in the muscle fibres, dense calcification may be found in the walls of the artery without significant narrowing of the vessel lumen. The focal accumulation of lipids in the subendothelial tissue of the intima causes an elevation of the intima which usually progresses and gradually leads to stenosis of the arterial lumen. Arterial stenosis probably does not become haemodynamically significant

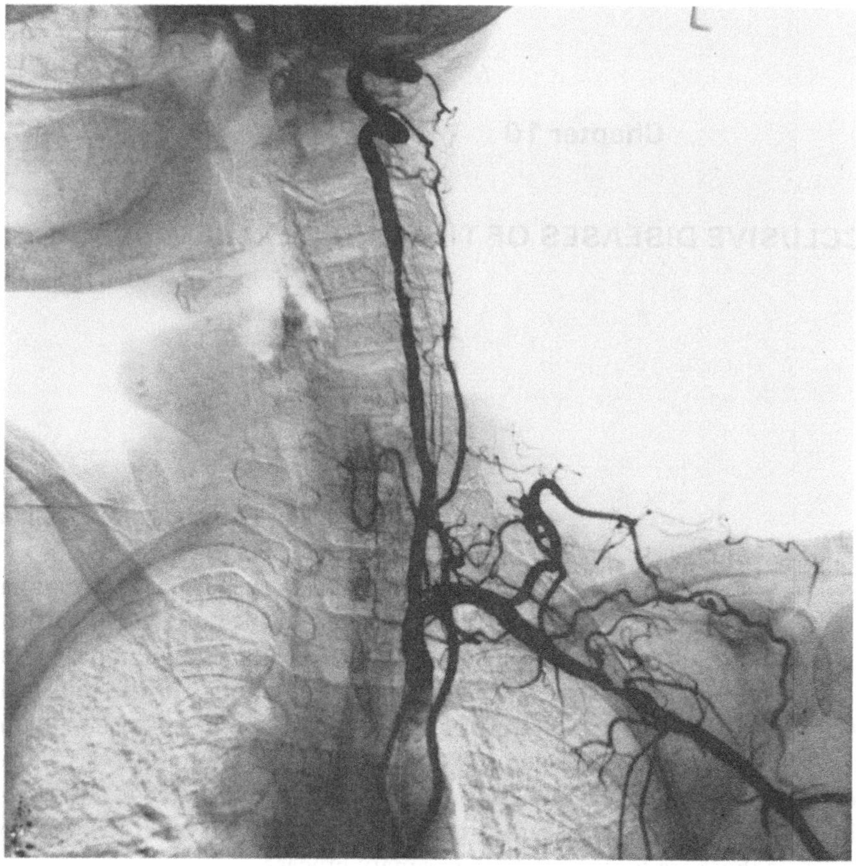

Fig. 140
Atheromatous changes and a severe stenosis of the left subclavian artery. The cathetertip is placed in the proximal part of the left subclavian artery.

until the cross-sectional area of the arterial lumen is reduced by more than 50% (Crawford *et al.*, 1962). The lumen is usually narrowed excentrically by atheroma confined to one side of the arterial wall.

In the course of the pathological process, the continuity of the intima can remain intact. A sudden increase in the degree of stenosis can result from intramural haemorrhage caused by rupture of a small vessel in the arterial wall or penetration of an enlarged atheromatous plaque through the endothelial lining of the intima leading to the formation of an ulcer and subsequent thrombosis.

Ulcerations through the endothelium may take place without significant narrowing of the arterial lumen. Atheromatous ulceration is however clinically important since it is a common source of emboli (Castaigne *et al.*, 1973).

10.1.1 Radiological Diagnosis of Arteriosclerosis

Arteriosclerosis obliterans is a disease which involves most of the arterial vascular system. It is usually associated with hypertension.

The diagnosis of arteriosclerosis of the hands can be made by plain films which may show calcifications of the arterial wall. If calcifications are not demonstrable on the plain films arteriosclerosis cannot be ruled out. Moreover radiologically demonstrable calcifications are not always evidence of severe arteriosclerosis obliterans, nor is the degree of calcification an indication of the degree of peripheral ischaemia. Thus, dense calcifications in the wall of an artery need not necessarily affect the lumen of the vessel (De Reus and Vink, 1955).

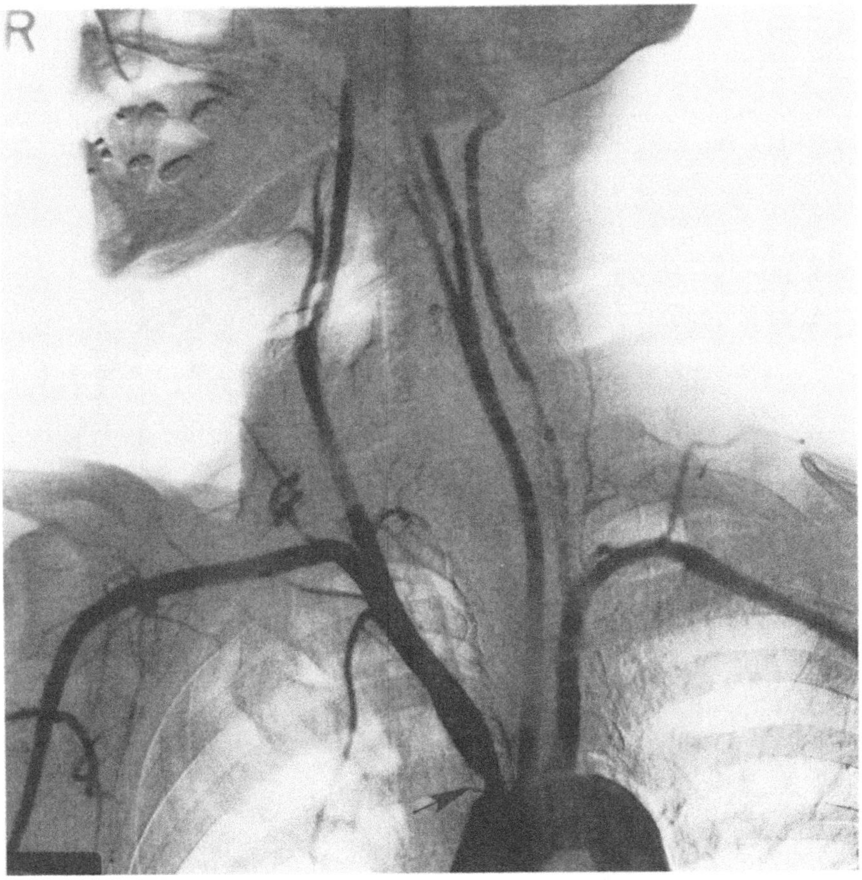

Fig. 141
Aortic arch aortography demonstrates an isolated smooth stenosis at the origin of the innominate artery (arrow).
The subclavian and axillary arteries are normal.

10.1.2 Analysis of Our Case Material

In reviewing our case material, in the period from 1970 to 1980 there were thirty-six patients with arteriosclerotic changes referred to our department for investigation of the arteries of the arm. The age of the patients varied from 40 to 76 years.

In all cases the visualization of the arteries of the upper arm was carried out by means of the transfemoral catheterization technique, placing the catheter selectively into the proximal part of the subclavian or innominate artery.

In twenty-four patients the same technique was used for visualization of the arteries of the forearm and hand by introducing the catheter into the distal part of the brachial artery as described and illustrated in section 3.5. These patients had mild circumscribed atheromatous changes of the great vessels of the upper limb which showed smooth outlines and did not significantly impair the arterial lumen. In eight of the 24 patients only an isolated slight narrowing of the subclavian or innominate artery was present (Fig. 141). This single, so-called annular, stenosis with smooth contours may be congenital or acquired through regular atheromatous deposits in the vascular wall (Anderson, 1966). The smoothness of the stenosis indicates that no thrombi are attached to the narrowed segment (van Andel, 1976). In all investigated cases there were no complications related to the examination technique. However in twelve patients, brachial angiography could not be performed by the catheterization technique because of severe atheromatous changes and multiple stenoses of the proximal vessels of the arm, as shown in Figure 140. These patients underwent 'cut-down' brachial arteriography for the visualization of the arteries of the forearm and hand.

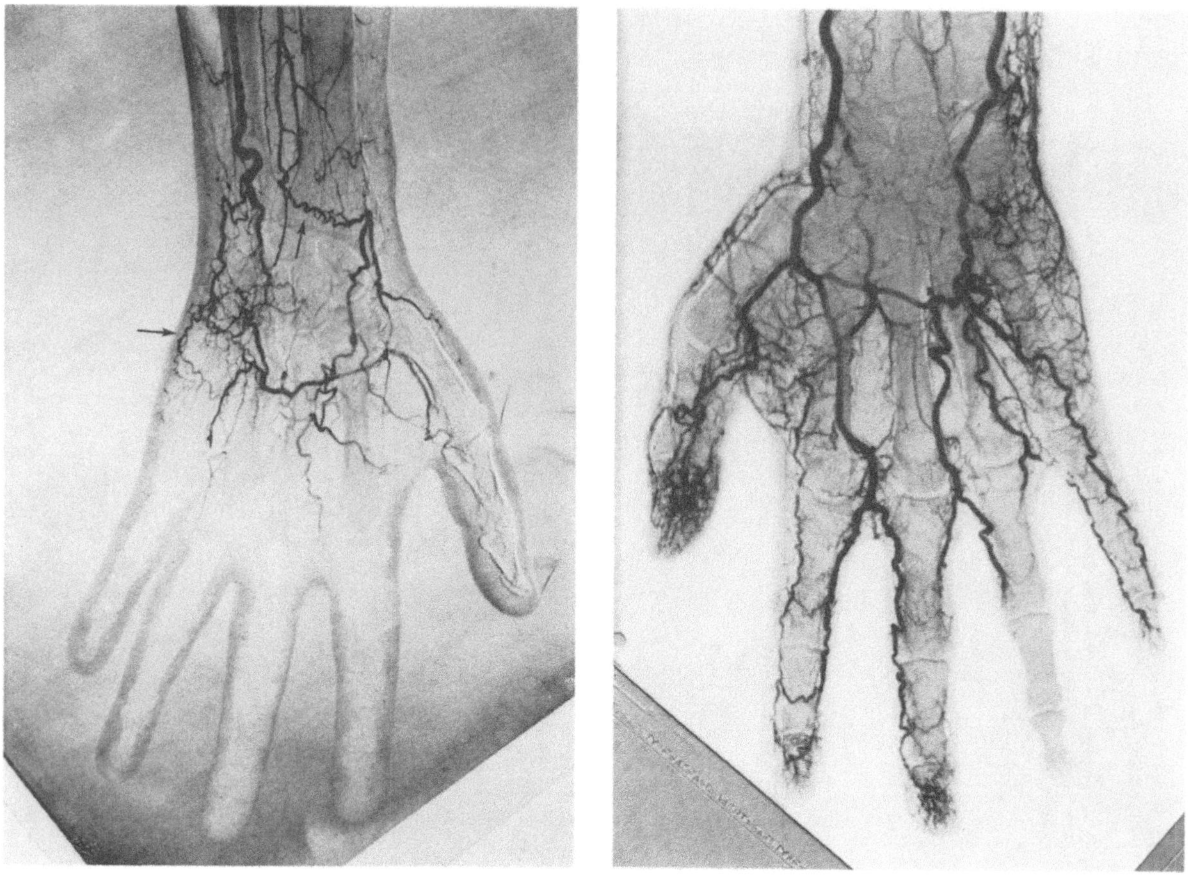

a b

Fig. 142
Arteriosclerosis of the hands of two different patients.
Severe arteriosclerotic changes in the arteries of the forearm (A) and hand (B).
The arteries show irregular constrictions, a tortuous course and multiple occlusions (arrows); 'corkscrew' collaterals are visible in Fig. 142A (arrows).

10.1.3 Conclusions

The angiographic signs of advanced arteriosclerosis obliterans of the arteries are well known. The arteries show circumferential smooth or irregular constrictions over short or long segments, elongation, tortuous course and kinkings. Multiple occlusions with direct or indirect collateral vessels are a common finding in arteriosclerosis. The collateral arteries which may develop are characterized by elongation, tortuosity and the 'corkscrew' pattern (Fig. 142). The latter type of collaterals was the most common finding on the arteriograms of the hands of our thirty-six patients.

Angiographic investigation of the arteries of the upper extremities of our arteriosclerotic patients was carried out by means of the transfemoral catheterization technique.

In arteriosclerotic patients selective catheterization of the arteries of the upper extremity should be performed with great caution, since there is a high potential risk of postcatheterization thrombosis. In order to prevent this, brachial artery catheterization should never be performed until the proximal vessels have been opacified and studied. If the subclavian and axillary arteries show atheromatous changes or stenoses, as illustrated in Figure 140, the catheter technique is not indicated for brachial and hand arteriography. In such instances direct brachial artery puncture or 'cutdown' arteriography is usually the method of choice.

When the only abnormality of the major vessels

of the upper limb is an isolated short constriction which has a smooth contour and does not significantly change the arterial lumen (Fig. 141), the catheter technique for opacification of the distal vessels may be used.

10.2 Steal Phenomena

10.2.1 Subclavian Steal

Literature

The term subclavian steal is used when either an obstruction or a severe stenosis of the subclavian artery at its origin causes reversed flow in the ipsilateral vertebral artery, often accompanied by cerebral arterial ischaemia. 'Brachial-basilar insufficiency' and 'vertebral grand larceny' are synonyms for the same condition.

Patients with subclavian steal may be asymptomatic; then the term subclavian steal phenomenon is used. However, for those cases where cerebral symptoms or complaints referable to the arm are present, the term subclavian steal syndrome is applied.

The basic pathological process in subclavian steal syndrome is an occlusion or a stenosis of the subclavian artery proximal to the origin of the vertebral artery. Occlusive disease at this site reduces the pressure in the subclavian artery distal to the obstruction. When the pressure at the subclavian end of the vertebral artery drops below the pressure in the basilar artery, the flow in the vertebral artery is reversed.

In 1961, Reivich, Holling, Roberts and Toole studied two patients with symptoms of cerebral ischaemia in whom a reversal of the blood flow through the left vertebral artery was demonstrated. In both cases the anatomical lesion producing the reversed flow was a stenosis of the left subclavian artery proximal to the origin of the vertebral artery. This observation was confirmed in experimental animals by producing reversal of blood flow in vertebral arteries after ligation of the subclavian arteries proximal to the origin of the vertebral vessels. The authors also showed that when the subclavian blood pressure is 10% less than the systemic arterial pressure, flow in the vertebral artery is reversed.

It is important to realize that a 50% reduction in the square of the lumen of an artery is necessary to produce a pressure gradient of 10% (Reivich *et al.*, 1961).

This peculiar pathological vascular pattern, called the *subclavian steal* by the editors of the New England Journal of Medicine in 1961, was first recognized by Luigi Contorni in 1960. He encountered this particular type of collateral circulation in a case of occlusion of the first portion of the left subclavian artery. In this case arteriography had revealed that collateral circulation to the left arm consisted of reversed flow from the right vertebral artery through the basilar system into the left vertebral and subclavian arteries. In the literature Contorni's arteriogram was the first objective demonstration of collateral vertebro-vertebral circulation in human pathology.

Mannick (1962) reported the first case of right subclavian steal syndrome. In 1964, Ethier reported the radiographical aspects of a case of bilateral subclavian stenosis in which there was reversal of flow in one vertebral artery and bidirectional flow in the other. Newton and Wylie (1964) presented the radiographical features of a case of occlusive disease of the innominate and left subclavian arteries with signs of reversed flow in both vertebral arteries and in the right carotid artery.

A description of the clinical aspects of the bilateral subclavian steal syndrome was given in 1965 by Collier and Hales. In the same year van Voorthuisen reported a case of left subclavian steal due to coarctation of the aortic arch. The stenosis of the aorta was localized between the origins of the left common carotid artery and the left subclavian artery.

Although this syndrome was recognized for the first time in 1960, the history of obliterative aortic arch diseases causing cerebral and upper extremity ischaemia goes back almost four centuries. In the second part of the sixteenth century Harvey described a patient with differential radial pulses which he attributed to the presence of a thoracic aortic aneurysm.

In 1664, when Thomas Willis studied the system which now bears his name, he was perfectly aware that a reversed flow can occur in the basilar and carotid arteries at the base of the brain since he had demonstrated this experimentally. In 1684 he hypothesized that 'The cerebral circulation at the base of the brain is anatomically arranged in such a manner that the entire brain could probably be perfused from either side'. This concept of cerebral blood supply is now widely accepted. In 1757 William Hunter described a patient in whom the left radial pulse could not be palpated after the development of an aortic aneurysm. In 1818 R. Harrison of Dublin became the first surgeon to ligate the first portion of the left subclavian artery in a 32-year-old man with an aneurysm in the distal portion of the same artery. The patient died four days after surgery from a secondary haemorrhage. Another nineteenth century surgeon, A. Smyth of New Orleans, was the first to successfully ligate the innominate artery in a patient suffering from aneurysm of the right subclavian artery. The operation was performed on May 15th, 1864. The post-operative course was normal until the 14th day, when a sudden major bleeding occurred from the aneurysm. As a tribute to the work of these two nineteenth century surgeons, Contorni proposed in an article in 1973 that this syndrome should bear their names: he called it the 'subclavian steal syndrome' or the 'Harrison-Smyth's Syndrome', but this term was not accepted in modern literature. In 1875 Broadbent noted at post mortum segmental atherosclerotic occlusion of the branches of the aortic arch in a patient who, when living, had exhibited bilateral loss of the radial pulses.

Hunt, in 1914, emphasized the role of occlusive disease of the extracranial cerebral arteries in the production of cerebral symptoms.

The pathophysiology and mechanism of the reverse flow in subclavian steal syndrome are now well established. In cases of proximal stenosis or total occlusion of the subclavian or innominate artery the vertebral artery is used as a collateral pathway, providing the corresponding upper extremity with blood at the expense of the cerebral circulation. Both stenosis and total occlusion proximal to the origin of the vertebral artery can result in collateral flow to the upper extremity on the side of the lesion.

Since the subclavian artery supplies the whole upper extremity a considerable amount of blood is diverted from the cerebral circulation to the arm. The vertebro-vertebral pathway is the largest source of supply to the affected arm, but it is not the only contributor to this collateral circulation. Other collateral pathways include various branches of the external carotid, vertebral, and proximal subclavian arteries. Moreover, the inferior thyroid artery, the intercostal arteries, the thyrocervical trunk and the internal mammary arteries may in some instances contribute to the collateral circulation.

In 1964 Newton and Wylie published excellent angiographic evidence of these various collaterals.

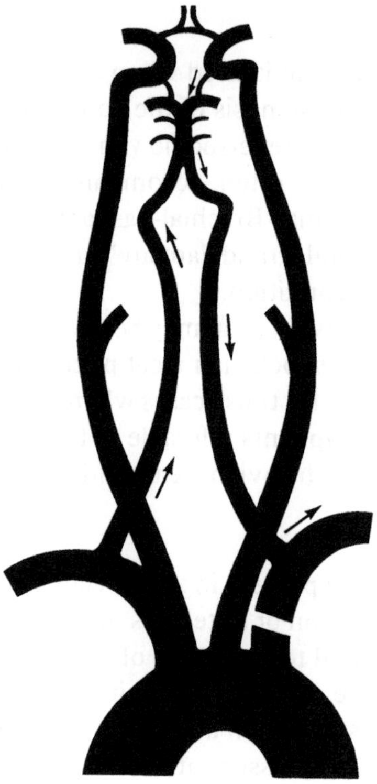

Fig. 143
Schematic diagram of collateral blood circulation by way of the internal carotid arteries through the posterior communicating arteries and the basilar-vertebral system.

Finally, significant collateral circulation can come from the internal carotid arteries by way of the posterior communicating artery and the basilar vertebral system (Fig. 143).

a. Aetiology

The conditions which often cause subclavian steal can be divided into the congenital and the acquired types.

The most common anomalies causing subclavian steal are obstruction of the aortic arch proximal to the ostium of the left subclavian artery as in infantile coarctation, tubular hypoplasia and interruption of the aortic arch. Congenital atresia and hypoplasia of the proximal part of the subclavian arteries and isolation of the left subclavian artery from the aortic arch as well as isolation of the right subclavian artery from the innominate artery are other common congenital abnormalities that could lead to subclavian steal (Bradley, 1966; Maranhao *et al.*, 1968; Becker *et al.*, 1971; Shuford *et al.*, 1971; Shaher *et al.*, 1972; Pifarré *et al.*, 1974).

The most common cause of the subclavian steal syndrome is acquired disease. In short, any intra- or extravascular process capable of causing stenosis or occlusion of the proximal subclavian artery can produce subclavian steal.

Arteriosclerosis is the most frequently reported cause of subclavian steal; occlusion of the proximal subclavian or innominate artery is usually caused by an arteriosclerotic plaque.

In the past, two relatively frequent conditions which often resulted in stenosis or occlusion of the innominate and subclavian arteries were aneurysm and arteritis secondary to the luetic aortic arch disease. Recently, it was established that, next to arteriosclerosis, traumatic and dissecting aneurysms, embolism, tumour thrombosis and 'nonspecific inflammatory' arteritis are the main pathological conditions which produce stenosis and occlusion of the branches of the aortic arch.

In 1972, an acute subclavian steal syndrome following blunt trauma to the chest was reported by Blesovsky *et al.*

Subclavian steal may also occur after certain vascular operations in the upper thorax. The Blalock-Taussig shunt and the Shumaker operative procedure for a coarcted aorta may create a vascular anatomy leading to vertebral steal which sometimes may become clinically significant (Shumaker, 1955; Folger and Shah, 1965).

Finally, Takayashu arteritis, kinking and adventitial inflammation around the ansa subclavia have been reported as occasional causes of subclavian steal.

b. Symptomatology

Patients with subclavian steal may be asymptomatic. However as a rule there will be cerebral symptoms or complaints pertaining to the arm. Why some patients with a steal phenomenon are symptomatic while other are not is not exactly known. The presence of cerebral symptoms depends not only on the amount of blood shunted away from the brain but also on the remaining cerebral circulation, which depends on the condition of the other cerebral vessels. When the posterior communicating arteries and the circle of Willis are not fully developed or the contralateral vertebral artery is hypoplastic or obstructed, cerebellar ischaemia may develop since the possibility of collateral cerebellar perfusion to compensate for the steal is not present. It has been postulated that anatomical variations in the circle of Willis may contribute to the symptoms of subclavian steal. Angiographic studies of Willis' circle have revealed that in 33% of the patients the posterior cerebral artery is fed by the internal carotid artery and that 11 to 43% of the population has a very large posterior communicating artery (Fisher, 1965). Such individuals probably would not develop cerebral symptoms from an isolated proximal subclavian occlusion. However, in most of the cases of subclavian steal reported in the literature involvement of the carotid system or multiple lesions of the other aortic branches was also present. The importance of the compensatory role of the carotid arteries in cerebral perfusion is now well established from angiographic and clinical observation.

Javid in 1960 reported that, in all of his patients with subclavian steal, compression of the common carotid artery resulted in loss of the ipsilateral radial pulse. This finding corroborates the great contribution to the circulation in the posterior fossa by the carotid and posterior communicating arteries following subclavian occlusion.

The degree of stenosis of the subclavian artery necessary to produce symptoms is not known, but it has been arbitrarily stated by some authors that surgery is indicated if 50 to 60 percent or more of the diameter of this vessel is shown to be occluded on roentgen examination, or if there is a significant lowering (more than 30 mm Hg) of the systolic blood pressure in the affected arm (Nemir *et al.*, 1965). The amount of steal varies and it may even be intermittent. Normal arterial flow through the arm varies between 100 and 200 cc per minute. After exercise or reactive hyperaemia, this flow may increase tenfold to exceed that of the cerebral circulation; that is why vertebrobasilar insufficiency symptoms are precipitated in some individuals by exercise of the involved arm.

The complaints in subclavian steal syndrome can be divided into neurological symptoms related to cerebrovascular insufficiency and symptoms related to brachial insufficiency. Cerebral symptoms and upper extremity claudication may occur alone or in combination. The most frequent symptoms are those of basilar insufficiency. The percentage of patients with cerebral symptoms associated with subclavian steal varies in the literature; probably about 50% have cerebral symptoms. Symptoms related to the arm persist in only 3% of the cases.

The chief persisting complaints in a classic subclavian steal syndrome are the neurological symptoms. Neurological manifestations may be caused by ischaemia or infarction of any structure dependent upon the vertebrobasilar system for its blood supply.

These include the upper spinal cord, the entire brain stem, cerebellum, thalamus, labyrinth, cochlea and the occipital lobes of the cerebral hemispheres.

Consequently, a mixture of signs and symptoms related to dysfunction of any or all of these structures can arise. Intermittent vertebrobasilar insufficiency is very often characterized by episodes of vertigo, nausea, headache, mono-, hemi-, para- or quadri-paresis, or paralysis, numbness of one to four extremities in any combination, numbness around the mouth, diplopia, dysphagia, dysarthria, and bilateral or unilateral homonymous hemianopsia (North *et al.*, 1962; Nemir Jr. *et al.*, 1965; Terpstra *et al.*, 1977).

Brachial insufficiency symptoms are less frequent in patients with subclavian steal syndrome. The arm complaints reported in the literature vary, but usually consist of intermittent or constant pain in the affected extremity, precipitated initially by increased activity of the arm. Paraesthesia, weakness, coolness, numbness and burning in the fingers, hand and occasionally the forearm represent transient symptoms referable to the arm.

c. Clinical Diagnosis

In 75% of the cases with subclavian steal, the lesion occurs on the left side. The average age of the patients ranges between 50 and 60 years, with a definite male predominance of about four to one (Ashby *et al.*, 1963).

The classical description would be one of episodes of vertebrobasilar insufficiency precipitated by exercise of the involved arm.

This usually occurs but is by no means constant; nevertheless, for this reason an exercise test should be used as a part of the physical examination in any case of suspected subclavian steal. Patients with clinical evidence of cerebral vascular insufficiency related to a particular position of the head may initiate symptoms by certain movements such as sharp extension or lateral rotation of the head.

Objective clinical findings in a classical case are significant difference in blood pressure between the two arms, decreased or absent radial pulse and subclavian bruit on the affected side. Difference in blood pressure between the two upper limbs is an important clinical feature of this syndrome. A difference in blood pressure of more than 20 mm Hg systolic should lead to suspicion of subclavian steal. Arterial pressure differentials of more than 40 mm Hg usually indicate a total subclavian block (Rosenburg, 1965).

The blood pressure may be unobtainable on the affected side, depending upon the severity of the occlusion and the collateral blood flow. The difference between the diastolic levels is less than that between the systolic levels.

Weakness or absence of a pulse in the ipsilateral limb is a rather constant physical finding in subclavian steal. Sometimes, if both radial pulses are equal upon palpation, the one on the affected side will be delayed; hence the importance of timing both radial pulses in such cases. The weak or delayed pulse in the ipsilateral subclavian artery may become even fainter or disappear after hyperextension or rotation of the neck. A systolic murmur may be heard over the ipsilateral pulmonary or supra-aortic area and it may be transmitted to the ipsilateral infraclavicular and supraclavicular spaces along the course of the subclavian artery. A subclavian murmur is present when stenosis exists.

d. Angiography

The most suitable angiographic procedure for demonstration of retrograde vertebral flow in sub-

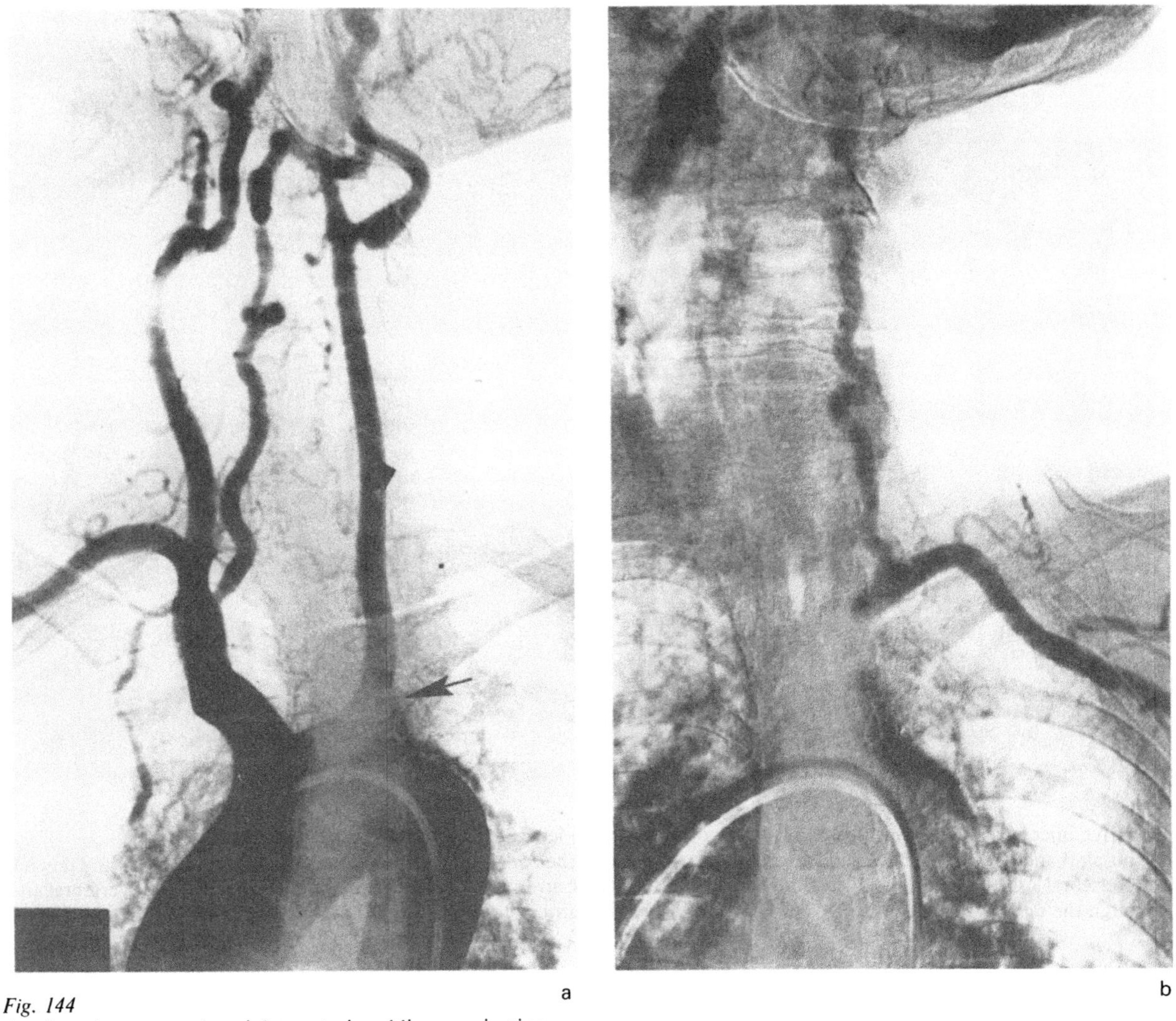

Fig. 144
Aortic arch aortography, right posterior oblique projection.
A. Two seconds after injection into aortic arch. Simultaneous opacification of the right subclavian artery and the carotid arteries. The left subclavian artery (arrow) is completely occluded approximately 1 cm distal to its origin.
B. Five seconds later. The distal left subclavian artery is opacified by retrograde flow in the left vertebral artery. There is an occlusion of the proximal intrathoracic portion of the subclavian artery.

clavian steal is aortic arch aortography, either by cine-angiography or by multiple serial films. Injection of contrast medium into the ascending aorta permits visualization of antegrade flow in the non-stenotic vessels immediately after injection, and the late films will demonstrate reversed flow down the vertebral artery into the subclavian artery of the affected side (Fig. 144).

Opacification of the occluded subclavian artery can also be achieved by selective injection into the vertebral artery on the contralateral side (Fig. 145). The contrast fluid passes up to the basilar artery and descends down the opposite vertebral artery into the occluded subclavian artery. With this selective study the small vertebro-vertebral collaterals become visible, as described by Newton and Wyle in 1964.

10.2.2 Bilateral Subclavian Steal Syndrome

Bilateral subclavian steal means complete occlusion or severe stenosis at the origin of both subclavian arteries with brachial vascularization via reversal of blood flow through the vertebrobasilar system. This syndrome is a rare condition. To date only eleven cases of bilateral subclavian steal syn-

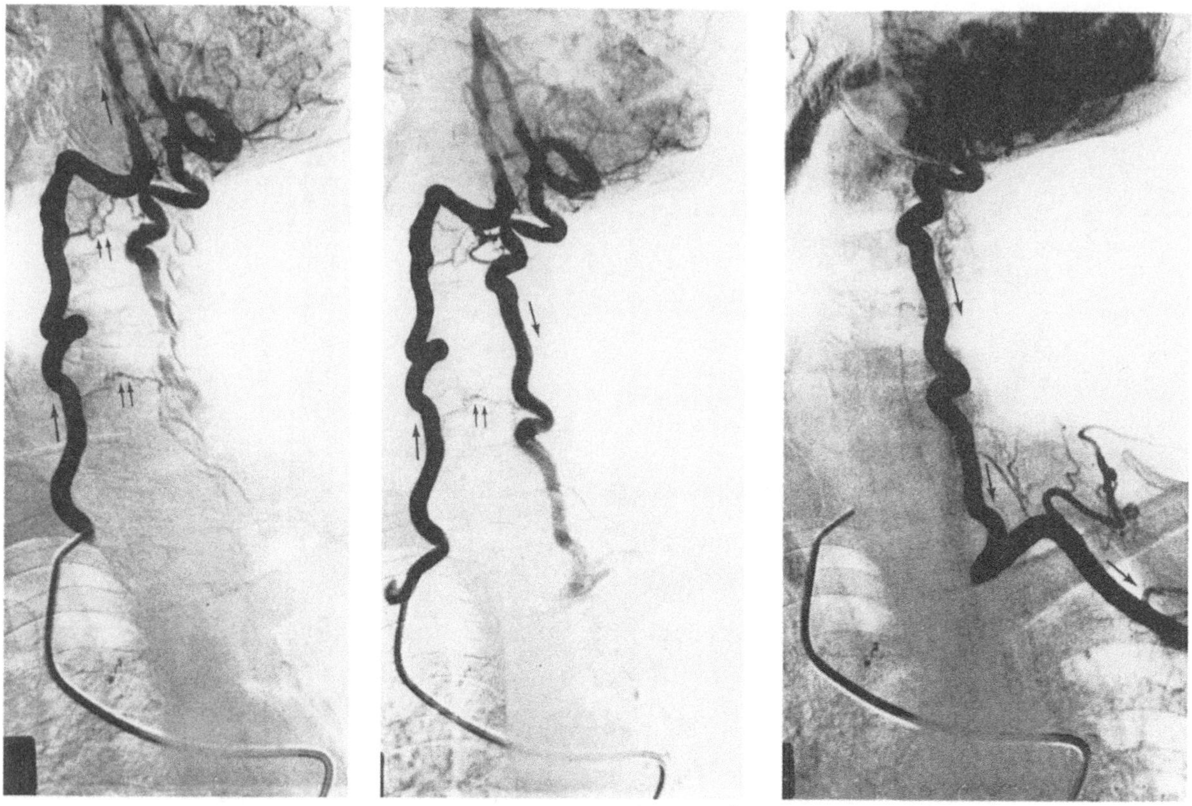

Fig. 145
Selective injection into the right vertebral artery of patient with left subclavian steal (same case as in Fig. 144).
A initial, B and C – later films in sequence demonstrate flow of the contrast medium up the right vertebral artery and down the left vertebral artery into the occluded left subclavian artery (large arrows). Collateral flow extends from the right vertebral artery through the radicular spinal arteries (double small arrows) to participate in the filling of the left vertebral artery.

drome have been reported in the literature (Collier *et al.*, 1965; Coder *et al.*, 1965; Müller *et al.*, 1967; Skalpe *et al.*, 1970; Riley, 1974; Avarelo *et al.*, 1976).

Arteriosclerosis is the most frequent cause of this syndrome, five of the published cases showed arteriosclerotic occlusion of the origin of both subclavian arteries. Other causes of this syndrome include Takayasu's arteritis, congenital stenosis of the subclavian arteries and stenosis associated with coarctation of the aortic arch.

The syndrome consists of reversal of blood flow in both vertebral arteries, usually resulting in cerebral ischaemia following exercise of the upper extremities. The patients presented with cerebral vascular insufficiency associated with asymmetrical blood pressure and pulses in the upper extremities.

Although patients with unilateral steal syndrome are occasionally asymptomatic, all cases of reported bilateral subclavian steal syndrome were symptomatic.

10.2.3 Innominate Steal Syndrome

In close analogy to the original case of subclavian steal reported by Reivich in 1961, a similar pattern characterized by occlusion or stenosis of the innominate artery and reversal of flow in the right vertebral artery was called the 'innominate steal syndrome' (Pratesi *et al.*, 1968).

Although the aetiological factors and most of the symptoms of this syndrome are the same as those of subclavian steal, the haemodynamic findings and clinical picture suggest that this syndrome is different from the subclavian steal. At present many authors call occlusion or severe stenosis of the innominate artery with retrograde flow in the right vertebral artery the 'innominate steal syndrome'.

According to Pratesi *et al.* (1968), when the right upper extremity is at rest or carries out moderate exercise, two different haemodynamic conditions may be set up:

1. The blood coming from the left vertebral artery traverses the right vertebral artery with reversal of flow, and goes on to fill the right subclavian and right carotid arteries, where the flow is normal. Such a haemodynamic situation corresponds to that observed by Bosniak (1963) and Blakemore *et al.* (1963). Furthermore, Blakemore *et al.* were able to show that the flow in the right carotid artery is greater than that in the subclavian artery on the same side (Blakemore *et al.*, 1963).
2. Blood passes up the left vertebral and left carotid arteries in the normal fashion. The right subclavian artery is filled by retrograde flow down the right vertebral and right carotid arteries. In such a haemodynamic situation, the intracranial right carotid territory is supplied via the circle of Willis.

The occurrence of one of these two possibilities depends fundamentally on the anatomical and functional state of the left vertebral artery, the posterior communicating arteries and the anterior communicating artery.

Clinical symptoms may be attacks of slight dizziness, episodes of right hemiparaesthesia and hemiparesis, occurring upon exercising of the upper right limb.

10.2.4 Analysis of Our Case Material

During the period 1970-1980 forty-one patients with 'steal syndromes' were investigated angiographically in our department. There were 18 males (44%) and 23 females (56%) with an average age of 53 years. Forty-four percent of patients were between 50 and 70 years of age (see Table XXX).

TABLE XXX

Age and Sex Distribution in 41 Patients with a 'Steal Syndrome'.

Age (Years)	*Males* Nr.	%	*Females* Nr.	%	*Total* Nr.	%
0-30	1	2.4	1	2.4	2	5.0
31-40	2	5.0	5	12.1	7	17.0
41-50	3	7.3	4	9.8	7	17.0
51-60	3	7.3	5	12.2	8	19.6
61-70	6	14.6	4	9.8	10	24.4
71-80	3	7.3	4	9.8	7	17.0
Total	18	43.9	23	56.1	41	100

TABLE XXXI

Distribution of Symptoms in 41 Adult Patients with a 'Steal Syndrome".

Distribution of Symptoms	*Frequency* *Nr.*	*Percent*
Only neurological symptoms	16	39.0
Both neurological and upper extremity symptoms	21	51.2
Only upper extremity symptoms present	4	9.8

All of the patients were symptomatic with complaints of vertebrobasilar insufficiency and intermittent claudication of the affected extremity. The average duration of the symptoms before radiological diagnosis was 16 months. One patient had noted neurological symptoms for more than three years. All symptoms are summarized in Table XXXI. Both neurological and upper extremity symptoms were present in 21 cases (51%), while 16 patients had only neurological symptoms (39%).

In total, neurological symptoms were present in 90 percent of our cases.

The most common neurological symptoms were dizziness and visual impairment. Less common were vertigo, syncope and paresis of one or more extremities. Occipital headache was present in a number of cases.

The most common upper extremity symptom was intermittent claudication. In one patient with the innominate steal syndrome, cyanosis of the fingertips of the right hand was noted, most probably as a result of peripheral arterial insufficiency.

Upon physical examination the most constant finding was a difference in blood pressure between the two upper extremities. The blood pressure on the involved side could not be measured in four cases. Systolic bruits in the supraclavicular region were not a constant finding; nevertheless they were present in the majority of cases. The distal pulses of the affected extremity were decreased or absent in almost all cases.

For the definitive diagnosis all patients underwent aortic arch angiography. In two patients with total occlusion of the left subclavian artery an additional selective arteriogram was obtained by placing a catheter in the proximal part of the right vertebral artery. These arteriograms clearly dem-

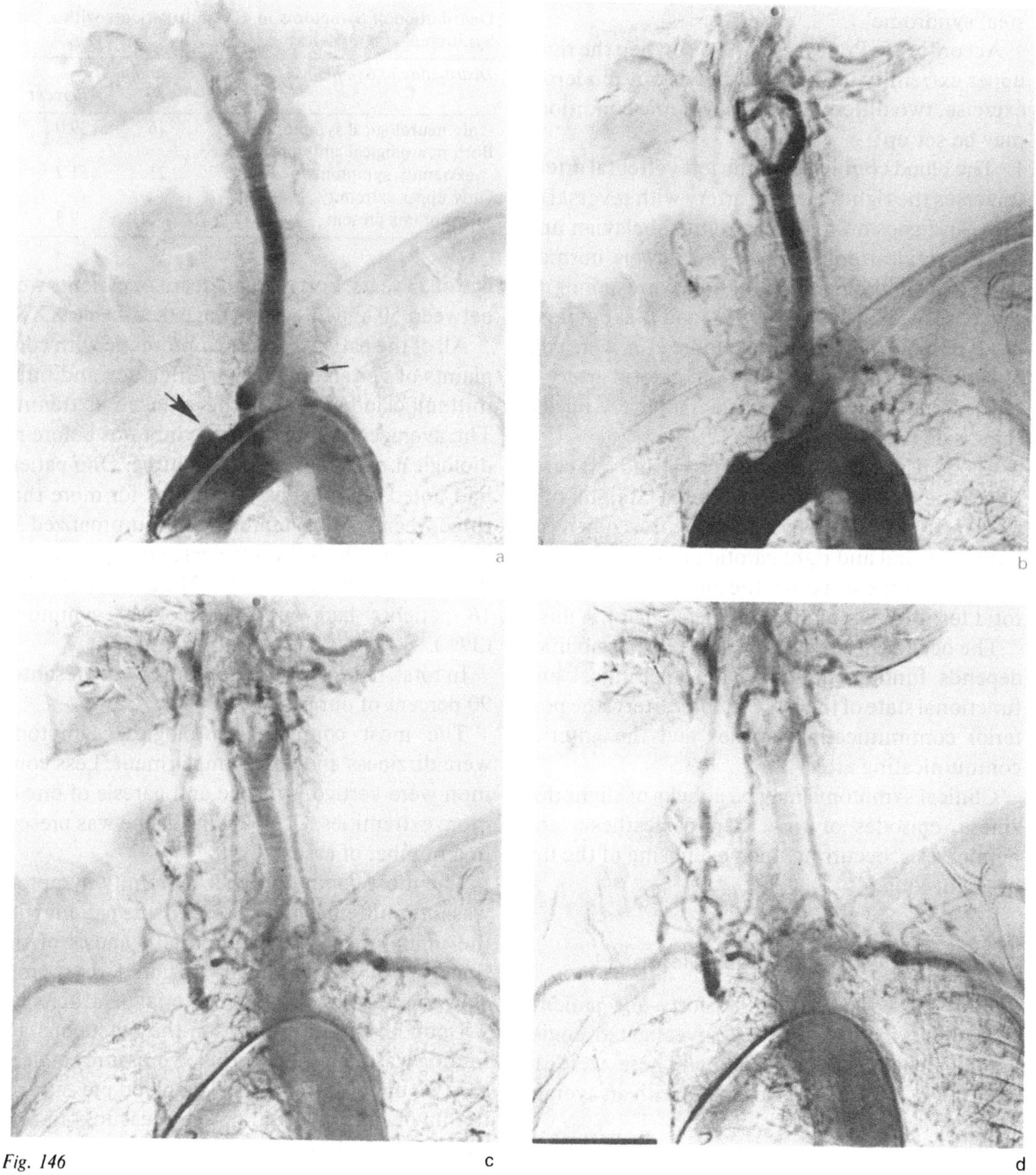

Fig. 146

Combination of innominate and left subclavian steal syndrome.

A. Film taken 1.5 seconds after beginning of contrast injection shows opacification of the left common carotid artery only and complete occlusion of the innominate artery (large arrow) and the left subclavian artery (small arrow) at their origin.

B. Two seconds after injection, the left vertebral artery is clearly visible, the distal portion is more densely opacified. The time and the appearance of this artery show the presence of a reversal of flow. Note also opacification with retrograde flow of the cervical portion of the right external and internal carotid arteries.

C. Film taken three seconds after injection demonstrates retrograde opacification of both vertebral arteries and the right carotid artery as well as antegrade flow in both subclavian arteries.

D. Film taken 4 seconds after injection demonstrates the same findings as in the previous figure. The arteries are more intensely opacified.

TABLE XXXII

Site of Obstruction in 41 Adults with a 'Steal Syndrome'.

Vessel	*Stenosis*		*Occlusion*		*Total*	
	Nr.	*%*	*Nr.*	*%*	*Nr.*	*%*
Aortic arch	1	2.4	–	–	1	2.4
Left Subclavian	9	22.0	21	51.2	30	73.2
Right Subclavian	5	12.2	3	7.4	8	19.6
Innominate	1	2.4	1	2.4	2	4.8
Total	16	39	25	61	41	100

onstrated the retrograde flow down the contralateral vertebral artery toward the left subclavian artery. Moreover, the arteriograms showed additional collateral vessels which usually are not visible on arch aortograms, even on subtraction films (Fig. 145).

The angiographic findings for our 41 patients are summarized in Table XXXII.

In one case a left subclavian steal syndrome was found to be due to coarctation of the aortic arch. The stenotic part of the arch was located between the origins of the left common carotid and the left subclavian arteries.

In two cases the cause of a right-sided steal syndrome was obstruction of the innominate artery. In one of these cases there was also complete occlusion of the left subclavian artery with the typical signs of subclavian steal on that side. This particular case of a bilateral steal deserves separate discussion (Fig. 146).

The patient, a 51-year-old man, had a history of frequently recurring episodes of vertigo and binocular visual blurring several times a day for a period of almost two years. The attacks, which lasted several minutes, were usually accompanied by numbness and tingling in the fingers of both hands. Full recovery occurred after each of these attacks. Physical examination revealed a brachial artery pressure of 80/60 mm Hg on the right and 95/75 mm Hg on the left side.

Decreased and delayed radial pulses were found on both sides, particularly on the right. Slight cyanosis of the fingertips of the right hand was observed. On auscultation, there were no systolic bruits audible over the carotid arteries or the left and right supraclavicular fossae. The first film of the angiographic study (Fig. 146) demonstrated occlusions of the first portions of the innominate and the left subclavian arteries. Later serial films showed filling of the right carotid and both vertebral arteries by retrograde flow and opacification of the subclavian arteries with antegrade flow. Numerous hypertrophic muscular branches, serving as collaterals, were opacified in the neck and upper thorax.

In another case of a bilateral subclavian steal syndrome the right subclavian artery was totally occluded and the left showed a severe stenosis at its origin.

This patient, a 64-year-old woman, complained of periodic coldness and numbness of both extremities and a claudication that precluded even such minimal activity as combing her hair. She also had neurological symptoms such as blurring of vision, vertigo and sometimes nausea. These symptoms had been progressive for about 18 months.

Further analysis of our material shows that in 24 cases (58.6%) complete occlusion of the subclavian artery was responsible for the syndrome (Table XXXII). The subclavian steal syndrome occurred on the left side only or in combination with an innominate steal in 31 cases (75.6%); in 10 cases (24.4%) the steal syndrome was either right subclavian or innominate.

10.2.5 Conclusions

The subclavian steal syndrome is the result of a localized obstruction of the subclavian or innominate arteries, proximal to the origin of the vertebral artery. It seems to be more common on the left side. Patients suffering from this syndrome have more frequent and more pronounced neurological symptoms than complaints pertaining to the arm. The symptoms are aggravated by exercise of the involved extremity.

The most constant physical findings in this syndrome are a significant blood pressure difference between the upper extremities and decreased or absent arterial pulses in the involved arm. Occlusion of an innominate artery produces the same symptoms as the subclavian steal syndrome, since in both cases cerebral vessels as well as those in the arm are involved.

Our case material consists of 41 patients with a slight female preponderance. In all cases a stenosis or occlusion of the subclavian or innominate artery was found. It was located on the left side in

75% of the cases, on the right in 25%. In two patients a bilateral steal syndrome was present and in one patient a combination of left subclavian steal and innominate steal.

10.2.6 Thyrocervical Steal Syndrome

Literature

A 'thyrocervical steal' is present in patients with total occlusion or severe segmental obliteration of the subclavian artery beyond the vertebral orifice. In its 'pure' form the stenosis is distal to the vertebral artery but proximal to the thyrocervical trunk (Fig. 147, large arrow) which means that the subclavian artery distal to the stenosis is filled by reverse flow through the branches of the thyrocervical trunk. This is possible because of anatomical connections between the muscular and perispinal branches of the vertebral and carotid arteries and the branches of the thyrocervical trunk in the neck (Fig. 147, small arrows).

The thyrocervical steal syndrome also occurs in patients with occlusive disease involving the subclavian artery as well as the vertebral artery on the same side. There are reports in the literature of this syndrome in patients with the subclavian steal syndrome who were treated surgically by ligation of the vertebral artery (Trevino, 1970). This syndrome can also be found after surgical damage to the vertebral artery and subsequent ligation in patients with subclavian steal on the same side, undergoing neck surgery for other reasons.

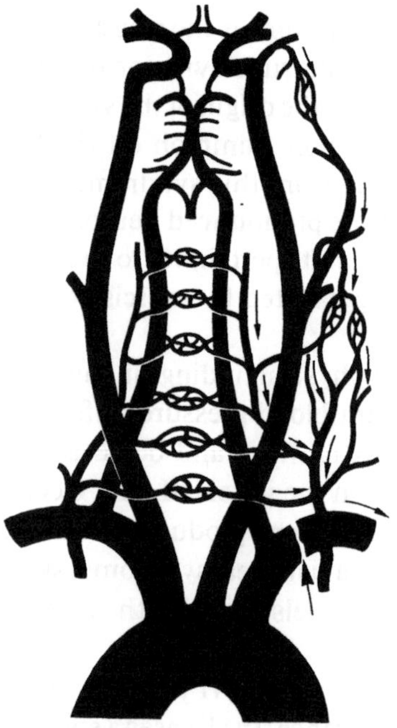

Fig. 147
Schematic diagram of collateral blood circulation in left thyrocervical steal syndrome.

In 1970 Newtons and Potts described the thyrocervical steal syndrome in a patient with anomalous origin of the left vertebral artery arising directly from the aortic arch and complete occlusion of the left common carotid artery and the left subclavian artery.

In this syndrome the arterial blood supply to the upper extremity is carried out by the collaterals of the vertebral and carotid arteries to the ascending branches of the thyrocervical trunk. The circulation in the thyrocervical trunk is reversed and flows down the subclavian artery beyond the site of the obstruction (Fig. 147 arrows). If the lumen of the subclavian artery is completely occluded, the blood flows to the arm via the lateral branches of the thyrocervical trunk in the normal direction, mainly through the transverse scapular artery and the suprascapular artery.

The arterial blood supply to the diseased arm is provided predominantly by the vertebral arteries. Both vertebral arteries have extensive perispinal collateral branches through which blood flows into ascending branches of the thyrocervical trunk on the involved side. The other major collateral pathway appears to be through the anastomoses between the occipital branch of the external carotid artery and the distal part of the ascending cervical artery of the thyrocervical trunk.

The degree of shunting varies in accordance with the degree of obstruction of the subclavian artery and the oxygen demand of the upper limb (Mueller and Hinck, 1967).

10.2.7 Analysis of Our Case Material and Report of a Case

The thyrocervical steal syndrome appears to be rare. In our material of 592 aortic arch arteriograms, taken during the period 1970-1980, we found this syndrome only twice. The angiographic findings of one of these cases are presented in Fig. 148.

The patient, a 74-year-old man, had had inter-

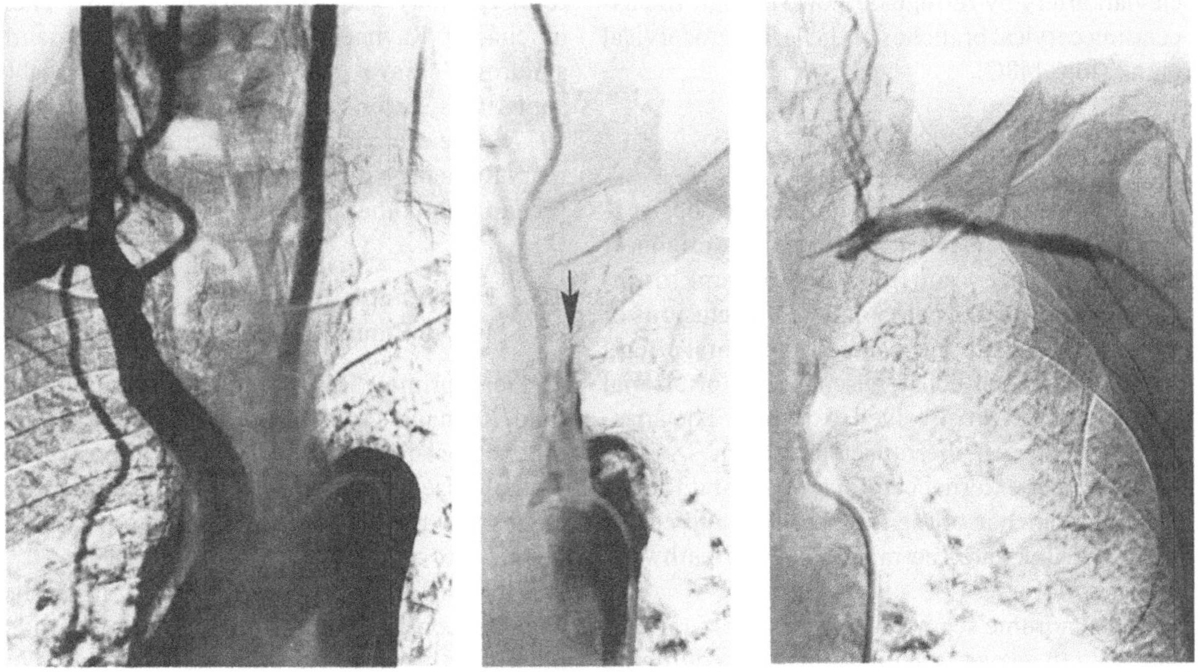

a b c

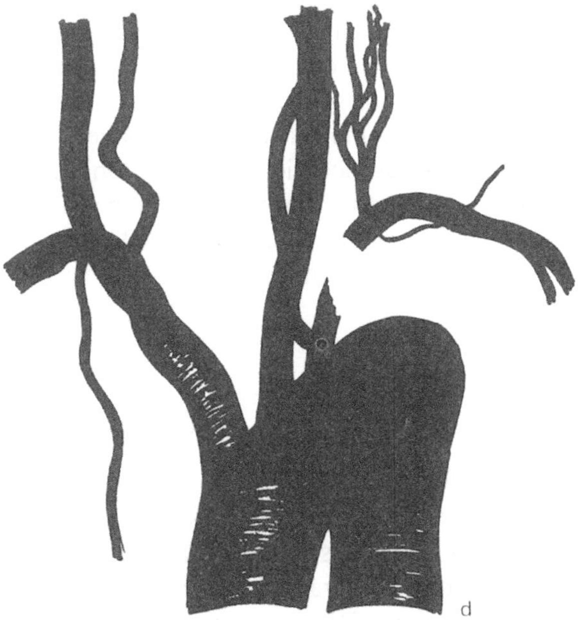

d

Fig. 148
Left Thyrocervical Steal Syndrome.
a. Injection into aortic arch demonstrates filling of both carotid and both vertebral arteries. No filling of the left subclavian artery.
b. Selective injection into the orifice of the left subclavian artery demonstrate a normal filling of the left vertebral artery. There is total occlusion of the left subclavian artery (arrow) just beyond of the vertebral orifice.
c. Later film in sequence demonstrates filling of the left subclavian artery, by retrograde flow through ascending cervical branches of the left thyrocervical trunk.
d. Schematic diagram of the angiographic findings in the case reported.
(Reproduced from J. M. Greep *et al.*, Pain in Shoulder and Arm, chapter 3. Martinus Nijhoff, The Hague, Boston, London 1979.)

mittent dizziness, occipital headaches, blurred vision and constant pain in the left arm for about two and a half years. Associated with these complaints were occasional discolouration and weakness of the left hand.

Significant physical findings included the following:

a. Systolic blood pressure: 36 mm Hg in the left and 165 mm Hg in the right arm.
b. Very weak almost non-palpable radial pulse on the left side, and
c. Slight atrophy of the musculature of the left extremity.

Thoracic aortography revealed complete occlusion of the left subclavian artery just beyond the origin of the vertebral artery (Fig. 148B arrow).

Late films demonstrated filling of the left subclavian artery by retrograde flow through the ascending cervical branches of the left thyrocervical trunk (Fig. 148C).

10.2.8 Conclusions

The thyrocervical syndrome is caused by obstruction of the subclavian artery between the origins of the vertebral artery and thyrocervical trunk, or appears as a result of a combination of occlusions of the subclavian and the ipsilateral vertebral artery. There are several collateral channels for arterial blood supply to the involved extremity. The anastomoses between the muscular branches of the vertebral and external carotid arteries and the ascending branches of the thyrocervical and costocervical trunks are the main collateral pathways in this syndrome.

The syndrome seems to be appear very rare. In the past ten years the syndrome was encountered in our material only twice, while in the same period 592 thoracic aortograms and 1,213 cerebral and 750 subclavian arteriograms were performed.

Aortic arch angiography is the most suitable radiological procedure for the diagnosis of this syndrome and demonstration of the collaterals. One of our two cases is discussed clinically and radiologically.

10.3 Vasospastic Disorders

Literature

The most common vasospastic disorders are characterized by episodes of digital colour changes in the form of sequential blanching of the digits (arteriospasm), induced by cold or emotional stress, followed first by bluish (cyanotic) discolouration (venous stasis) and then by redness (reactive hyperaemia) of the digits. These changes are known as Raynaud's symptoms. They were first described by the French physician Maurice Raynaud in 1862. In addition to these symptoms, discomfort and dysaesthesia in the affected extremities may be present.

Despite general agreement about the vasospastic nature of these symptoms and their association with exposure to cold and emotional stimuli, clinical categorization has caused confusion. The terms primary and secondary Raynaud's phenomena, or Raynaud's 'disease' and 'Raynaud's syndrome' have been used interchangeably, sometimes inconsistently (Rösch and Porter, 1977). Therefore a clear distinction between primary Raynaud's disease and Raynaud's syndrome secondary to other processes is important.

10.3.1 Raynaud's Disease
(syn: Primary Raynaud's phenomenon)

The term primary Raynaud's disease is used when mild Raynaud's symptoms are present without other associated diseases. Absence of obstructive arterial disease and other systemic alterations makes the prognosis of this symptom complex favourable.

Primary Raynaud's disease is uncommon. It is usually seen in young 'healthy' women, and is most often bilateral. The attacks are episodic, symmetrical and almost always manifested in the hand (although the feet may also be affected). The symptoms are precipated by cold and emotional stress. The clinical course is usually benign, and severe changes in the blood supply to the affected digits are uncommon (Metzler and Silver, 1979). On extremely rare occasions the nutritional disturbances may lead to acronecrosis of the digits, a very painful condition characterized by a prolonged and poor healing tendency (Terpstra *et al.*, 1977).

10.3.2 Raynaud's Syndrome
(syn: Secondary Raynaud's phenomenon)

The term Raynaud's syndrome or secondary Raynaud's phenomenon is used usually to refer to Raynaud's symptoms occurring as a consequence of a disease. It is characterized by greater severity and progression of the symptoms, significant organic arterial disease and a poor prognosis (Allen and Brown, 1932; Porter *et al.*, 1975; Lemmens, 1979).

The causes of secondary Raynaud's phenomenon may be classified into four main groups:

1. Peripheral arterial occlusions (arteriosclerosis, embolism, injury, thromboangiitis obliterans).
2. Arterial and neural lesions (thoracic outlet syndrome).
3. Intoxication (ergot, heavy metals).

4. Systemic disease (scleroderma, disseminated lupus erythematosus, rheumatoid arthritis, dermatomyositis and thrombocytopenic purpura).

The diagnosis of Raynaud's syndrome is made by clinical and laboratory examination and arteriography.

10.3.3 Differential Diagnosis

Since Raynaud's symptoms can be the first manifestations of a serious underlying disease, some authors recommend that no case must be classified as primary Raynaud's disease until all investigations have been completed and a considerable period (approximately two years) of careful follow-up has passed. (Allen *et al.*, 1962).

Gifford Jr. and Hines (1957) are of the opinion that by using certain clinical criteria (Table XXXIII) it is possible to distinguish Raynaud's disease from Raynaud's phenomenon in up to 95% of the cases.

TABLE XXXIII

Clinical Criteria of Raynaud's Disease.

1. Episodes of Raynaud's symptoms, precipitated by cold or emotional stress.
2. Duration of the symptoms at least two years.
3. Absence of other primary diseases.
4. Involvement of the hands and/or the feet, but always bilaterally.
5. Absence of gangrene or limited to small areas on the fingertips.

Recent studies with detailed immunological evaluation suggest that most patients with Raynaud's symptoms, even the young 'healthy' females, have an autoimmune disease or other immunological abnormalities and therefore should be classified as having Raynaud's syndrome (Porter *et al.*, 1975; Rösch and Porter, 1977).

10.3.4 Angiography

The opinions in literature differ about the usefulness of angiography in primary vasospastic disorders. While some authors consider it valuable, particularly for exclusion of organic vascular changes or evaluation of the results of various forms of therapy, others consider it unimportant for the diagnosis and management of Raynaud's disease. Different recommendations have been made concerning the procedure for brachial artery angiography in patients with Raynaud's disease: general anaesthesia, stellate block, administration of large doses of vasodilator, hand warming, heated angiographic rooms and oral administration of alcohol. All these have been used to minimize the risk of vasospasm. A direct puncture of the brachial artery is not recommended since the puncture very often causes severe spasms in patients with Raynaud's disease.

Our angiographic procedure for patients with Raynaud's disease does not differ from that used for other conditions. The angiograms are performed under local anaesthesia and the percutaneous transfemoral approach is used for introduction of the catheter.

When the catheter is positioned in the distal brachial artery, the vasodilator tolazoline is administered intra-arterially in a dose of 20 to 30 mg before injection of the contrast medium. Whenever the vasospastic symptoms are very severe and clinically evident as pale and cold hands then, before the intra-arterial injections of vasodilator and contrast medium, the hand is warmed by placing it in warm water for several minutes. When the temperature rises the skin colour changes. This vasodilatory response to higher skin temperature is physiological; however, it varies from patient to patient, occurring later in those with severe Raynaud's syndrome.

10.3.5 Angiographic Findings

It is known that in primary Raynaud's phenomenon the wall of the arteries appears normal in the early phase of this condition. When vasospasm continues for longer periods, changes take place in the arterial wall which may lead to peripheral occlusions (Bergan *et al.*, 1971). Thus the angiographic findings are dependent on the stage of the disease. In the early stage, the arteriogram appears normal or demonstrates spasm of the arteries (Fig. 149). In advanced stages the arteriogram may reveal occlusions of the distal digital arteries.

In our material on primary Raynaud's disease a few cases with vasospastic disorders were seen

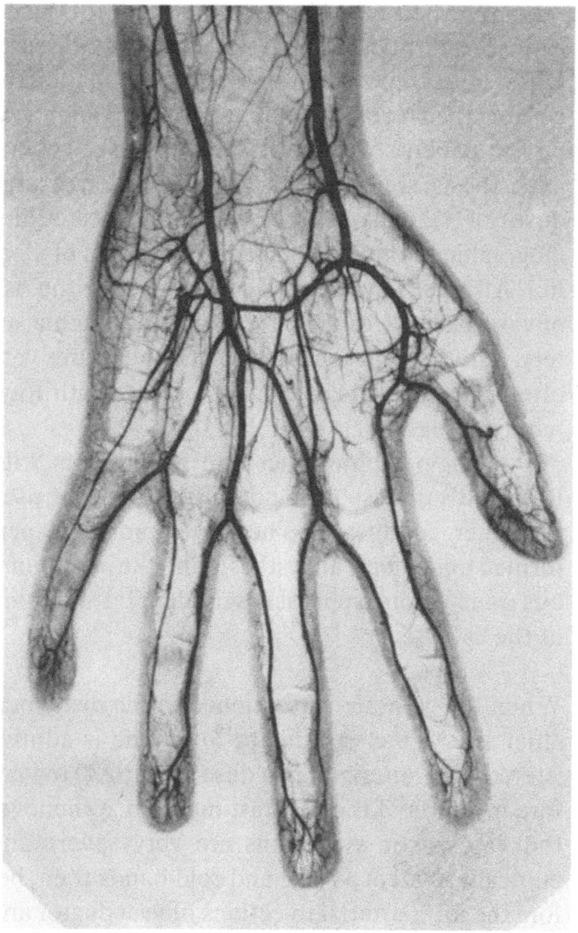

Fig. 149
Hand arteriogram of young female patient with clinical diagnosis of primary Raynaud's phenomenon demonstrates spastic proper digital arteries in the fourth and fifth fingers on the ulnar side and spastic side-branches of all digital arteries. There are no peripheral occlusions.
The arteriograms were obtained after heating the hand for 5 minutes in warm water and intra-arterial administration of 30 mg tolazoline, prior to the injection of contrast medium.

(Fig. 149). There were no cases with definite occlusions of the digital arteries.

10.3.6 Conclusions

The angiographic technique for investigation of the arteries of the hand in patients with primary and secondary vasospastic disorders does not differ from that used for other conditions. The method includes transfemoral catheterization of the distal brachial artery under local anaesthesia and use of vasodilators before injection of the contrast medium. When vasospastic symptoms are severe and clinically evident the usual dose of 20 mg tolazoline should be increased to 30 mg per extremity. In some instances, for better vasodilatation of the small peripheral arteries, an external warming of the hand is necessary. For this reason, before the injection of vasodilator and contrast medium the hand is placed in warm water for several minutes.

In patients with primary vasospastic disease the arteries of the hand appear normal on arteriograms, unless acronecrosis of the digits is present.

Cases with secondary Raynaud's phenomenon are discussed in the chapters on embolism, scleroderma, thromboangiitis obliterans, occupational trauma and thoracic outlet syndrome.

10.4 Arterial Embolism and Thrombosis of the Upper Extremities

10.4.1 Literature on Arterial Embolism

There are many publications about acute embolic occlusions of the cerebral and visceral vessels, aortic bifurcation and the main arteries of the lower extremities. However, publications dedicated entirely to acute occlusions of the arteries of the upper extremities are rare, and practically all of them are based on no more than 10 to 15 cases. In recent literature two publications have appeared describing a large number of acute embolic occlusions of the arteries of the upper limb. In 1977 Savelyev *et al.* published a remarkable number of 260 cases of acute arterial emboli in the upper extremities. The report covered a period of 35 years of experience with this disease. The second publication of 28 cases of embolic occlusions of the upper extremity arteries was presented in 1975 by Hodgkinson and Tracy.

Other large series reported in the literature in the last 30 years are summarized in Table XXXIV.

Arterial emboli are known to occur much less frequently in the upper limb than in the lower limb. This can be concluded from the analysis of previous reports given in Table XXXIV. From the summary of these reports it can be seen that embolic arterial occlusions involved the upper extremities in 15.3 percent of the cases, the most frequent site being the brachial artery (50.4%) (see Table XXXV).

Depending upon their origin, the emboli in the

TABLE XXXIV

Relative Incidence of Upper Limb Emboli.
Reported in the Literature since 1950.

Author	*Total number of embolisms*	*Upper limb emboli Nr.*	*percentage*
Haimovici (1950)	279	46	17.0
Daley *et al.* (1951)	393	39	10.0
Warren *et al.* (1954)	232	59	18.6
McGarity *et al.* (1960)	86	16	18.6
Young *et al.* (1963)	114	21	18.4
Cranley *et al.* (1964)	214	29	13.6
Martin *et al.* (1969)	88	12	13.6
Thompson *et al.* (1970)	188	27	14.4
McGowan and Mooneeram (1973)	174	22	16.6
Total	1768	271	15.3

The average incidence of upper extremity arterial embolism is 15.3%.

upper limb can be classified into three categories:
1. Emboli originating from the heart.
2. Emboli originating from a diseased proximal arterial tree, and
3. Emboli of unknown aetiology (undetermined).

Emboli in the peripheral arteries most commonly originate from the heart. In the series of Savelyev *et al.* (1977) cardiac diseases were the cause of the embolism in the arteries of the upper extremity in 92.58 percent of the cases. Mural thrombus secondary to fibrillation of the left atrium was the source of almost half of the total number of emboli originating from the heart. Next in frequency was rheumatic heart disease, mainly mitral stenosis, which in his series accounted for one-third of the cases. The third large group was myocardial infarctions which occurred less than one month previously (Sheinin and Inberg, 1967). In about 10 percent of the cases of Savelyev *et al.* (1977), a myocardial infarction with mural thrombus was the cause of peripheral embolization in the upper extremity. The first symptoms of a so-called 'silent' myocardial infarction may be peripheral arterial embolism (Lary and Takats, 1954).

In the past, the cause of atrial fibrillation in nearly 64 percent of the patients was found to be a rheumatoid heart disease. Embolism of the peripheral arteries was usually more common in women than in men, because of the higher incidence of rheumatoid heart disease in women. However, in the last 20 years this has changed. At the present time the patients are usually older and the majority have arteriosclerotic heart disease, which in turn has become the most common cause of atrial fibrillation (Stephens *et al.*, 1971).

Other less common sources of cardiac emboli are subacute bacterial endocarditis, fungal endocarditis, ventricular aneurysm, atrial myxoma, idiopathic hypertrophic subaortic stenosis (Kawarda *et al.*, 1973) and the release of prosthetic valve material (Pluth and Danielson, 1974).

TABLE XXXV

Location of Acute Embolic Occlusion in the Arteries of the Upper Limb.

Artery	*1. Series of Savelyev et al. (1977) in percentage (260 cases)*	*2. Series of Hodgkinson and Tracy (1975) in percentages (28 cases)*	*3. Present series (1980) in percentage (11 cases)*	*Average of percentage*
Subclavian	18.0	17.8	9.1	15.0
Axillary	25.1	25.0	18.2	22.7
Brachial	55.3	32.2	63.6	50.4
Radial	1.2	17.9	9.1	9.4
Ulnar	0.4	7.1	–	2.5
Total	100	100	100	100

The second category of emboli consists of those which originate from a diseased proximal part of the same arterial tree. This group includes emboli which arise from ulcerated atherosclerotic plaques, traumatized arteries, true or false aneurysms and a compressed subclavian artery at the thoracic outlet as well as emboli associated with surgical procedures, such as brachial arteriotomy (Cross and Ellis, 1966), cannulation of the radial artery (Michaelson and Walsh, 1970) and catheterization of an artery (Sachatello *et al.*, 1974). Other emboli in this group are bacterial emboli associated with a systemic illness and septicaemia, or bacterial emboli which appear 'down stream' from a nidus of infection in the wall of an artery, such as mycotic aneurysm (Merry *et al.*, 1972). Finally emboli originating from malignancy in an arterial wall are also included here (Till and Faiburn, 1947; Liggett and Kartchner, 1979).

The third category of emboli are those without a known causative factor or those with an assumed aetiology, for example, the emboli which occur in young women after the use of oestrogen-containing oral contraceptive pills (O'Connor and Pollock, 1975). Catheter-generated thrombi may cause embolization of a distal artery during a diagnostic procedure or may be scraped off during catheter withdrawal. Oversized catheters, multiple catheter changes, prolonged duration of the study, and lack of heparin administration correlate directly with increased embolic incidents. Arterial wall damage with subsequent formation of emboli is also related to the technique and manner of catheterization and to the experience and gentleness of the examiner.

10.4.2 Clinical Manifestations

The clinical symptoms of acute arterial embolization of the upper extremity are dependent on the site and extent of the occlusion. Emboli involving the subclavian, axillary or brachial artery above the deep brachial artery may lead to severe ischaemia of the limb with loss of function and consequent gangrene. In such cases the collateral circulation may be threatened by the embolus itself or by the proximal or distal propagating arterial thrombosis which may develop (Hodgkinson and Tracy, 1975). Emboli in the subclavian artery can cause death, if they lodge at the origin of the vertebral artery (Clauss, 1971), or if associated thrombosis leads to embolization of the vertebral or right carotid artery (Shucksmith, 1963).

Small emboli in the distal brachial artery or its branches are much less limb-threatening since a rich collateral network of arteries exists around the elbow.

Normally peripheral embolism is easily recognizable clinically, because of the sudden onset of pain in the extremity followed by coldness, pallor, paraesthesia, numbness and varying degrees of paralysis with loss of pulses distal to the involved site.

At times, however, onset may be insidious and differentiation from arterial thrombosis may be impossible without arteriography. Occasionally, the early stage of acute deep thrombophlebitis is accompanied by such marked vasospasms and pain that the diagnosis of arterial embolism is considered until further studies clarify the situation (Thompson, 1974).

10.4.3 Angiography

In the past some authors considered preoperative angiography in cases with embolic disease contraindicated (Wagner 1957, McCook *et al.*, 1959).

Other authors recommended angiography only in ambiguous cases, especially for patients with a known embolic disease and atypical sensory or motor disturbances of the limb (Wessler *et al.*, 1958).

Today angiography is considered to be absolutely indicated in each case of acute arterial obstruction. It has even been suggested that the procedure should be repeated within several hours of surgery to evaluate the effect of the surgical treatment.

Although, in most instances, the site of the embolus can be determined fairly precisely by Doppler examination and by the physical signs and symptoms, angiography should be performed in most of the cases to establish the definitive diagnosis as well as the exact localization of the site and the extent of the embolic occlusion. Another advantage of angiography is the information obtained regarding collateral circulation and pre-existing arterial disease. In atherosclerotic patients and when an embolus is located in the subclavian or the axillary artery, precautions must be taken if

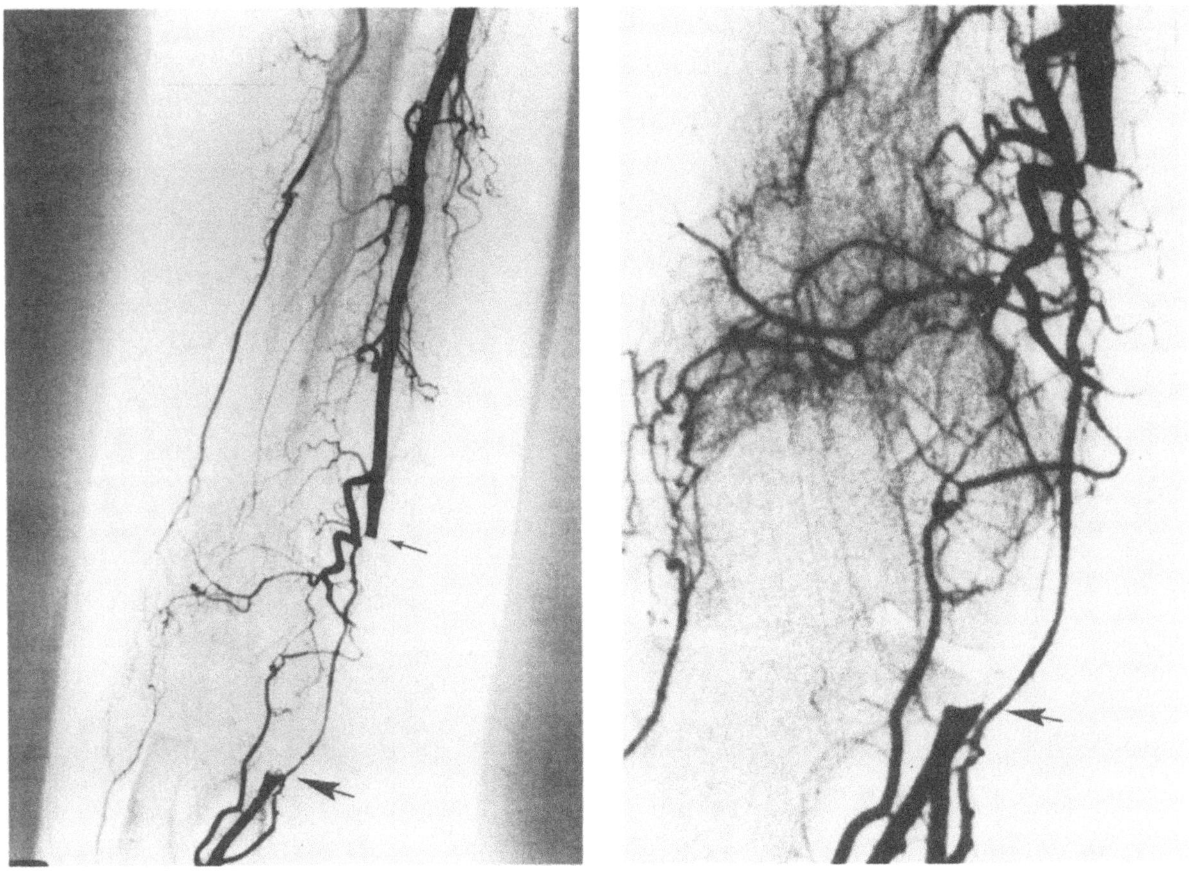

a b

Fig. 150

A. Recent embolus in right brachial artery occluding the distal portion of the vessel.
A sudden break in contrast column with a horizontal cutoff at the proximal margin of the occlusion (small arrow).
The distal margin of the occlusion is crescent-shaped (concave) due to the round shape of the distal end of the clot (large arrow).

B. Magnified picture of the same case.
Patient with hypertension and myocardial infarction in history.

a selective catheterization technique is to be used, as described in 9.7.1.

10.4.4 Analysis of Our Case Material

Between 1970 and 1980 eight acute cases of arterial emboli in the upper extremity were evaluated angiographically in our department. Patients with posttraumatic peripheral emboli and patients with thoracic outlet syndromes were not included in this series.

TABLE XXXVI

Site of Embolism in Our Series of Eight Patients.

Artery	*Right*		*Left*		*Total*	
	Nr.	*%*	*Nr.*	*%*	*Nr.*	*%*
Subclavian	1	9.1	–	–	1	9.1
Axillary	1	9.1	1	9.1	2	18.2
Brachial	4	36.5	3	27.1	7	63.6
Radial	–	–	1	9.1	1	9.1
Ulnar	–	–	–	–	–	–
Total	6	54.5	5	45.5	11	100

The mean age of the patients was 61 years (range between 26 and 85 years). Males and females were affected with approximately equal frequency. There was no significant preference of the emboli for either arm; right-sided embolic occlusions were slightly predominant (see Table XXXVI).

The majority of the emboli (64%) was located in the region of the brachial artery, particularly in its distal part (Table XXXVI); the next most common site was the axillary artery (18%). In two patients an embolus was seen in both axillary arteries and in one patient in the subclavian as well as the radial artery. In ten out of eleven embolizations the em-

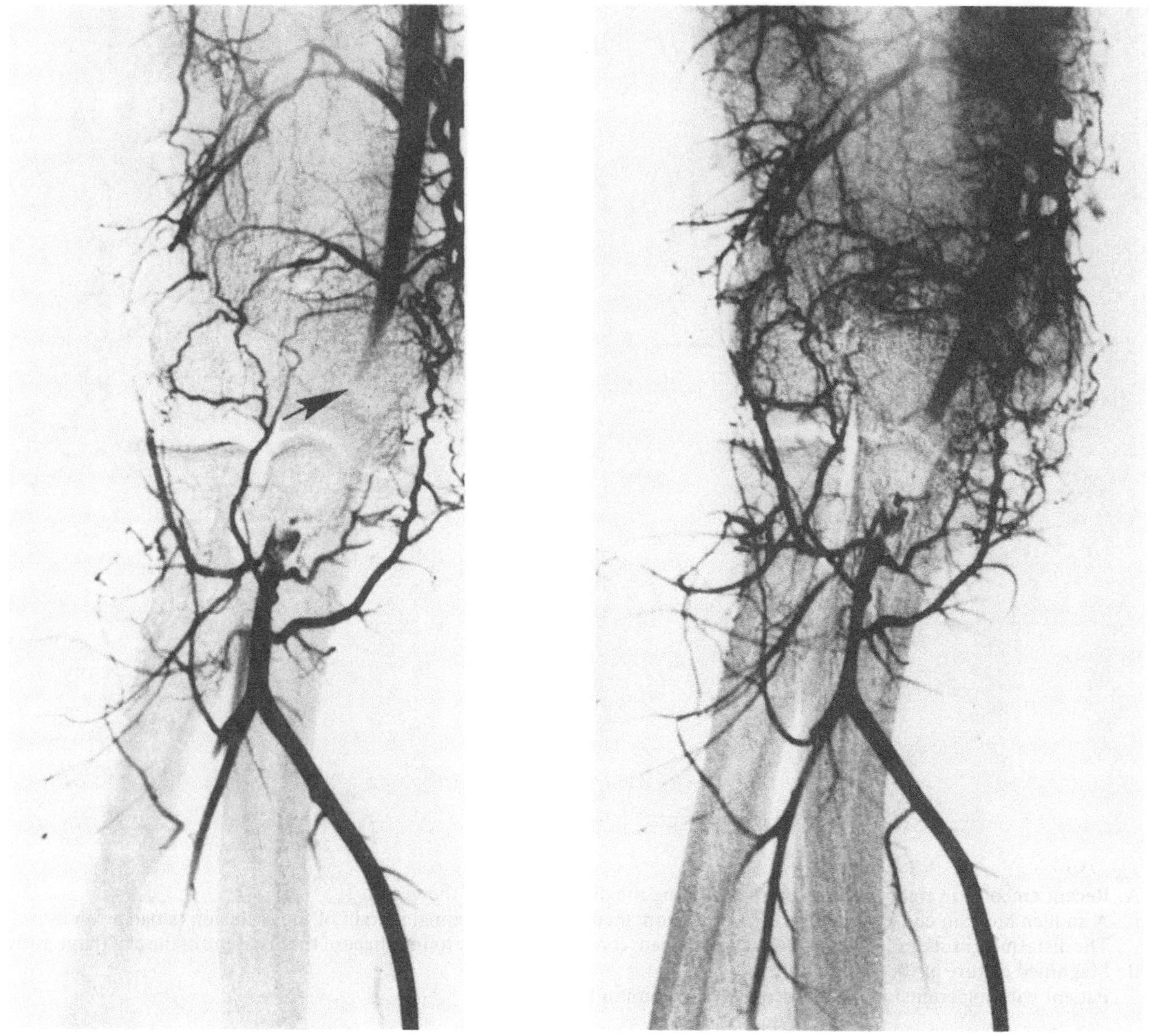

Fig. 151 a b

A. Embolic obstruction of the distal brachial artery with a conical termination of the contrast column at the proximal margin of the occlusion (arrow). The diagnosis confirmed on surgery.
Note decreased density of the contrast medium at the same site due to spasm.

B. Repeated arteriogram after injection of 20 mg. vasodilator (Priscol) shows disappearance of the spasm and better filling of the collateral arteries.

bolus had completely occluded the lumen of the artery (Fig. 150).

Most of the patients had a history of rheumatic valvular disease or arteriosclerotic heart disease. In the youngest patient, a 26-year-old female, brachial artery obstruction occurred four hours after selective catheterization of the subclavian artery at the same site.

From the arteriograms of cases with confirmed acute arterial embolism it can be concluded that embolic occlusions produce a variety of angiographic patterns.

A recent embolus which obstructs the vessel completely can be seen as a sudden break in the contrast medium, producing an abrupt horizontal cut-off or less frequently a concave shape in the distal portion of the artery (Fig. 150). The collateral circulation in these cases is often poorly developed possibly due to the suddenness of the occlusion. In cases where the collateral vessels are wide enough to feed the occluded vessel distal to the embolus, the distal end of the clot can be visualized. The contrast column usually shows a crescent-shaped lower margin, caused most probably by the

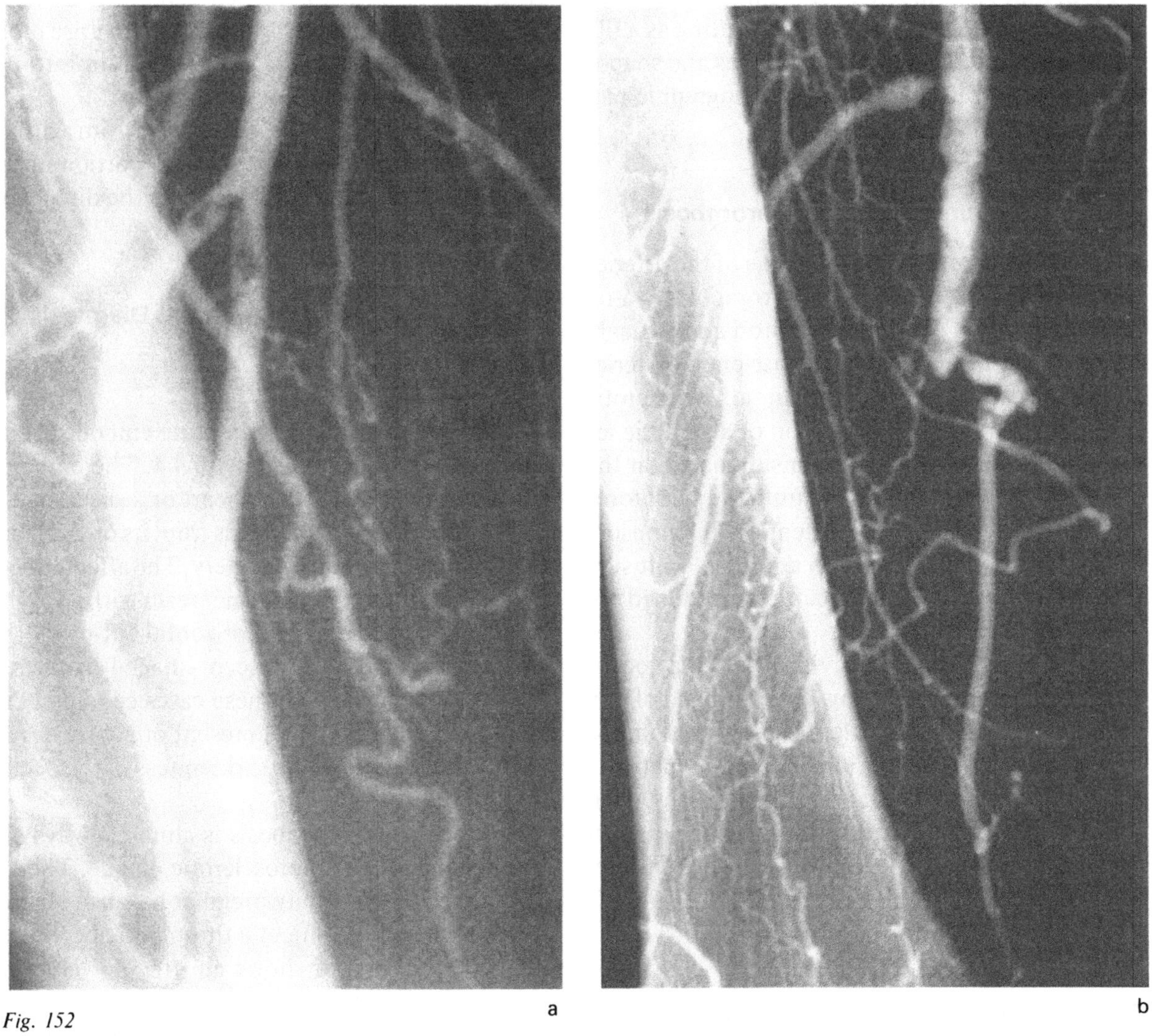

Fig. 152

A. Arterial Embolism.
An impacted embolus at arterial bifurcation causes a filling defect shaped like a saddle. The proximal artery and the side branches appear normal.

B. Arterial Thrombosis.
The affected artery shows diffuse arteriosclerotic changes. The thrombotic occlusion causes a typically irregular tapering termination of the contrast column.

Note marked collateral network distal to the occlusion.

rounded lower end of the embolus itself (Fig. 150B, arrow). In such cases the size of the embolus can be determined on arteriograms. Moreover the occluded non-visualized part of the artery in this type of embolus may have a convex upper and lower margin, indicating the rounded shape of the proximal and distal ends of the clot.

This crescent-shaped pattern, which was seen in most of our cases, usually appears when the embolus obstructs the vessel totally and there is no associated spasm of the occluded artery. When the occlusion is combined with spastic vascular changes the angiographic pattern usually shows conical tapering of the column of contrast medium in the terminal part of the occluded artery. Occasionally a relative decrease in the density of the contrast medium immediately proximal to the occluded portion of the artery may be observed (Fig. 151A, arrow).

Other common angiographic patterns of emboli noted on our arteriograms were an intraluminal rounded, sharply defined filling defect which did not totally occlude the artery or an irregular filling defect in the lumen of the artery.

Sometimes an embolus can be impacted at the point of an arterial bifurcation, presenting as a filling defect in the lumen of both arteries and shaped like a saddle (Fig. 152A). This angiographic pattern was seldom observed.

10.4.5 Literature on Arterial Thrombosis

Compared with embolic occlusions of the arteries of the upper extremity arterial thrombosis is a relatively common condition (Weston and Ardagh, 1974). Acute thrombosis of the peripheral arteries is usually superimposed on an atherosclerotic plaque. As a rule, total occlusion of a stenotic arteriosclerotic artery occurs so insidiously that the patient is unaware of the event until the symptoms of claudication demand his attention (Thompson, 1974). Occasionally, however, a sudden occlusion may cause all the clinical features described for acute embolism.

Thrombosis of the subclavian artery may occur as a result of compression by a fibrous band of cervical rib at the thoracic outlet. Acute symptomatic thrombosis may also be precipitated in patients with underlying peripheral vascular diseases when hypotension develops for any reason, such as massive gastrointestinal haemorrhage, acute infarction, cardiac arrhythmias or congestive heart failure (Thompson, 1974).

10.4.6 Clinical and Radiological Diagnosis

The clinical recognition of arterial thrombosis is often achieved without difficulty by physical examination and Doppler ultrasonic study. An acute thrombotic occlusion, especially in patients with arteriosclerotic disease, gives rise to symptoms of sudden ischaemia in the affected limb. In such instances it is often difficult to decide whether the acute ischaemia is due to an embolus in an arteriosclerotic artery or to an acute thrombotic occlusion. Angiography in these cases is considered to be valuable for differentiation between these two conditions (Weston and Ardagh, 1974).

On an arteriogram a thrombotic occlusion of an artery, if not of traumatic origin, is usually accompanied by arteriosclerotic changes in the vessel. Distal to the occlusion collaterals are present in most cases.

According to Zeitler (1974) two types of collateral vessels can be distinguished: direct and indirect.

Direct collaterals are branches which arise proximal to the occluded segment and drain into the same artery distal to the occlusion.

Indirect collaterals, however, arise from a different vessel and drain into the distal portion of the occluded artery or are connected to the direct collateral branches.

10.4.7 Radiological Differential Diagnosis Between Embolic and Thrombotic Occlusions

The angiographic signs of an acute embolic occlusion have been described in 10.4.4. The embolus which originates from the heart or a diseased artery is transported distalwards from its origin, usually to a normal peripheral artery. The affected segment of the artery, if it does not react with a spasm, is indicated by an abrupt horizontal cut-off of the contrast column or a crescent-shaped pattern at the site of occlusion. In these cases collateral circulation is frequently not present or poorly developed, possibly due to the suddenness of the occlusion.

Acute arterial thrombosis is almost always superimposed on an atherosclerotic plaque. The affected artery is generally irregular because of arteriosclerosis. At the site of a thrombotic occlusion the contrast column shows an irregular tapering (Fig. 152B). The presence of an existing atheroma is often obvious. Distal to the thrombotic occlusion collaterals are usually present, arising proximal to the affected segment or from branches of an adjacent vessel.

10.4.8 Conclusions

Acute embolism must be considered in arterial occlusion of sudden onset in an otherwise normal artery. On the arteriogram an embolic occlusion is usually characterized by an abrupt block of the contrast column with a transverse distal margin or a concave lower margin caused by the rounded upper end of the embolus. Collaterals are usually absent or poorly developed.

Arterial thrombotic occlusions are recognized by the irregular tapering of the occluded segment and are usually combined with moderate or well-developed collaterals.

These arteriographic signs of embolic and thrombotic occlusion are in our experience characteristic. Arteriography is undoubtedly of great value in assessing the exact location of the occlusion and its extent but may also help in the diagnosis of and differentiation between these two conditions, although the latter is not always possible.

10.5 Fibromuscular Hyperplasia

Literature

Fibromuscular hyperplasia usually involves medium-sized arteries. It is seen most frequently in the renal arteries, predominantly in young women. In 1964 it was suggested by Palubinskas and Ripley that this disease might involve any other medium-sized artery of the body. The first case of fibromuscular hyperplasia of a renal artery was reported by Leadbetter and Burkland in 1938. The vascular changes occurred in the ectopic right kidney of a five-year-old boy with hypertension. Since that time many other authors have published numerous cases of fibromuscular hyperplasia of the renal arteries (Boyd and Lewis, 1938; Perry, 1945; Goodman, 1952; McCormack *et al.*, 1958; Yendt *et al.*, 1960; Palubinskas and Wylie, 1961; Kincaid, 1961; Sutton *et al.*, 1963). Until 1963 fibromuscular hyperplasia was described exclusively in renal arteries. Later the lesion was identified in other arteries.

In 1964 fibromuscular hyperplasia of the coeliac artery was reported by Palubinskas and Ripley. The next year (1965) the first proven case of fibromuscular hyperplasia localized in the internal carotid arteries was published by Connet and Lansche. Additional reports on fibromuscular hyperplasia in abdominal and carotid arteries and in other extrarenal arteries have appeared during the past fifteen years; they include involvement of the external iliac, femoral, popliteal, posterior tibial and peroneal arteries (Wylie *et al.*, 1966; Clairborne, 1970; Perry, 1972; Price and Vawater, 1972; Stewart *et al.*, 1973; Stanley *et al.*, 1975).

The first case of fibromuscular hyperplasia of an artery in an upper extremity was reported in 1965 by Dobell and Pirozynski. They described a stenosis of the axillary artery caused by fibromuscular changes in the arterial wall. Two additional cases of fibromuscular hyperplasia of the axillary artery were published by Garrett *et al.* in 1967 and by Saha *et al.* in 1975.

The only case of brachial artery fibromuscular hyperplasia was reported by Sortland and Sjaastad in 1977 in a 64-year-old man who had suffered diffuse left-sided arm pain for one year. In this case the diagnosis of fibromuscular hyperplasia of the left brachial artery was established by angiography. The arteriograms demonstrated angiographic changes considered to be typical of fibromuscular hyperplasia.

A biopsy of the diseased vessel was not taken and the diagnosis was not verified histologically.

There are three types of idiopathic fibrous and fibromuscular dysplasia of the arteries, which can be distinguished according to the pathological changes in the different layers of the arterial wall.

When the pathological process involves the tunica intima, the term intimal fibroplasia, or intimal fibrous stenosis is used. If only the tunica media is affected, the term 'medial fibromuscular stenosis' is applied, and if the pathological process involves predominantly peri-arterial (adventitial) tissue, then it is called a 'peri-arterial fibrous stenosis' or periarterial fibroplasia (McCormack, 1961; Hunt *et al.*, 1962; Pinedo, 1972).

Of these entities, medial fibromuscular stenosis, or the so-called fibromuscular hyperplasia, is by far the most common type; the other two are quite rare. Microscopically this lesion shows proliferation of smooth muscle fibres and fibrous tissue in various proportions.

The cause of these lesions of the arteries has not yet been established. There is general agreement that they do not resemble arteriosclerosis (Kincaid, 1966).

Microscopically fibromuscular hyperplasia is characterized by rings of hyperplasia of the fibrous and muscular elements of the media, with alternating zones of medial destruction and fragmentation resulting in small mural aneurysms. These alternating zones of fibromuscular thickening and defects in the media and elastic tissue give the affected artery a corrugated irregular internal surface, which produces a characteristic pattern on arteriograms.

10.5.1 Clinical Manifestations

The main symptoms of fibromuscular stenosis of an important brachial artery is ischaemic pain, chronic or upon exertion depending on the degree of circulatory impairment. Microemboli may form because of the irregular inner surface of the diseased artery and the turbulent flow. In such cases all signs and symptoms of distal ischaemia may be present. Physical examination may reveal decreased or absent distal pulses.

10.5.2 Angiography

Since a typical, nearly pathognomonic angiographic pattern of fibromuscular hyperplasia exists, selective angiography of the diseased arteries is the most reliable method for diagnosing this condition. The definitive diagnosis, however, is achieved by examination of a biopsy specimen. On rare occasions spastic contractions of an artery may cause a similar pattern, which usually disappears after intra-arterial administration of vasodilator drugs.

The angiographic findings in fibromuscular hyperplasia are characteristic. Because of the corrugated inner surface of the affected artery, the arteriogram shows the so-called 'sausage string' or 'string of beads' pattern. There are characteristic ring-like stenoses which are not always symmetrical. The segments of the artery between the rings are usually dilated, and are not always the same size and shape. Sometimes small aneurysms are seen.

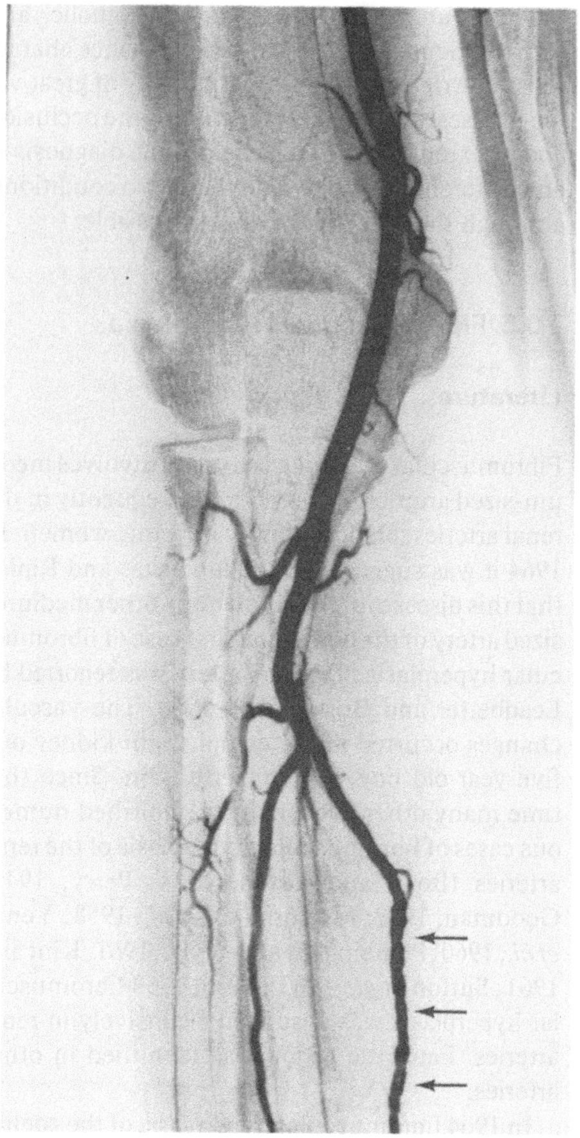

Fig. 153
Fibromuscular Hyperplasia af the Ulnar Artery.
The right brachial arteriogram demonstrates involvement of the proximal ulnar artery. Typical ring-like stenotic parts are visible (arrows) resembling a 'sausage string'. The remaining arteries are normal.

10.5.3 Our Case Material

To date no cases of fibromuscular hyperplasia of the ulnar artery have been reported in the literature. The following case history represents the first known proven case of fibromuscular hyperplasia of the ulnar artery.

A 46-year-old man, a professional truck driver, had suffered progressive pain in his right hand for 6 months. The pain was chronic with acute exacerbations. The middle, fourth and fifth fingers were the most painful. Exposure to cold aggravated the symptoms and caused numbness and more pain in the last three fingers. He had also noted progressive weakness of the right arm over about a six-month period.

Physical examination revealed a hypertension of 180/110 Hg mm. The radial and ulnar pulses on the left side and the radial pulse on the right were normal. The ulnar pulse of the right arm was not palpable.

Thoracic aortography and selective catheterization of both the subclavian and brachial arteries was performed by the transfemoral route. The right ulnar artery had the 'string of beads' pattern characteristic of fibromuscular hyperplasia (Fig. 153). The most distal part of this artery was occluded. A repeat arteriogram was carried out following intra-arterial injection of tolazoline hydrochloride, but the angiographic changes persisted. Selective arteriography of the left upper extremity revealed no abnormalities.

The diseased distal part of the right ulnar artery was resected and the diagnosis was confirmed histologically.

10.5.4 Conclusions

Fibromuscular hyperplasia appears not only in the renal arteries but also in other arteries of the body. The proliferative changes in the tunica media of the arterial wall can cause a characteristic angiographic pattern. The diagnosis can be proven by biopsy.

A verified case of fibromuscular hyperplasia of the right ulnar artery is described; This localization has not yet been reported in the literature.

10.6 Thromboangiitis Obliterans
(Buerger's disease)

Literature

Thromboangiitis obliterans was originally described in great detail by Leo Buerger in 1908.

The essential feature of thromboangiitis obliterans is progressive peripheral limb ischaemia, always terminating in gangrene. The disease is relatively rare and is seen particularly in male cigarette smokers, with onset in the third and fourth decades of life. Women and nonsmoking men rarely develop this syndrome. The aetiology of the disease is unknown.

According to Buerger (1920), thromboangiitis obliterans is an aspecific, idiopathic, segmental inflammatory-obliterative disease involving primarily the small and medium-sized vessels of the extremity. The appearance of such lesions outside of the extremities is rare. Cerebral arterial changes and mesenteric arterial thrombosis have been reported in association with Buerger's disease (Asang and Mittelmeier, 1957).

The pathological process starts in the small arteries of the extremities. The lower extremities are involved more frequently; in 42% of the cases the arteries of the upper limb are involved, alone or together with the arteries of the lower limb (Schinoya *et al.*, 1974).

Since 1933 many investigators have expressed scepticism concerning the definition of thromboangiitis obliterans. The question was raised as to whether Buerger's disease is an entity separate from arteriosclerosis or an arteriosclerotic disease with secondary distal arterial thrombosis (Livingston, 1933; Fisher, 1957; Gore and Burrows, 1958; Wessler *et al.*, 1960).

Some investigators have shown that thromboangiitis obliterans is a separate clinicopathological entity (Barker, 1962; McKusick *et al.*, 1962).

Buerger's disease is a nonspecific inflammation associated with thrombosis of the vessels of the extremities. The occluded vessels are contracted and indurated. The arteries and veins may be bound into a rather firm cord and cannot be separated easily.

Microscopically, in the first acute stage, the lumen of the affected vessels is occluded by a thrombus. The artery shows inflammation involving all coats of the vessel wall, except the internal elastic lamina.

The second, or intermediate, stage is one of healing.

In the third stage, the intima is thickened and the lumen occluded by connective tissue. The inflammation has disappeared and fibrous tissue has formed in the adventitia, binding together the arteries and veins. These findings distinguish thromboangiitis obliterans from arteriosclerosis and arteritis in which damage to the internal elastic lamina can be present.

In his various publications Buerger differentiated thromboangiitis obliterans from Raynaud's disease, scleroderma, arteriosclerosis and diffuse vasculitis. He also noted that the minute arteries, arterioles and capillaries are free of disease, that normal 'skip'areas in an involved vessel can occur and that the degree of perivascular reaction is extremely variable, even along the course of one vessel. (Buerger, 1939)

10.6.1 Clinical Manifestations

The clinical symptoms of thromboangiitis obliter-

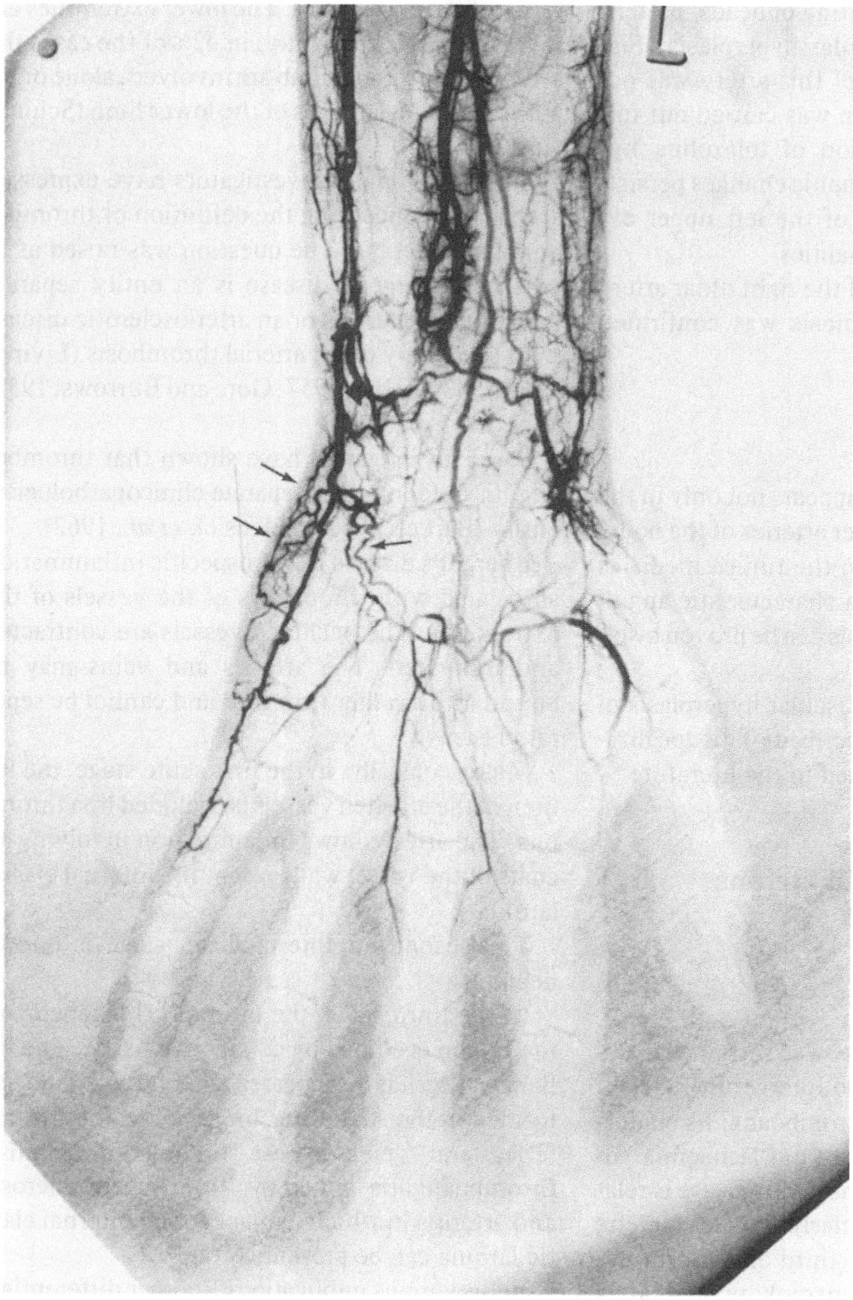

Fig. 154
Thromboangiitis Obliterans (Buerger's disease).
The arteriogram demonstrates multiple segmental occlusions of the arteries of the forearm. Narrowed lumen throughout the whole length of the metacarpal arteries from the second and third interosseous spaces and complete occlusions of all digital arteries. Note the unusually rich network of collaterals around the occluded arteries in the forearm and some 'corkscrew' collaterals in the hypothenar (arrows).

ans of the upper limb include persistent ischaemia of one or both hands, coldness, blanching, cyanosis, atrophy of the skin and a highly characteristic pallor of the skin upon elevation of the hands and redness upon hanging (Eguro and Goldner, 1973). Intermittent claudication and severe pain indicate the degree of ischaemia of the extremities; ultimately gangrene may occur. The arterial lesions are frequently accompanied by superficial or deep thrombophlebitis of the affected extremity.

10.6.2 Angiography

The angiographic examination of patients with thromboangiitis obliterans has a certain value, although diagnostically the angiographic pattern of diseased vessels is not entirely specific (Janevski, 1979). In the earliest literature little attention was paid to the angiographic patterns of thromboangiitis obliterans. Angiography was regarded only as a helpful tool for opacification of the diseased vessels to determine the site for biopsy. This situation has changed, since more angiograms have been used to evaluate cases of Buerger's disease. Recent publications give angiography a more important role in the diagnosis of Buerger's disease (McKusick *et al.*, 1962; Szilagyi *et al.*, 1964).

10.6.3 Analysis of Our Case Material

The angiograms of those patients for whom the diagnosis was confirmed by a biopsy from the occluded segments of the vessels were analysed.

In the period 1970-1980 twenty-nine patients were referred to our department for angiographic investigation with a clinical diagnosis of thromboangiitis obliterans of the upper extremity.

Five patients with clinical and angiographic signs characteristic of Buerger's disease were excluded from consideration since their biopsy material was not representative and the histological diagnosis of thromboangiitis obliterans doubtful.

In 14 patients the clinical diagnosis was confirmed by histological examination. In all cases both arms were involved. The patients were males and many of them heavy smokers. The age varied between 20 and 45 years old.

In all cases the arteriograms demonstrated:

1. Multiple distal segmental occlusions localized predominantly in the hand and forearm with absence of arteriosclerotic changes. The proximal parts of the occluded vessels and the apparently uninvolved vessels showed smooth arterial walls with normal calibre or a progressive but regular decrease in the arterial lumen towards the occluded segments (Fig. 154). These arteriographic features were seen on all arteriograms of our 14 cases (28 hands).
2. On fourteen hand arteriograms (50%) the metacarpal, some common volar and the proper digital arteries had a slightly narrowed lumen throughout their entire length.
3. The collateral circulation was established primarily through multiple very small vessels surrounding the occluded segments of the arteries. They represent the so-called direct type of collateral circulation. These small collaterals emanating from distal occluded vessels with the configuration of tree roots or a spider's legs have a peculiar appearance. They terminate in the soft tissue or fill the distal uninvolved segments of the arteries (Fig. 155). This type of collaterals was found in severe cases of Buerger's disease.

The collaterals arising from an adjacent non-occluded artery (indirect collaterals) or from the involved artery but proximal to the occlusion (direct collaterals) have a typical tortuous course are known in the literature as 'corkscrew' collaterals. This second type of collaterals was present on more than 70 percent of our arteriograms. We believe that both types of collateral are rather pathognomonic for thromboangiitis obliterans.

4. Another angiographic sign observed especially in the early stage of thromboangiitis obliterans is the corrugated pattern involving a short segment of a peripheral artery and called the 'rippling' sign. On our arteriograms it was usually found in the distal portion of the digital arteries and was frequently combined with occlusion of some neighbouring arteries (Fig. 156). At this site the 'rippling' sign has not yet been described in the literature. It might represent recanalization of a thrombus or a preocclusive stage of an affected artery. The sign may be specific for the early stage of thromboangiitis obliterans.

The above-mentioned angiographic signs have also been observed by other investigators (Martorell, 1967; McKusick *et al.*, 1962; Szilagyi *et al.*, 1964).

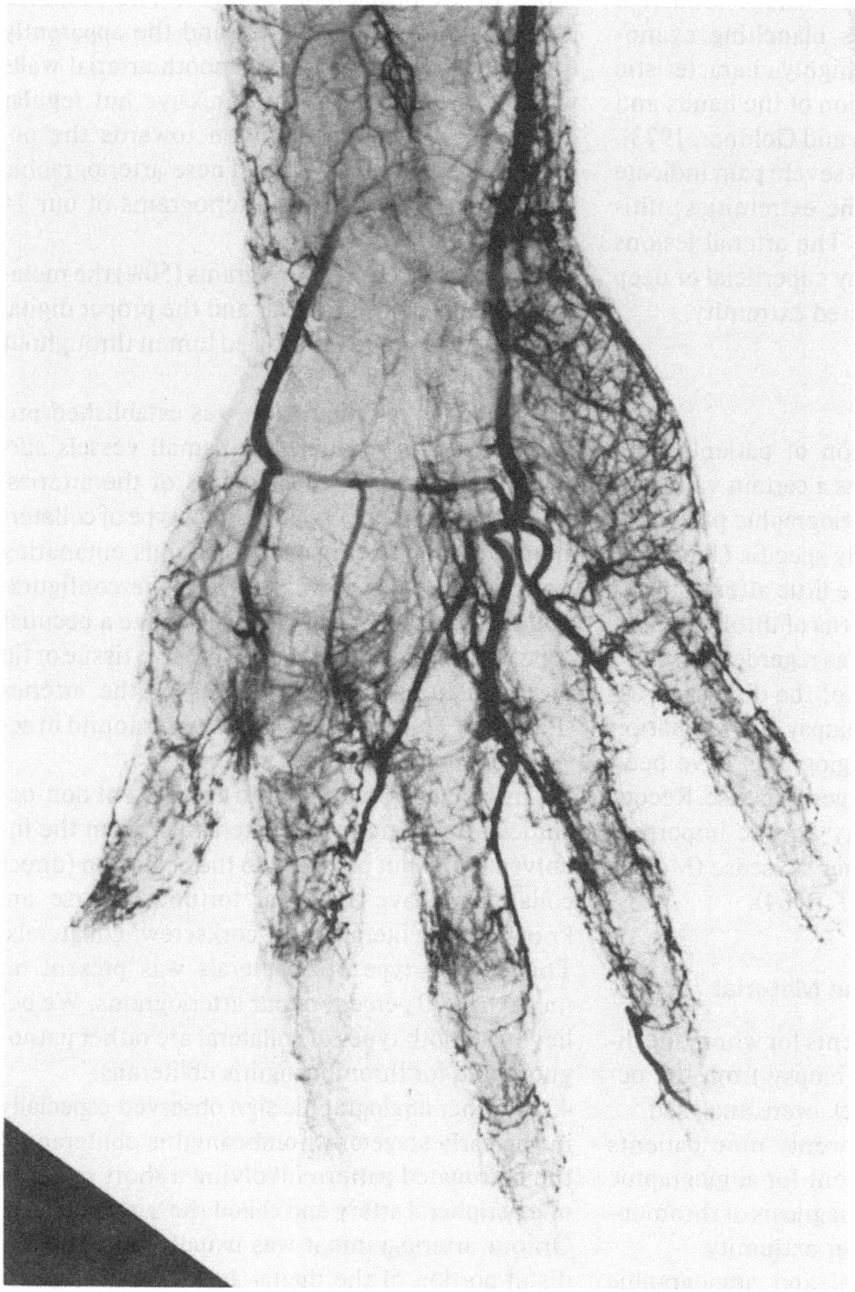

Fig. 155
Right hand arteriogram of patient with thromboangiitis obliterans shows segmental occlusions of the radial and proper digital arteries with multiple very tiny collateral vessels around the occluded segments.
These collaterals which resemble tree roots or spider's legs are regarded as rather characteristic of Buerger's disease.
The proximal uninvolved segments of the arteries appeared normal.

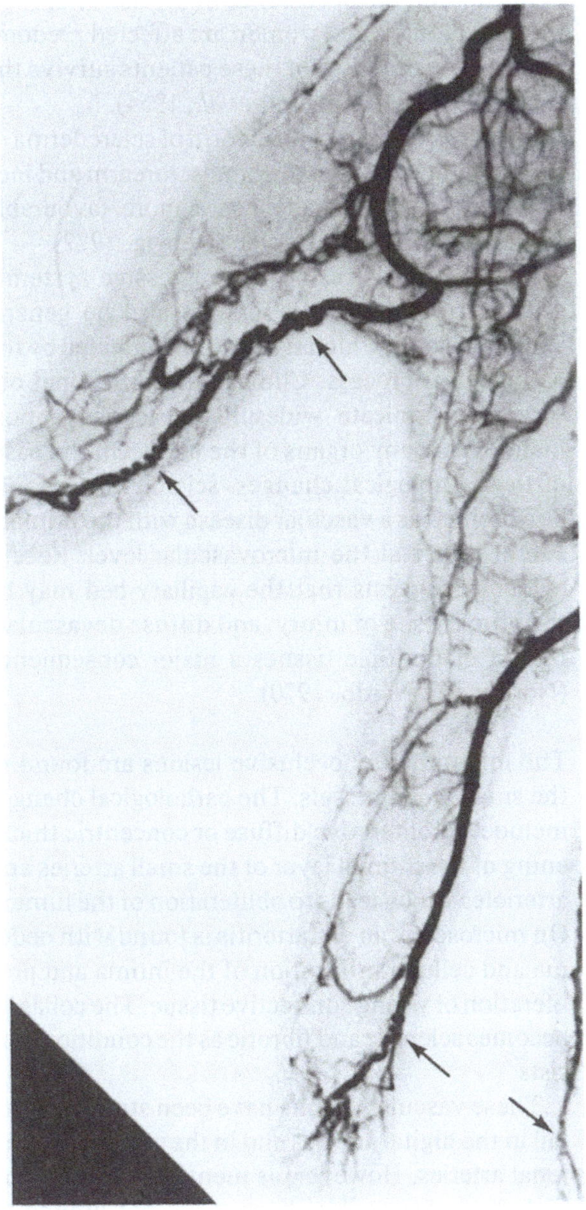

Fig. 156
Digital arteries in early stage of thromboangiitis obliterans show corrugated or 'rippling' pattern of most peripheral segments (arrows).
Note also complete occlusion of the arteria indicis radialis and a segmental occlusion of the second arteria princeps pollicis with 'corkscrew' collaterals.

10.6.4 Differential Diagnosis of Thromboangiitis Obliterans and Arteriosclerosis Obliterans

The arterial occlusions described above are also found in arteriosclerosis obliterans, but in our experience the segmental character of the occlusive lesions and the typical collateral network are rather specific for thromboangiitis obliterans. Another difference between thromboangiitis obliterans and arteriosclerosis obliterans is the fact that in thromboangiitis obliterans the uninvolved vessels and the segments between the occlusions in involved arteries appeared completely normal. Arteriosclerosis, however, is in general a diffuse process which involves most of the vessels of the upper extremity. Arteriosclerotic vessels are usually narrowed with an irregular lumen and a tortuous course (Fig. 142B). They never show smooth tapering like the preoccluded segment of the involved vessels in thromboangiitis obliterans. The tortuosity and irregularity of the arteriosclerotic walls are the main angiographic differences between these two entities. Nevertheless, arteriosclerosis obliterans remains the main problem in the radiological differential diagnosis of thromboangiitis obliterans.

10.6.5 Conclusions

In the last ten years in Sint Annadal Hospital the clinical diagnosis of thromboangiitis obliterans was made in 29 cases; however the diagnosis was confirmed by histological examination in only 14 cases. The arteriograms of the hands of those patients with histologically confirmed Buerger's disease were analysed.

Arteriography revealed the characteristic segmental pattern of involvement and usually also peripheral distribution of the lesions. The collaterals distal to the occlusions in our opinion are fairly pathognomonic for this disease. The indirect collaterals or those emanating from the proximal nonoccluded segment of an artery often exhibit a corkscrew pattern. The second type of collaterals is those found in advanced stages of the disease.

They originate at the sites of occlusion, are multiple and very small in calibre. Radiating from the occluded segments of the arteries these collaterals resemble the roots of a tree or spider's legs.

Another angiographic sign observed in cases in an early stage of the disease, the so-called 'rippling sign', was usually found in the distal portion of the digital arteries. This localization has not yet been reported in the literature. It might represent recanalization of a thrombus or a preocclusive stage in an affected artery.

From our series of 28 arteriograms of the hand of patients with proven Buerger's disease it can be concluded that the segmental character of the occlusions, the typical pattern of the collaterals and the 'rippling' sign are the most characteristic angiographic features in Buerger's disease. In addition, an attempt is made to differentiate thromboangiitis obliterans from arteriosclerosis obliterans based on angiographic findings.

10.7 Collagen Diseases

Systemic diseases associated with connective tissue disorders include scleroderma, rheumatoid arthritis, dermatomyositis, lupus erythematosus, periarteritis nodosa and thrombocytopenic purpura.

10.7.1 Scleroderma

Literature

Scleroderma occurs in two forms:
1. Localized scleroderma (scleroderma morphea) and
2. Diffuse scleroderma (progressive systemic sclerosis or scleroderma progressiva).

As the names imply, the two forms of scleroderma are distinct entities and a transition between the two probably does not exist (Helwig, 1972).

Localized scleroderma is characterized by circumscribed or linear lesions of the skin with central hypopigmentation and hyperpigmented borders. The affected areas of the skin are smooth plaques which are thickened, indurated and fixed. Scleroderma morphea occurs in children and adults. The signs and symptoms of systemic disease are absent in this form of scleroderma.

Diffuse scleroderma is a progressive systemic disease of unknown aetiology which involves large areas of the surface of various parts of the body. The face and hands are usually severely affected. In addition to the skin the disease can affect the subcutaneous tissue, the skeletal muscles and any visceral organ, such as the oesophagus, lung, kidney, bowel, spleen, pancreas, heart, thyroid, central nervous system and synovium.

In children the occurrence of diffuse scleroderma is rare. In adults, women are affected predominantly, and only 50% of these patients survive the first five years (Leinwand *et al.*, 1954).

Acrosclerosis is a clinical form of scleroderma in which involvement of the hands, forearm and face is prominent; it usually has a more favourable course than the diffuse type (Helwig, 1972).

Not only is the cause of progressive systemic sclerosis unknown, but there is also no general agreement as to which tissue is first affected by the pathological process. Clinical and functional observations indicate widespread vascular abnormalities in many organs of the body. On the basis of the pathological changes, scleroderma should be classified as a vascular disease with the primary site of injury at the microvascular level. Recent evidence suggests that the capillary bed may be the primary site of injury, and diffuse devascularization of multiple tissues a major consequence (Norton and Nardo, 1970).

The inflammatory occlusive lesions are found in the small blood vessels. The pathological changes include a proliferative diffuse or concentric thickening of the intimal layer of the small arteries and arterioles which leads to obliteration of the lumen. On microscopy an endarteritis is found with oedema and cellular infiltration of the intima and proliferation of young connective tissue. The collagen becomes sclerotic and fibrotic as the condition persists.

These vascular lesions have been studied in detail in the digital arteries and in the pulmonary and renal arteries. However, as mentioned before, the pathological vascular changes are not limited to these vessels. They have been reported in almost every arterial bed.

According to Goetz (1945) who investigated scleroderma of the digital arteries of the extremities, there is a marked hypertrophy of the tunica media which causes an irregular narrowing of the vascular lumen and segments of total obstruction.

Microscopically, thick sections of palmar skin biopsies reveal perivascular infiltration early in the course of the disease (Leinwand *et al.*, 1954). In later stages of scleroderma a marked decrease in the number of skin capillaries has been demonstrated. The entire dermis has been noted to be avascular and large dilated capillaries are often apparent clinically as telangiectases. (Montgomery, 1967).

Pathological changes in the oesophagus of patients with scleroderma were first described by Rake in 1931. They include inflammatory atrophic and fibrotic changes in all structures of the oesophageal wall. Atrophy of the smooth muscle is responsible for ineffective peristaltic contractions or complete aperistalsis of the oesophagus (Saladin *et al.*, 1966).

The pathological changes in the arterioles of the lung of patients with scleroderma were first described by Matsui (1928) and later by other authors. The most common lesion was a concentric fibrosis of the intima of the arterioles, a change which is considered to be the most specific pathological finding of scleroderma.

The kidneys are particularly predisposed, the interlobular arteries of the renal parenchyma being mainly involved. Hypertrophy of the intima of these vessels causes narrowing and occlusion of the vessels with subsequent formation of focal cortical infarcts.

Clinical manifestations of vascular disease in the extremities, oesophagus and lungs are common throughout the patient's illness. Symptoms of renal involvement, however, are rarely present until late in the course of the disease. When patients with scleroderma do develop signs of renal impairment, a fulminant uraemic syndrome often appears which progresses rapidly and if not treated follows a rapid lethal course in 90 percent of the cases. (Levine and Boshell, 1960; Norton and Nardo, 1970; Cannon *et al.*, 1975).

Abnormalities of the large vessels in patients with scleroderma are uncommon. When present, they probably result from involvement of the small vessels in the arterial wall (vasa vasorum). Panaortitis has been reported in several cases of systemic sclerosis (Recant and Lacy, 1964; Sackner, 1966).

A case of carotid arteritis in a patient with scleroderma leading to cerebral infarctions was reported by Lee and Haynes in 1967. Coronary arteries in patients with scleroderma are usually normal (Sackner, 1966; Weiss *et al.*, 1943).

a. Clinical Signs of Scleroderma Progressiva

If the lesions of systemic scleroderma are limited to the hands and skin of the face, then symptoms similar to those of Raynaud's disease are present: the patient complains of painful, cold, damp and cyanotic hands. The digits may show acrocyanosis and as the condition progresses, trophic ulcerations on the fingertips may develop. (Leinwand *et al.*, 1954; Dabich *et al.*, 1972).

The skin of the face appears atrophic, shiny, indurated and fixed, because of a diffuse devascularization of the skin and marked proliferation of connective tissue in the dermis and the subcutaneous tissue.

b. Angiography

There is practically no literature on angiography in scleroderma of the hands. In 1966 von Schober and Klüken described four patients with scleroderma of the hands whereby arteriography was undertaken only on one side. The second series was published by Dabich *et al.* in 1972. Their study includes a correlation of the clinical, arteriographic and plethysmographic findings in 31 patients with scleroderma of the hands. For visualization of the arteries the technique of percutaneous puncture of the brachial artery was used. They described narrowings and occlusion of the affected arteries but did not find any specific diagnostic sign of scleroderma on their arteriograms.

In our experience the technique for arteriography of the hand for patients with scleroderma need not differ from that used for patients with other condition. The only difference might be to consider the use of higher doses of tolazoline in some instances.

Other technical details of arteriography will be discussed in the analysis of the case material.

c. Analysis of Our Case Material

Between 1970 and 1980 twenty-two patients with a clinical diagnosis of scleroderma were referred to our department for angiographic evaluation of the arteries of the hands. All patients had complaints of Raynaud's phenomenon and clinical evidence of involvement of the skin of both hands. In ten patients, the skin of the palm and fingers was indurated and tight to a variable degree. In one patient, with a seven-year history of scleroderma, ulcerations on the fingertips of both hands were present (Fig. 157).

This analysis is restricted to the hand arteriograms of the 12 patients from whom skin biopsies were taken and the diagnosis verified pathohisto-

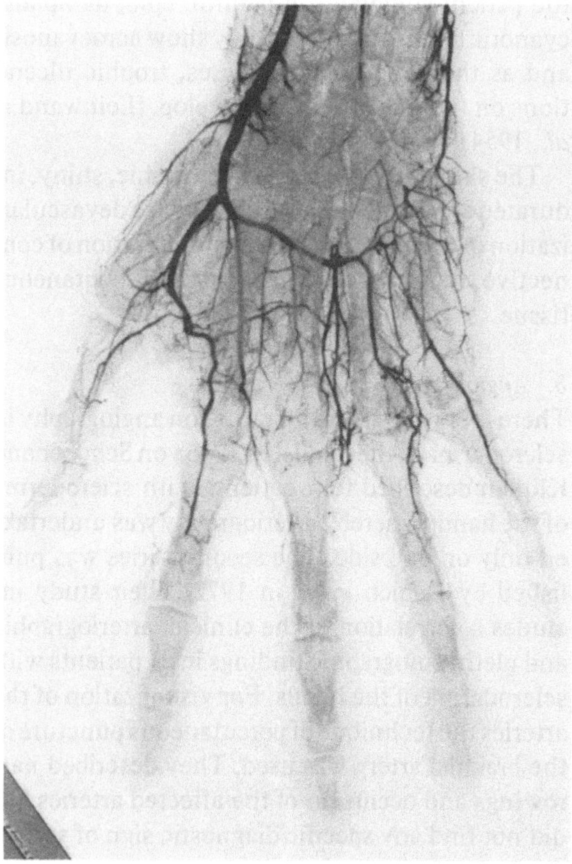

Fig. 157
Hand arteriogram of patient with scleroderma.
All arteries of the hand and digits are small in calibre. There is total occlusion of the distal ulnar artery, the superficial volar arch and all common and proper digital arteries. Sparse, tiny collaterals are visible in the webs of the fingers. Collateral filling of the digital arteries distal to the occlusions is not present. The metacarpal arteries show tapering and multiple irregular stenoses.

logically. There were 8 females and 4 males, with an average age of 49 years (between 30 and 61 years). Both hands of all patients were examined. The arteriograms were obtained by transfemoral selective catheterization of the brachial artery and administration of 20 mg tolazoline intra-arterially before injection of the contrast medium. In two cases the arteriograms were repeated after administration of an additional dose of 20 mg tolazoline per hand. It is important to emphasize that in the interpretation of arteriograms an organic occlusion should be diagnosed when it persists until the end of the arterial phase of a series.

Presence of anastomotic collateral vessels to the site distal to an occlusion should be considered as a corroborative sign of organic arterial obstruction.

The arteriographic findings of all arteriograms are summarized in Table XXXVII.

The arteriograms demonstrated organic arterial occlusions in all patients. The lesions were most frequent in the proper digital arteries of the third, fourth and fifth digits, but other vessels were often involved. Both hands were almost equally affected. The ulnar artery and the superficial volar arch were totally occluded on ten arteriograms. These cases were accompanied by occlusion of more than two common volar digital arteries. In addition to occlusions, multiple focal stenoses were observed in the common and proper digital arteries. One of the most impressive arteriographic findings was a nearly total absence of collaterals. In a few cases, a very small, not very well-developed collateral network was observed. The absence of a compensatory collateral circulation distal to the occlusions may be a characteristic angiographic feature of scleroderma.

In more advanced cases with complete occlusion of almost all digital arteries, the proximal nonoccluded vessels showed more pronounced irregularities and narrowing. In spite of the extensive pathological changes in the distal arteries of the hand, the draining veins appeared to be normal in the areas where they were visualized. On 24 arteriograms of the hands of our 12 patients with scleroderma, the radial artery and the deep volar arch were never occluded.

This observation has not yet been reported in the literature.

10.7.2 Lupus Erythematosus

Literature

Systemic lupus erythematosus is a generalized disease of unknown aetiology involving collagen tissue throughout the body. Actually it is considered to be an autoimmune disease. It occurs more commonly in females. The peak of incidence lies between 15 and 50 years. The course is characterized by a multiplicity of skin and visceral lesions. Symptoms may be fever, polyarthritis, enlargement of lymph nodes, cutaneous lesions of the face, pleural and pericardial involvement and renal glomerulonephritis. In typical cases the initial skin

TABLE XXXVII

Clinical and Arteriographic Findings on Hand Arteriograms of 12 Patients with Scleroderma; Total occlusion +. Occlusion of two proper digital arteries ++.

Patient				*Arteries of the hand*				*Common vol. digit. art.*				*Proper digital arteries*				
Nr.	*Age (years)*	*Sex*	*Hand*	*Radial*	*Ulnar*	*Superfic. arch*	*Deep arch*	*I*	*II*	*III*	*IV*	*I*	*II*	*III*	*IV*	*V*
1	51	F	R										+	++	+	
			L									+	++	++		+
2	50	F	R		+	+			+	+	+	+	++	++	++	++
			L		+	+			+	+	+	+	++	+	+	++
3	57	F	R									+	+	++		
			L									+	++	+	++	+
4	49	M	R		+	+				+	+		+	++	++	+
			L											++		+
5	61	M	R		+	+			+	+	+	+	+	++	++	++
			L		+	+			+	+		+	++	++	++	++
6	36	F	R						+	+		+	+	++	++	++
			L		+	+			+	+	+	+	++	++	++	++
7	30	F	R						++				+	++		+
			L										+	++		+
8	61	F	R						+	+			+	++		
			L		+	+		+	+	+	+	+	++	++	++	++
9	39	F	R					+					++	+	+	
			L		+									++	+	+
10	60	M	R		+	+			+	+	+		++	+	++	+
			L		+	+			+	+	+		++	+	+	+
11	49	F	R										+			+
			L										+	++		+
12	45	M	R									+	++			+
			L									+			+	+

lesion is a butterfly-shaped erythematous patch across the bridge of the nose which spreads rapidly.

The vascular lesions are most common and severe in the kidney, but they may be present in any organ of the body. The pathological process is characterized by a fibrinoid degeneration of collagen tissue in the small arteries and arterioles. In advanced cases a complete fibrinoid necrosis of all coats of the arteries may occur. Marked thickening of the intima causes pronounced narrowing of the arterial lumen. Fibrinoid necrosis and elastic tissue disruption may combine in focal areas to produce multiple aneurysms, similar to those seen in periarteritis nodosa.

a. Angiographic Signs

The arteriographic findings are not specific. Multiple sites of narrowing and occlusion of the small and large vessels is all that may be seen. Sometimes multiple aneurysms at arterial bifurcations are seen. We did not perform angiography of the upper extremity in cases with proven lupus erythematosus.

10.7.3 Rheumatoid Arthritis

Literature

Rheumatoid arthritis is a systemic disease characterized by progressive involvement of the joint synovial membrane, soft tissue, bone, cartilage and blood vessels. The arteries are involved in 8.8 percent of the cases (Sokoloff *et al.*, 1951). It occurs more often in women than in men. The radiographic changes of rheumatoid arthritis in the digital arteries have been described by many authors (Laws *et al.*, 1963; Scott *et al.*, 1967; Marshall 1968).

a. Angiography

The angiographic findings are not specific. They include spasm, narrowing and total occlusion of the digital arteries.

Marshall (1968) noted that narrowing of the digital arteries was frequently localized proximal to the occluded segments. The occlusions were associated with destructive and erosive skeletal changes surrounded by hyperaemic areas that could be seen in the capillary phase of the arteriograms. This dense network of capillaries in the areas most affected by the rheumatoid process may be considered as a pathognomonic angiographic sign (Soila, 1964). Arterial occlusions were more common in males and occurred in all fingers with the same frequency (Marshall, 1968).

These changes have only been seen in adults with chronic rheumatoid arthritis. In 1973 a case of digital arterial thrombosis and vasculitis in a patient with juvenile rheumatoid arthritis was reported by Carson. Juvenile rheumatoid arthritis is rarely accompanied by vasculitis.

Dermatomyositis and *thrombocytopenic purpura* are rare conditions. The arteriographic changes in these diseases are not specific.

No cases of proven rheumatoid arthritis of the arteries of the arm were referred to our department for angiographic investigation.

10.7.4 Conclusions on Arteriography in Collagen Diseases of the Hand

The arteriograms of the hand of 12 patients with histologically verified diagnosis of scleroderma were analysed. Occlusions of the peripheral arteries were found in all cases. As a rule the occlusions were seen in the proper digital arteries of the second, third and fifth fingers. Less commonly these occlusions were found in the thumb and ring finger, the ulnar artery, the common volar digital arteries and the superficial volar arch.

A characteristic finding on all 24 arteriograms of our patients was a lack of involvement of the radial artery and the deep volar arch. Another typical angiographic sign was an unusually sparse collateral circulation distal to the occlusions. The sparse collaterals were tiny and very short and were not able to fill the distal segment of the occluded arteries. Although these characteristics were present on almost all analysed arteriograms, the establishment of the diagnosis scleroderma on the basis of angiography alone cannot yet be justified. For a definitive diagnosis histological examination of the diseased arteries is mandatory.

Finally, to complete this section on collagen diseases, the clinical and angiographic aspects of lupus erythematosus and rheumatoid arthritis were discussed briefly with reference to the literature. No cases of these diseases were referred to our department for angiography of the hand.

10.8 Conclusions on Angiography in Acquired Vascular Diseases

The aetiology of acute and chronic ischaemia of the hand and fingers in acquired vascular diseases is variable.

Acute ischaemia is characterized by sudden onset of the symptoms. Arterial thromboembolism is the main cause of acute ischaema of the upper limb. Peripheral emboli usually originate from the heart. A mural thrombus secondary to fibrillation of the left atrium is the source of almost half of the total number of emboli originating from the heart. Other cardiac sources of emboli are mitral stenosis, myocardial infarction, ventricular aneurysm, severe heart failure and, rarely, atrial mixoma, endocarditis and artificial valves.

The second group of emboli which may cause acute ischaemia of the hand and fingers is arterial in origin. They include emboli from aortic aneurysms, ulcerated arteriosclerotic plaques and post-traumatic arterial aneurysms as well as those which arise as a complication of thoracic outlet syndrome, after surgery of a proximal artery of the arm or after catheterization of an artery.

In patients with episodic digital ischaemia Raynaud's disease and Raynaud's syndrome must be considered.

Classical Raynaud's disease is characterized by bilateral involvement, no history of any other organic disease or trauma and a high incidence in young women. The symptoms are precipitated by cold and emotional stress and the course of the disease is usually benign.

Raynaud's phenomenon, however, is an expression of many entities. In order to discover the underlying disease it is often necessary to follow the patient for at least two years, during which time it is presumed that an associated disease not apparent at the onset of the vasospastic disorder will become evident.

For patients with chronic hand and digital ischaemia several diagnostic possibilities must be considered. Chronic recurring trauma may produce thrombosis and occlusion of the arteries of the palm and fingers or occlusion of small digital arteries and arterioles. Such ischaemic lesions with or without skin necrosis are found in individuals subjected to occupational trauma, e.g. mechanics, farmers, bricklayers, metalworkers, operators of pneumatic drills and even typists; in the latter the changes are located only in the fingertips. A careful history is indispensable for diagnosis of these conditions; the nature of the work performed by the patients or their hobbies must be determined.

Thromboangiitis obliterans is another possible cause of chronic hand and digital ischaemia. This disease presents clinically as Raynaud's phenomenon, but is always associated with migratory phlebitis. It usually occurs in heavy smokers. The lower extremities are more commonly involved.

On arteriograms there is a characteristic segmental pattern of arterial involvement and typical collaterals; in the early stage of thromboangiitis obliterans a corrugated pattern along a short distal segment of the digital arteries was observed. This so-called 'rippling sign' might represent a specific sign for thromboangiitis obliterans.

Other less common diseases associated with hand and digital ischaemia include scleroderma, systemic lupus erythematosus, dermatomyositis, polyarthritis nodosa, rheumatoid arthritis and fibromuscular hyperplasia. Except for the latter the majority of these conditions are characterized by bilateral ischaemia and associated systemic changes.

Fibromuscular hyperplasia may also appear in the arteries of the upper extremity. A histologically verified case of this disease in the right ulnar artery is described. This location has not yet been reported in the literature.

In systemic sclerosis the arteriograms of the hand of all of our patients showed no occlusion of the radial artery and the deep palmar arch. The occlusions and stenoses were primarily observed in the proper digital arteries and less frequently in the ulnar artery, the superficial palmar arch and the common volar digital arteries. The collateral circulation distal to the occluded arteries was unusually sparse.

Filling of the distal segment of the occluded arteries through collaterals was not seen on any arteriogram.

Although there are fairly characteristic signs, the diagnosis of scleroderma should not be based on the arteriogram alone.

The definitive diagnosis of scleroderma and other collagen diseases is established by histological examination of skin and muscle biopsy material.

REFERENCES

10.1 Arteriosclerosis

ANDERSON, W. A. D.: *Pathology, 5th ed. C. V. Mosby Co., Mo., 1966.*

ANDEL VAN, G. J.: Percutaneous Transluminal Angioplasty Excerpta Medica, Amsterdam-Oxford. *American Elsevier Publ., Co., Inc., New York, 1976.*

BOYD, W.: A Text book of Pathology. *8th ed. Lea & Febiger, Philadelphia, 1970.*

CASTAIGNE, P., F. LHERMITTE, J. C. GAUTIER, R. ESCOUROLLE *et al.*: Arterial Occlusions in the vertebro-basilar system, a study of 44 patients with post-mortem data. *Brain 96: 133-154, 1973.*

CRAWFORD, E. S., D. W. WUKASCH and M. E. DEBAKEY: Hemodynamic changes associated with carotid artery occlusion: an experimental and clinical study. *Cardiovascular Res. 1: 3-10, 1962.*

DE REUS, H. D. and M. VINK: The diagnosis and surgical treatment of peripheral obliterating arterial diseases. *Arch. Chir. Neerlandicum, 7: 105-123, 1955.*

DOERR, W.: Spezielle pathologische Anatomie-1. *Springer Verlag, Berlin, Heidelberg, New York, 1970.*

MEYER, W. W.: Spezielle Pathologie der Arteries. *In G. Herberer et al., Angiologie, Grundlagen, Klinik and Praxis, 2nd ed. p. 60 Georg Thieme Verlag, Stuttgart, 1974.*

MOOSSY, J.: The Pathology of Neurovascular Disease. *In R. G. Siekert, editor: Cerebrovascular surgery report for the Joint Council Subcommitee on Cerebrovascular Diseases and Stroke of the National Heart and Lung Institute, 1970.*

SCHORNAGEL, H. E.: Pathologische anatomie van vaatzieken bij het ouder worden. *Ned. T. Geneesk., 111; 1789–1793, 1967.*

10.2 Steal Phenomena

ASHBY, R. N., B. G. KARAS and A. H. CANNON: Clinical and roentgenographic aspects of the subclavian steal syndrome. *Amer. J. Roentg., 90: 535-545, 1963.*

AVARELO, F. and B. T. KATZEN: Bilateral Subclavian Steal Syndrome. *Amer. J. Roentg., 127: 668-669, 1976.*

BECKER, A. E., M. J. BECKER and J. E. EDWARDS: Congenital Anatomic Potentials for Subclavian Steal. *Chest, 60: 4-13, 1971.*

BLAKEMORE, W. S., W. H. HARDESTY, J. E. BEVILACQUA and T. A. TRISTAN: Reversal of blood flow in the right vertebral artery accompanying occlusion of the innominate artery. *Ann. Surg. 161: 353-356, 1963.*

BLESOVSKY, A., V. ČOLANČEVSKI, J. FERGUSON and W. URQUHART: Acute Subclavian Steal Syndrome following blunt thoracic trauma. *Thorax, 27: 492-495, 1972.*

BOSNIAK, M. A.: A collateral pathway throughout the Vertebral arteries associated with obstruction of the innominate and proximal Subclavian arteries. *Radiology, 81: 89-91, 1963.*

BRADLEY, W. G.: Congenital Aortic Arch Abnormalities with the 'Subclavian-Steal' Pattern and Blood Flow. *Brit. Heart J., 28: 718-720, 1966.*

BROADBENT, W. H.: The absence of pulsation in both radial arteries, the vessels being full of blood. *Trans. Clin. Soc. London, 8: 165-168, 1875.*

CODER, D. M. and R. L. FRYE: Symptomatic bilateral 'Subclavian Steal'. *Mayo Clin. Proc. 40: 473-476, 1965.*

COLLIER, D. and D. R. HALES: Bilateral Subclavian Steal. *California Medicine, 103: 348-350, 1965.*

CONTORNI, L.: Il circole collaterale vertebro-vertebrale nell' obliterazione dell' arteria subclavia alla sua origine. *Minerva Chir. 15: 268-271, 1960.*

CONTORNI, L.: The true story of the 'Subclavian Steal Syndrome' or 'Harrison and Smith's Syndrome'. *J. Card. Surg., 14: 408-417, 1973.*

EDITORIAL: New Vascular Syndrome-Subclavian Steal. *New. Eng. J. Med. 265: 912-913, 1961.*

ETHIER, R.: Observations on Retrograde Vertebral Artery Blood Flow. *Am. J. Roentgenol., 91: 1245-1253, 1964.*

FISHER, C. M.: The circle of Willis: Anatomical variations. *Vasc. Dis. 2: 99-104, 1965.*

FOLGER, G. M. Jr. and K. D. SHAH: Subclavian steal in patients with Blalock-Taussig anastomosis. *Circul. 31: 241-252, 1965.*

HARVEY, W.: Anatomical studies on the motion of the heart and the blood. *Leake translation, Springfield, Ill, Charls C. Thomas, 1931.*

HARRISON, R.: The Surgical anatomy of the arteries of the human body. *Hodges and Smith Ed., Dublin 1829.*

HUNTER, W.: The history of an aneurysm of the aorta with some remarks on aneurysm in general. *Medical Observations and Inquiries. London, 1: 323-357, 1757.*

HUNT, J. R.: The role of the Carotid Arteries in Causation of Vascular Lesions of Brain With Remarks on Certain Special Features of Symptomatology. *Am. J. Med. Sc., 147: 704-709, 1914.*

JAVID, H.: Occlusive Disease of Branches of the Aortic Arch. *S. Clin. N. Amer., 40: 111-114, 1960.*

MANNICK, J. A., C. G. SUTER and D. M. HUME: The 'Subclavian Steal Syndrome': a further documentation. *J.A.M.A., 182: 254-258, 1962.*

MARANHAO, V., A. S. GOOCH, S. G. G. ABLAZA, *et al.*: Congenital Subclavian Steal Syndrome Associated With Right Aortic Arch. *Brit. Heart. J., 30: 875-878, 1968.*

MÜLLER, J. H. and W. MUNSTER, Doppelseitiges Subclavian steal syndrome. *Fortschr. Geb. Röntgenstr. Nuklear. Med., 107: 554-555, 1967.*

MUELLER, R. L. and V. C. HINCK: Thyrocervical Steal. *Am. J. Roentg. 101: 128-129, 1967.*

NEMIR, P. Jr., S. BAHABOZORGUI and D. E. WAGNER: Brachial-basilar insufficiency and the subclavian steal syndrome. *J. Thor. Cardiovasc. Surg., 50: 534-544, 1965.*

NEWTON, T. H. and E. J. WYLIE: Collateral circulation associated with occlusion of the proximal subclavian and innominate arteries. *Amer. J. Roentg. 91: 394-405, 1964.*

NORTH, R. R., W. S. FIELDS, M. E. DE BAKEY *et al.*: Brachial-basilar Insufficiency Syndrome. *Neurology, 12: 810-820, 1962.*

PRATESI, F., M. CAPELLINI, M. MACCHINI, A. NUTI *et al.*: The Innominate Steal. *Vasc. Dis., 5: 214-225, 1968.*

PIFARRÉ, R. and R. G. ROUSE: Congenital subclavian steal syndrome: Anatomy, Physiology, Pathology and Surgical correction. *Chest, 66: 299-301, 1974.*

REIVICH, M., H. E. HOLLING, B. ROBERTS and J. F. TOOLE: Reversal of flow through the vertebral artery and its effect on cerebral circulation. *New. Engl. J. Med., 265: 878-885, 1961.*

ROSENBURG, J. C. and F. C. SPENCER: Subclavian Steal Syndrome: Surgical treatment of three patients. *Amer. Surg. 31: 307-312, 1965.*

RILEY, J. C.: Bilateral Subclavian Steal. *Rocky Mt. Med. J., 71: 151-154, 1974.*

SHAHER, R. M., P. PATTERSON, A. STRANAHAN, T. OLDER *et*

al.: Congenital pulmonary and subclavian arteries steal syndrome. *Amer. Heart J., 84: 103-109, 1972.*

SHUMAKER, H.: Surgical treatment of coarctation of the aorta; Further experiences with use of subclavian arteries. *Amer. J. Surg., 89: 1235-1242, 1955.*

SHUFORD, W. H., R. G. SYBERS, R. C. SCHLANT: Subclavian Steal Syndrome in right aortic arch with isolation of the left subclavian artery. *Amer. Heart Jour., 82: 98-104, 1971.*

SKALPE, I. O. and G. S. SEMB: Congenital bilateral 'Subclavian Steal' blood flow pattern. *Scan. J. Thor. Cardiovasc. Surg. 4: 153-158, 1970.*

SMYTH, A. W.: Successful operation in a case of subclavian aneurysm. *New. Orleans Med. Rec. 1: 4-6, 1866.*

SMYTH, A. W.: A case of successful ligature of the innominate artery. *New Orleans, Med. Surg. J., 22: 446-450, 1869.*

TAKAYASHU, M.: *Acta Soc. Ophth. Jap. 12: 554- 1908.*

TERPSTRA, J. L., H. J. P. BEERSTECHER, M. N. VAN DER HEYDE, en L. TH. STUBBÉ: Arteriële en veneuze pathologie. *Stafleu's Wetenschappelijke Uitgeversmaatschappij B. V., Leiden, 1977.*

TREVINO, R. J.: Thyrocervical Steal Syndrome. *Arch. Otolaryng., 92: 177-180, 1970.*

VOORTHUISEN VAN, A. E., T. DE ROO en P. A. G. M. BEELEN: Omkering van de bloedstroom in de arteria vertebralis en het 'Subclavian Steal syndrome'. *Ned. T. Geneesk. 109: 1705-1716, 1965.*

WILLIS, T.: Practice of Physick. *S. Pordage, London, pt 6: 59-1684.*

10.3 Vasospastic Disorders

ALLEN, E. V. and G. E. BROWN: Raynaud's disease. A critical review of minimal requisites for diagnosis. *Am. J. Med. Sci. 183: 187-200, 1932.*

ALLEN, E. V., N. W. BARKER and E. A. HINES: Peripheral Vascular Disease. *Ed. 3. W. B. Saunders Co. Philadelphia, 1962.*

BERGAN, J. J., J. CONN Jr. and O. TRIPPEL: Severe Ischemia of the Hand. *Ann. of Surg. 173: 301-307, 1971.*

GIFFORD, Jr. R. W. and E. A. HINES: Raynaud's disease among women and girls. *Circulation, 16: 1012-1021, 1957.*

LEMMENS, H. A. J.: Nomenclature of Ischemic handsyndromes, In Raynaud's Phenomenon. *Ed. by H. Heidrich, TM-Verlag, 19-24, 1979.*

LEMMENS, H. A. J.: Angiographic Findings in Ischemic Handsyndromes, In Raynaud's Phenomenon. *Ed. by H. Heidrich, TM-Verlag, 131-134, 1979.*

METZLER, M. and D. SILVER: Vasospastic Disorders. *Postgrad. med. 65: 79-84 and 87-88, 1979.*

RAYNAUD, A. G. M.: De l'asphyxie locale et de la gangrene symmétrique des extrémités. *Rignoux, Paris, 1862.*

RAYNAUD, M.: New Researches on the Nature and Treatment of local asphixia of the Extremities (Barlow. T. translator). *New Sydenham Society, London, 1888.*

RÖSCH, J. and J. M. PORTER: Hand angiography of Raynaud's syndrome. *Fortschr. Röntgenstr., 127: 30-37, 1977.*

PORTER, J. M., R. L. SNIDER, E. J. BARDANA, J. RÖSCH, L. R. EIDEMILLER: The diagnosis and treatment of Raynaud's phenomenon. *Surgery, 77: 11-23, 1975.*

TERPSTRA, J. L., H. J. P. BEERSTECHER, M. N. VAN DER HEYDE en L. TH. STUBBÉ: Arteriële en veneuze pathologie. *Stafleu's Wetenschappelijke Uitgeversmaatschappij B.V., Leiden, 1977.*

10.4 Arterial Embolism and Thrombosis of the Upper Extremities

CLAUSS, R. H.: Remedial Arterial Disease. *Grun and Stratton, New York, 1971.*

CRANLEY, J. J.: R. J. KRAUSE, E. S. STRASSER, C. D. HAFNER, T. J. FOGARTY: Peripheral arterial embolism: Changing concepts. *Surgery, 55-57, 1964.*

CROSS, D. F. and J. G. ELLIS: Occurrence of the Janewey lesion in micotic aneurysm. *Arch. Inter. Med. 118: 588-589, 1966.*

DALEY, R.; T. W. HATTINGLEY, C. L. HOLT, E. F. BLEND and P. D. WHIT: Acute arterial Embolism. *Am. Heart J. 42: 566-570, 1951.*

HAIMOVICI, H.: Peripheral arterial embolism: Study of 330 unselected cases of embolism of extremities. *Angiology 1: 20-36, 1950.*

HODGKINSON, D. J. and G. D. TRACY: Upper Limb Emboli: A Reappraisal. *Aust, N. Z. J. Surg. 45: 139-143, 1975.*

KAWARDA, Y., M. NAJMI, T. MATSUMOTO: A case report of arterial emboli in a male secondary to idiopathic hypertrophic subaortic stenosis. *Vasc. Surg. 7: 276-283, 1973.*

LARY, B. G. and G. TAKATS: Peripheral Arterial Embolism after Myocardial Infarction. *J.A.M.A., 155: 10-14, 1954.*

LIGGETT, C. and M. KARTCHNER: Peripheral Arterial Tumor Embolism by Malignant Tumors. *West. J. Med. 130: 72-75, 1979.*

MARTIN, P.: On arterial embolism of the limbs. *Brit. J. Surg. 56: 882-884, 1969.*

MCCOOK, J., E. UQUET, P. LIANES, P. BRUCIET, D. CHARLES *et al.*: Peripheral Arterial Embolism. *Angiology, 10: 165-167, 1959.*

MCGARITY, W. C., W. D. LOGAN and F. W. COOPER: Peripheral Arterial Embolism. *Surg. Gynecol. Obst. 106: 399-405, 1958.*

MERRY, M., J. DUNN, R. WEISMANN and E. D. HARRIS: Popliteal Mycotic Aneurysm presenting as septic arthritis and purpura. *J.A.M.A., 221: 58-60, 1972.*

MCGOWAN, W. A. L. and R. MOONEERAM: A Review of 174 patients with arterial embolism. *Brit. J. Surg. 60: 894-896, 1973.*

MICHAELSON, E. D. and R. F. WALSH: Osler's node- a complication of prolonged arterial cannulation. *N. Eng. J. Med. 283: 472-473, 1970.*

O'CONNOR, J. and J. G. POLLOCK: Acute Arterial Occlusion and the contraceptive pill. *J. Cardiovasc. Surg. 16: 176-180, 1975.*

PAGE, C. P., C. O. HAGOOD Jr. and W. T. KEMMERER: Management of postcatheterization: Brachial artery thrombosis. *Surgery, 72: 619-623, 1972.*

PLUTH, J. R. and G. K. DANIELSON: Poppet Embolism in cloth-covered silastic poppet valves. *Mayo Clinic. Proc. 49: 811-814, 1974.*

SACHATELLO, C. R., C. B. ERNST and W. O. GRIFFEN Jr.: The Acutely Ischemic Upper Extremity: Selective Management. *Surg. 76: 1002-1009, 1974.*

SAVELYEV, V. S., I. I. ZATEVAKIN and N. V. STEPANOV: Artery Embolism of the Upper Limb. *Surgery, 81: 367-375, 1977.*

SCHEININ, T. M. and M. V. INBERG: Management of Peripheral Arterial Embolism. *Ac. Chir. Scand. 133: 517-521, 1967.*

SHUCKSMITH, H.: Arterial Embolism of the Upper Limb. *Brit. Med. J., 2: 835-837, 1963.*

STEPHENS, G. L., E. L. SCOFIELD and V. N. MATHUR: Peripheral Arterial Embolism. *J. Kentucky Med. Assoc., 69: 587-589, 1971.*

THOMAS, J. M.: Spontaneous Bilateral Brachial Artery Thrombosis. *Angiology, 25: 156-157, 1974.*

THOMPSON, J. E.: Acute Peripheral Arterial Occlusions. *N. Eng. J. Med. apr. 25: 950-952, 1974.*

THOMPSON J. E., A. S. WESTON, L. SIGLER *et al.*: Arterial embolectomy after acute myocardial infarction: a study of 31 patients. *Ann. Surg. 171: 979-986, 1970.*

TILL, A. S. and E. A. FAIBURN: Massive Neoplastic Embolism. *Brit. J. Surg., 35: 86-89, 1947.*

WAGNER, F. B.: Arteriography in peripheral vessels. *Angiology, 8: 402-404, 1957.*

WARREN, R., R. R. LINTON and J. G. SCANNELL: Arterial Embolism; recent progress. *Ann. Surg., 140: 311-117, 1954.*

WESTON, T. S. and J. W. ARDAGH: Arteriography in Peripheral Arterial Embolism. *New. Zeal. Med. Journal, june 26: 1066-1067, 1974.*

WESSLER, S.; S. G. SHEPS, M. GILBERT and M. C. SHEPS: Studies on peripheral occlusive disease III. Acute arterial occlusion. *Circulation, 17: 512-516, 1958.*

YOUNG, J. R.; A. W. HUMPHRIES, V. G. DEWOLFE, F. A. LEFEVRE: Peripheral Arterial Embolism. *J.A.M.A. 185: 621-624, 1963.*

ZEITLER, E.: Röntgenmorphologie. Interpretation von Arteriogrammen in Angiologie, In: HEBERER, R. RAU and W. SCHOOP: Angiologie. *Grundlagen, Klinik und Praxis, 2nd ed. p. 269, Georg Thieme Verlag, Stuttgart, 1974.*

10.5 Fibromuscular Hyperplasia

BOYD, C. H. and L. G. LEWIS: Nephrectomy for arterial hypertension: Preliminary report. *J. Urol., 39: 627-635, 1938.*

CLAIRBORNE, T. S.: Fibromuscular Hyperplasia. *Am. J. Med., 49: 103-105, 1970.*

CONNETT, M. C. and J. M. LANSCHE: Fibromuscular Hyperplasia of the Internal Carotid Artery. *Ann. Surg. 162: 59-62, 1965.*

DOBELL, A. R. C. and W. J. PIROZINSKI: Fibromuscular stenosis of the axillary artery. *Can. J. Surg. 8: 288-291, 1965.*

GARRETT, H. E., S. HADASH and M. E. DEBAKEY: Fibromuscular Hyperplasia of the left axillary artery. *Arch. Surg. 94: 737-738, 1967.*

GOODMAN, H. L.: Malignant hypertension with unilateral renal-artery occlusion. *N. Eng. J. Med., 246: 8-12, 1952.*

HUNT, J. C.; E. G. HARRISON; O. W. KINCAID *et al.*: Idiopathic fibrous and fibromuscular stenosis of the renal arteries associated with hypertension. *Proc. Staff Meetings Mayo Clin., 37: 181-184, 1962.*

KINCAID, O. W. and G. D. DAWIS: Symposium on Hypertension associated with renal artery disease: Renal Arteriography in hypertension. *Proc. Staff. Meet. Mayo Clin. 36: 689-701, 1961.*

KINCAID, O. W.: Renal Angiography. *Chicago, Year Book Med. Pub. inc. 6: 102-146, 1966.*

LEADBETTER, W. F. and C. E. BURKLAND: Hypertension in unilateral renal disease. *J. Urol. 39: 611-626, 1938.*

MCCORMACK, L. J., J. B. HAZARD and E. F. POUTASSE: Obstructive lesions of the renal artery associated with remediable hypertension (Abstr). *Am. J. Path. 34: 582-586, 1958.*

MCCORMACK, L. J. Vascular changes in hypertension *Med. Clin. N. Amer., 45: 247-253, 1961.*

PALUBINSKAS, A. J. and H. R. RIPLEY: Fibromuscular Hyperplasia of the Extrarenal Arteries. *Radiology, 82: 451-455, 1964.*

PALUBINSKAS, A. J. and E. J. WYLIE: Roentgen Diagnosis of Fibromuscular Hyperplasia of the Renal Arteries. *Radiology, 76: 634-639, 1961.*

PERRY, C. B.: Malignant Hypertension cured by unilateral nephrectomy. *Brit. Heart. Jour. 7: 139-142, 1945.*

PERRY, M. O.: Fibromuscular disease of the Carotid Artery. *Surg. Gynaecol. Obstet., 134: 57-60, 1972.*

PRICE, R. A. and G. F. VAWATER: Arterial Fibromuscular Dysplasia in infancy and childhood. *Arch. Path. 93: 419-426, 1972.*

PINEDO, H. M.: Renovasculaire hypertensie. *Proefschrift, Rijksuniversiteit Leiden, pp. 35-52, 1972.*

SAHA, S. P., D. R. GOFF Jr., S. E. STEPHANSON Jr.: Arm Ischemia to Fibromuscular Hyperplasia of the Axillary Artery. *Sout. Med. Jour. 68: 645-646, 1975.*

SORTLAND, O. and O. SJAASTAD: Fibromuscular Hyperplasia of the Brachial Artery. *J. Oslo City Hosp. 27: 25-26, 1977.*

STANLEY, J., L. G. BRUCE, E. L. BOVE, V. SOTTIURAI and W. J. FRY: Arterial Fibrodysplasia. *Arch. Surg., 110: 561-566, 1975.*

STEWART, R. A. PRICE, R. NEBESAR and S. R. SCHUSTER: Progressive peripheral fibromuscular hyperplasia in an infant. *Surgery, 73: 374-380, 1973.*

SUTTON, D., F. J. BRUNTON, E. C. FOOT and J. GUTHRIE: Fibromuscular, fibrous and nonatheromatous renal artery stenosis and hypertension. *Clin. Radiol. 14: 381-391, 1963.*

WYLIE, J. E., F. M. BINKLEY and A. J. PALUBINSKAS: Extrarenal Fibromuscular Hyperplasia. *Am. J. Surgery, 112: 149-155, 1966.*

YENDT, E. R., W. K. KERR, D. R. WILSON and Z. F. JAWORSKI: The diagnosis and treatment of renal hypertension. *Am. J. Med. 28: 169-187, 1960.*

10.6 Thromboangiitis Obliterans

ASANG, E. and H. MITTELMEIER: Die systematisierte Endangiitis obliterans (Zugleich ein Beitrag zur Pathogenese der Arteriosclerose). *Arch. Kreisl., 26: 143-148, 1957.*

BARKER, N. W.: The case for retention of the diagnostic category 'thromboangiitis obliterans'. *Circulation, 25: 1-12, 1962.*

BUERGER, L.: Association of migrating thrombophlebitis with thromboangiitis obliterans. *Internat. Clin. s. 193: 84, 1909.*

BUERGER, L.: Pathology of thromboangiitis obliterans. *Med. Rec. 97: 431, 1920.*

BUERGER, L.: Thromboangiitis obliterans. Concepts of pathogenesis and pathology. *J. Internat. Chir. 4: 399, 1939.*

EGURO, H. and J. L. GOLDNER: Bilateral Thrombosis of the Ulnar Arteries, in the Hands. *Plast. Reconstr. Surg., 52: 573-578, 1973.*

FISHER, C. M.: Cerebral thromboangiitis. *Medicine, 36: 169, 1957.*

GORE, I. and S. BURROWS: Reconsideration of pathogenesis of Buerger's disease. *Am. J. Clin. Pathol. 29: 319, 1958.*

JANEVSKI, B.: Thromboangiitis obliterans (Buerger's disease) in 'Pain in Shoulder and Arm' *Edited by Greep et al. Martinus Nijhoff Pub. The Haque, Boston, London, 3: 41-42, 1979.*

LIVINGSTON, W. K.: Skin temperature studies III. Case report. Thrombosis of the arteries of the extremities, brain, heart and kidney, with general discussion of vascular disease. *West. J. Surg. 41: 21, 1933.*

MARTORELL, F.: Angiologia. *Salvat, Barcelona, 1967.*

MCKUSICK, V. A., W. S. HARRIS, O. E. OTTESON, R. M. GOODMAN and W. M. SHELLEY: Buerger's disease: A distinct clinical and pathological entity. *J.A.M.A. 181: 5, 1962.*

SHIONOYA, S., I. BAN, Y. NAKATA, J. MATSUBARA, K. SHINJO, M. HIRAI *et al.* Diagnosis, pathology and treatment of Buerger's disease. *Surgery, 75: 695-700, 1974.*

SZILAGYI, D. E., F. J. DE RUSSO and J. P. ELLIOT Jr.: Thromboangiitis obliterans: angiographic correlations. *Arch. Surg. 88: 824-835, 1964.*

WESSLER, S., S. C. MING, V. GUREWICH and D. G. FREIMAN Critical evaluation of thromboangiitis obliterans. *New. Engl. J. Med. 262: 1149-1160, 1960.*

10.7 Collagen Diseases

CANNON, P. J., M. HASSAR and D. B. CASE *et al.*: The relationship of hypertension and renal failure in scleroderma (progressive systemic sclerosis) to structural and functional abnormalites of the renal cortical circulation, *Medicine 53: 1-9, 1975.*

CARSON, R. A.: Digital artery thrombosis and vasculitis in juvenile rheumatoid arthritis. *Canadian Med. Assoc. Jour., 109: 384-386, 1973.*

DABICH, L., J. J. BOOKSTEIN, A. ZWEIFLER, and C. J. D. ZARAFONETIS: Digital Arteries in Patients with Scleroderma. *Arch. Int. Med. 130: 708-714, 1972.*

GOETZ, R. H.: The pathology of progressive systemic sclerosis (Generalized scleroderma) *Clin. Proc. 4: 337-392, 1945.*

HELWIG, E. B.: Disorders of connective tissue and mucinoses in Dermal Pathology. *Edited by Graham et al., Harper & Row, Pub. New York, 35: 757-790, 1972.*

LAWS, J. W., J. G. LILLIE and J. T. SCOTT: Arteriographic appearances in rheumatoid arthritis and other disorders. *Br. J. Radiology, 36: 477-493, 1963.*

LEE, J. E. and J. M. HAYNES: Carotid arteritis and cerebral infarction due to scleroderma. *Neurology, 17: 18-22, 1967.*

LEINWAND, I., A. W. DURYEE and M. N. RICHTER: Scleroderma (Based on a study of over 150 cases). *Ann. Int. Med., 41: 1003-1041, 1954.*

LEVINE, R. J. and B. R. BOSHELL: Renal Involvement in progressive systemic sclerosis (scleroderma). *Ann. Int. Med. 52: 517-529, 1960.*

MARSHALL, T. R.: Radiographic Changes in Rheumatoid Arthritis in Digits. *Radiology, 90: 121-123, 1968.*

MATSUI, S.: Über die Pathologie und Pathogenese von Scleroderma universalis. *Mitt. Med. Fak. Tokyo, 31: 55-116, 1928.*

MONTGOMERY, H.: Dermatopathology. *Hoeber Medical Division, Harper and Row Pub. Inc, New York, 1967.*

NORTON, W. L. and J. M. NARDO: Vascular Disease in Progressive Systemic Sclerosis (scleroderma). *Ann. Int. Med., 73: 317-324, 1970.*

RAKE, G.: On the Pathology and Pathogenesis of Scleroderma. *Bull. J. Hopkins Hosp. 48: 212-218, 1931.*

RECANT, L. and P. LACY: Clinical Pathological Conference on Scleroderma. *Amer. J. Med. 36: 301-304, 1964.*

SACKNER, M. A.: Scleroderma. *Grune & Stratton Inc. New York, 1966.*

SALADIN, T. A., A. B. FRENCH, C. J. D. ZARAFONETIS and H. M. POLLARD: Oesophageal Motor Abnormalities in Scleroderma and Related Disease. *Am. J. Dig. Disease, 11: 522-535, 1966.*

SCHOBER VON, R. und N. KLÜKEN: Angiographische Befunde bei Sclerodermia Progressiva. *Röntgenfortschritte, 105: 239-244, 1966.*

SCOTT, J. T., R. A. EL SALLAB and J. W. LAWS: The digital artery design in rheumatoid arthritis-further observations. *Br. J. Radiol., 40: 748-754, 1967.*

SOILA, P.: Some Features of Angiographic Findings in Rheumatoid Arthritis and Scleroderma. *Ac. Rheum. Scand. 10: 189-192, 1964.*

SOKOLOFF, L., S. L. WILENS and J. J. BUNIM: Arteritis of striated muscle in rheumatoid arthritis. *Am. J. Pathology, 27; 157-159, 1951.*

WEISS, S., E. A. STEAD and J. V. WARREN *et al.*: Scleroderma Heart Disease. *Arch. Int. Med. 71: 749-776, 1943.*

SUMMARY

The literature on the arteriographic examination of the upper extremity is fragmentary. This book provides a description of the technical and medical aspects of this type of arteriography and an extensive analysis of the angiographic anatomy and pathology of a large patient series.

Although the history of arteriography starts shortly after the discovery of roentgen rays, this field did not become highly developed until the past decade, when important technical and pharmaceutical advances as well as the development of vascular surgery made such growth possible.

The examination of most of the patients discussed in this book was carried out by means of the transfemoral catheterization technique according to Seldinger under local anaesthesia. In a few cases direct brachial arteriography was performed after surgical exposure of the brachial artery. Numerous technical details are considered, such as premedication, contrast media, anticoagulation, choice of catheter, etc. Complications of the vascular examination were rare, the most important being bleeding at the puncture site; the frequency of this complication for all angiographic examinations performed in the Radiology Department of St. Annadal Hospital was 0.5%.

Optimal visualization of the anatomical details of the arteries of the hand is only possible if spasms can be avoided. For this reason the use of a vasodilator is indicated. It was demonstrated that a spasm can lead to diverse constrictions with quite different radiological characteristics. Selected on the basis of data in the literature several drugs were tested in a group of 25 patients, leading to the choice of Tolazoline for further study. The optimum dosage and the best timing for the subsequent injection of contrast medium were determined from 50 arteriograms. The conclusions of this investigation were that a dosage of 20 mg is optimal for brachial arteriography, that Tolazoline must be administered very slowly (for example, in 120 secs.) and that arteriography must not be started until at least 30 secs. after termination of the administration of Tolazoline. No side-effects were seen when this vasodilator was used in this dosage.

For a better understanding of the numerous variations in the anatomy of the vascular system, a short description of the embryological development of the vascular system of the arm is presented in Chapter 5.

Chapter 6 contains an extensive analysis of the anatomical variations in the arterial vessels, as seen on 323 aortic arch aortograms and 750 selective arteriograms of the upper extremity. An analysis of the sites and branching of the vessels arising from the aortic arch showed that 8 patterns can be distinguished which occur with a frequency ranging from 73% to 0.3%. The most common type of branching pattern can be further subdivided into 3 groups, based on the position of the left common carotid artery with respect to the two other major branches of the aortic arch. The variations in calibre and length of the largest branch of the aortic arch, the innominate artery, as well as their eventual relationship to various types of aortic arch were determined. The calibre of the vertebral arteries was also found to differ markedly. In only 28% of the cases were the two arteries of equal calibre, whereas relative differences were noted on 232 arteriograms.

Subsequently the anatomy of the branches of the subclavian artery was analysed in detail. All branches of the subclavian artery localized in the region of the shoulder were studied to determine their point of origin; in this manner a large number of variations could be described. The axillary artery also exhibits many variations, some of which can be important for the execution of an arteriogram because partial filling of the peripheral vessels can be achieved when the catheter is placed in a certain position. In the upper arm many differences in calibre, origin and course of the branches of the brachial artery can be found; this can be important for an understanding of the collateral systems that develop when one of the arteries is injured. An interesting variation is when the radial artery arises from the axillary artery; this was seen in 5.2% of the patients. A high bifurcation of the brachial artery was encountered in 19.2% of the cases.

Many variations in the anatomy of the vascular system occur in the lower arm; as a result, 1 to 4 arteries may contribute to the circulation in the hand.

The anatomical variations in the arteries of the hand were studied on 500 arteriograms; all were examined by the subtraction technique. The deep volar arch appears to vary markedly in development and shape; the numerous variations can be separated into a group with a complete arch and a group with an incomplete arch. In both groups 4 subtypes could be distinguished, whereby several of these subtypes also showed specific variations. The superficial volar arterial arch also exhibits many differences, both in the nature and calibre of the afferent vessels and in shape. For the complete arch, 4 types of radio-ulnar arch were demonstrated in addition to an arch formed by the ulnar and the median arteries and one consisting of all three vessels. The incomplete superficial volar arch was so variable that 19 different patterns could be identified and four general categories formed.

This is the first time that such a detailed classification system has been published.

The chapters seven, eight, nine and ten cover the pathology of the arterial vascular system of the upper extremity, beginning with the traumatic lesions which can differ markedly in nature and localization. Traumatic lesions can be caused by either acute or chronic trauma. Next, a number of congenital vascular disorders are considered. The thoracic outlet compression syndrome is described in detail, including special methods of examination for radiodiagnosis. Of the degenerative vascular diseases, arteriosclerosis and its many manifestations is the most important.

Special types of radiological disorders, such as the steal syndrome of the subclavian artery, the innominate artery and the thyrocervical trunk, are discussed. Raynaud's disease, thromboembolitic diseases, fibromuscular hyperplasia, thromboangiitis obliterans and collagen diseases are also considered.

An important question which receives considerable attention in this chapter on pathology is whether the angiographic patterns can be indicative of the underlying pathological process. It was found that in some cases the angiographic characteristics of various pathological disorders are similar but that there are also several arteriographic patterns that form a strong indication for a specific diagnosis. For instance, it appeared that when scleroderma develops in the hand, the radial artery and the deep volar arch are never involved.

The size and diversity of the patient series are such that this survey of the angiographic pathology of the upper extremity can be considered practically complete.

INDEX OF SUBJECTS

9789400975965